Functional Human Movement

Functional Human Movement: measurement and analysis

Edited by

Brian R. Durward PhD MSc MCSP
Senior Lecturer

Gillian D. Baer MSc MCSP
Lecturer

Philip J. Rowe PhD BSc (Hons)
Area Research Co-ordinator and Lecturer

*Department of Physiotherapy, Queen Margaret College,
Leith Campus, Duke Street, Edinburgh EH6 8HF*

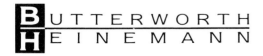

OXFORD   AUCKLAND   BOSTON   JOHANNESBURG   MELBOURNE   NEW DELHI

Butterworth-Heinemann
Linacre House, Jordan Hill, Oxford OX2 8DP
225 Wildwood Avenue, Woburn, MA 01801-2041
A division of Reed Educational and Professional Publishing Ltd

 A member of the Reed Elsevier plc group

First published 1999

British Library Cataloguing in Publication Data
A catalogue record for this book is available from the British Library

Library of Congress Cataloguing in Publication Data
A catalogue record for this book is available from the Library of Congress

ISBN 0 7506 2607 0

Composition by Genesis Typesetting, Rochester, Kent
Printed and bound in Great Britain by The Bath Press, Somerset

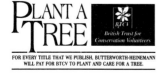

PLANT A TREE

FOR EVERY TITLE THAT WE PUBLISH, BUTTERWORTH-HEINEMANN
WILL PAY FOR BTCV TO PLANT AND CARE FOR A TREE.

Contents

Preface

The primary aim of physical rehabilitation is to manage the problems associated with abnormal functional movement. This management process requires the therapist to assess the individual, design an appropriate treatment or educational programme and evaluate the outcome. To carry out these tasks effectively it is necessary to understand functional movement and to be able to measure it. Therefore, the ability to measure functional movement is a primary requirement for professionals engaged in physical rehabilitation.

It is recognized that functional human movement is carried out in a range of complex social, psychological and cultural situations. Our understanding of the functional problems experienced by patients must be interpreted in the light of their particular environment, context and requirements. Nevertheless the restoration or management of functional movement remains a central part of the physical rehabilitation process, and therefore the outcome measures associated with physical rehabilitation should include sensitive, accurate and precise measures of human movement.

In our experience, the literature related to functional human movement reveals a range of difficulties and omissions. The literature is fragmented and difficult to obtain, there is often a lack of agreement in the definitions, terms and methods used, and descriptions of functional movements are varied and inconsistent. The literature is often written from a range of professional, academic and clinical perspectives other than that of the physical rehabilitation professional. For those intending to measure functional human movement, there is a lack of guidance regarding the scientific principles to be applied, the practices and procedures to be employed when measuring movement, and the techniques to be used when analysing and reporting the data.

Despite these difficulties, there is a growing recognition amongst health care professionals that an understanding of human movement can provide a scientific basis for clinical practice. As a result, there has been a growth in the number of publications reporting human functional movement. This process began with gait, but has since been extended to include an increasingly diverse range of tasks, all of which can be recognized as essential components of daily life.

From our professional perspective, there is a need to develop an understanding of these functional tasks, how they might be assessed and the way in which they are affected by illness and disease. We need to evaluate our role in the management of the patient's functional problems and to base our intervention on scientific understanding of functional human movement. With the drive for evidence-based practice and the need to demonstrate clinical effectiveness, these requirements are now a priority for those involved in physical rehabilitation.

In developing this book we have endeavoured to assist in the process of developing an understanding of the scientific basis for the measurement of functional human movement. The book comprises three sections. Section 1 presents, in three chapters, the general principles and practices associated with the measurement of movement, appropriate measurement parameters and a review of currently available motion analysis systems.

The second section consists of a series of reviews of specific functional tasks. Each chapter contains a description of the task, associated numeric data drawn from the literature and a review of the scientific methods used to record it. Many chapter authors have concluded with an analysis of the current 'state of the art' method for measuring that task, and an indication of the future developments required. Collectively these chapters provide an overview of the knowledge, techniques and issues involved in the measurement of human functional movement.

The third and final section contains a brief review and analysis of the field in general from the perspective of the editors. This analysis indicates the limitations of current knowledge and understanding, and discusses the direction of future developments in the measurement of functional human movement.

This book is intended as an introduction to the field for those who wish to understand or measure functional human movement. We envisage that this text will be of use in both undergraduate and postgraduate courses. In addition, we have attempted to consider the needs of clinicians who want to improve their understanding and evaluate their practice and the researcher embarking on a study which seeks to investigate functional human movement.

The preparation of this book has served to clarify many of the problems and issues we have encountered during our involvement in this area; however, many still remain. For us, the field of functional human movement is an intriguing, challenging and demanding topic. We hope this book will provoke and subsequently facilitate others to join us in exploring the potential for the study of human movement to contribute to the development of physical rehabilitation.

B. R. Durward
G. D. Baer
P. J. Rowe

Contributors

Gillian D. Baer, MSc, MCSP

Gillian Baer is a lecturer in the Department of Physiotherapy, Queen Margaret College, Edinburgh. She initially trained at the Middlesex Hospital School of Physiotherapy. After working as a physiotherapist at the National Hospital for Neurology and Neurosurgery in London she completed a Master's degree in Rehabilitation at Southampton University, where she investigated rising to stand in stroke patients. Since 1994, she has been responsible for the Neurological and Investigation of Human Performance modules for undergraduate and postgraduate students. Her current research includes the investigation of recovery profiles for different classifications of stroke, and the development of simple movement measurement techniques for use in the clinical setting.

Valerie A. Blair, BSc, MSc, BA, PhD

Valerie Blair qualified as a physiotherapist from The Queen's College in Glasgow. After working as a physiotherapist specializing in orthopaedics and spinal injuries, she completed a MSc and PhD in Bioengineering at the University of Strathclyde in Glasgow, undertaking projects in gait analysis and upper limb function. She has taught undergraduate and postgraduate physiotherapy students at Queen Margaret College in Edinburgh and Glasgow Caledonian University, and currently works as the Clinical Effectiveness Co-ordinator for the South Ayrshire NHS Hospitals Trust.

Brian R. Durward, MSc, PhD, MCSP

Brian Durward is senior lecturer in the Department of Physiotherapy, Queen Margaret College, Edinburgh. After training at the Glasgow Royal Infirmary School of Physiotherapy he worked in a number of hospitals in Glasgow, including the Institute of Neurological Sciences at the Southern General Hospital. Since completing a Master's degree in Bioengineering in 1984 he has worked in Edinburgh as a lecturer in the Department of Physiotherapy. He has also completed a PhD in Bioengineering with the University of Strathclyde in Glasgow, in which he investigated the movements of rising to stand and sitting down in stroke patients. He is currently responsible for the undergraduate physiotherapy programme and is the supervisor of two research students. His research interests include the development of physiotherapy outcome measures for stroke rehabilitation.

William J. Hardcastle, MA, PhD

William Hardcastle is Professor of Speech Sciences and Head of the Department of Speech and Language Sciences at Queen Margaret College, Edinburgh. From 1974 until 1993 he worked in the Department of Linguistic Science at Reading University, where he was Professor of Speech and Director of the Speech Research Laboratory. He has published books and articles in a number of different areas of speech science, including the mechanisms of speech production and sensorimotor control in both normal and pathological speech. He has been President of the International Association of Clinical Phonetics and Linguistics since 1991.

Adrian Lees, BSc, PGCE, PhD

Adrian Lees is currently Professor of Biomechanics and Head of the Centre for Sport and Exercise Sciences at Liverpool John Moore's University. He gained his degree in Physics and his PhD in Biomechanics from Leeds University. He has taught and researched biomechanics for nearly 20 years. He has contributed to many national and international conferences, and has published widely on a variety of topics in sport and exercise biomechanics. These topics include biomechanical techniques, gait analysis, biomechanical analysis of sports, joint biomechanics, biomechanics of injury, and the biomechanics of muscle performance and training.

Christine M. Myles, BSc (Hons), Grad. Dip. Phys., MCSP

Christine Myles is currently the Depuy International Research Fellow at Princess Margaret Rose Orthopaedic Hospital, Edinburgh, and is also on the staff of Queen Margaret College, Edinburgh. As a Research Physiotherapist, she has been involved in a number of research projects related to movement analysis and, in particular, the assessment of orthopaedic patients using electrogoniometry. She is currently undertaking a PhD with the Bioengineering unit of the University of Strathclyde, Glasgow.

A. C. Nicol, BSc, PhD

Sandy Nicol graduated in Mechanical Engineering from the University of Strathclyde in 1972 and joined the Bioengineering Unit to investigate the biomechanics of the elbow joint, leading to a PhD in 1977. This work resulted in the development of the Souter–Strathclyde prosthesis, followed by the development of flexible electrogoniometers to monitor joint motion. Biomechanics methods have been applied to all the joints of the upper and lower limbs, and have involved rheumatoid, hemiplegic, normal and athletic activities. His postgraduate teaching in the Bioengineering Unit has involved the supervision of 55 MSc and 45 PhD research programmes, together with distance learning biomechanics courses in the UK, Hong Kong and Singapore.

Philip J. Rowe, BSc (Hons), PhD

Philip Rowe is a lecturer and Research Fellow in the Department of Physiotherapy, Queen Margaret College, Edinburgh. He initially trained as a mechanical engineer at the University of Birmingham. Subsequently he carried out a PhD in Bioengineering at the University of Strathclyde in Glasgow, in which he investigated the rehabilitation of patients undergoing hip replacement. Since 1988, he has worked in Edinburgh and been responsible for the Biomechanics and Movement Science programmes for both undergraduate and postgraduate students. He is research co-ordinator within the Department and is involved in the supervision of a number of research students, primarily in the areas of orthopaedics, manual therapy and neurology.

A. Spaepen graduated in 1973 from the Department of Mechanical Engineering at the Katholieke Universiteit Leuven (Belgium). He worked as a research assistant at the Biomechanics Laboratory and received his PhD in 1980 from the same university. Since 1983 he has been a fully active member of the Faculty of Physical Education and Physiotherapy at KU Leuven, where he started the Laboratory of Ergonomics and Occupational Biomechanics in 1985. Since then, his main topics of research have been related to the quantitative use of EMG in movement analysis in general and more specifically, in occupational tasks, to the forward analysis of human movement (mainly gait) and to the use of assistive technology for persons with a disability.

Ann F. VanSant, PhD, PT

Ann VanSant is a Professor of Physical Therapy at Temple University, Philadelphia, where she teaches courses in life-span motor development, neurologic physical therapy and research. She is actively engaged in research related to life-span motor development, and is editor of *Pediatric Physical Therapy*, the official journal of the Section on Pediatrics of the American Physical Therapy Association.

Paulette van Vliet, B App Sc (Physiotherapy), MSc, PhD

Paulette van Vliet is Research Physiotherapist in the Division of Stroke Medicine, Nottingham City Hospital NHS Trust. She is involved in research into the development and evaluation of physiotherapy treatment of stroke patients, and occasionally teaches movement science-based analysis and treatment of stroke patients' movement to postgraduate physiotherapists.

James C. Wall PhD

James Wall is a Professor of Physical Therapy at the University of South Alabama where he teaches biomechanics, research methods and human learning. He is also an Adjunct Professor of Behavioral Studies and Educational Technology in the college of Education. His research interests focus on developing clinically useful techniques for the assessment of mobility and balance, and in the use of computer-based instructional materials. He is currently writing a workbook and laboratory manual based on the techniques he has developed for measuring gait together with a computer program that allows students to input the data collected with these techniques and obtain the calculated results and graphs.

W. De Weerdt

Willy De Weerdt is Professor at the University of Leuven, Faculty of Physical Education and Physiotherapy. He is a member and currently head of the Department of Rehabilitation Sciences. His main field of research is in the evaluation and rehabilitation of patients with stroke, Parkinson's disease, spasticity, urinary incontinence, vestibular dysfunction and balance disorders, estimation of the burden of disease, and time use and cost-effectiveness in rehabilitation after stroke. Most research topics are PhD projects.

Acknowledgements

As editors, we would especially like to thank all the contributors to this text. Our task in pulling the many strands together was made easier due to the willingness and enthusiasm of each contributor.

The staff of the Department of Physiotherapy at Queen Margaret College, Edinburgh must also be acknowledged for their tolerance and understanding.

Special thanks are due to Professor Pat Salter for his encouragement and motivation. In addition, special thanks are due to Professor J. P. Paul of the Bioengineering Unit, University of Strathclyde, for his continued support of our research endeavours.

The role of the undergraduate, postgraduate and research students at Queen Margaret College is recognized; it was our inability to answer their many searching questions that formed a major stimulus to start this work. Much appreciation is also due to the many subjects whose data has formed this book and who gave generously of their time, often in difficult circumstances.

We thank Rob Sellar, our typical Scottish school leaver, for his comments regarding clarity and accuracy. Thanks are also due to Dick Erskin for his assistance with photographic material.

Finally, we must thank our respective families for their continued support throughout this project.

1 Measurement issues in functional human movement

B. R. Durward, G. D. Baer and P. J. Rowe

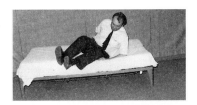

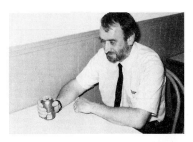

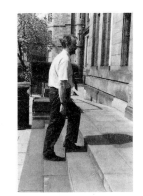

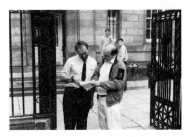

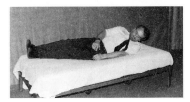

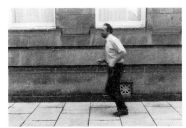

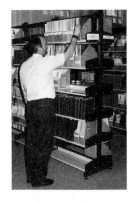

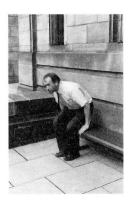

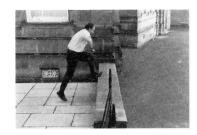

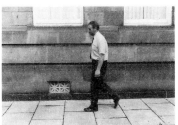

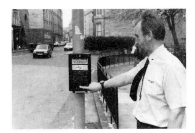

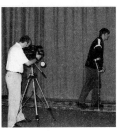

Introduction

The purpose of this chapter is to outline the main conceptual issues surrounding the measurement of functional human movement. The functional context will be defined, and the importance of understanding functional movement from both a general and clinical perspective will be explored. The implications of a scientific approach to measurement will be considered. In most cases, these measurement issues relate to the application of measurement systems capable of producing quantitative data, although some qualitative issues are addressed.

Functional human movement – the context

Within this book, the term 'functional human movement' relates to a range of purposeful movements associated with common task-related activities. Although human movement can be described or measured from various perspectives, including anatomical, biomechanical or physiological approaches, the essential feature of this text is the direct relationship between the measurement of movement and specific human functional tasks. For example, rather than analyse the function of the gleno-humeral joint from a purely anatomical or biomechanical perspective, the focus is shifted to the need to understand the joint's movement associated with the temporal and spatial features of tasks such as reaching and grasping. This study of human movement, with a functional task-related focus, requires the integration and unification of knowledge and understanding from a wide range of disciplines.

The functional human movements listed in Figure 1.1 can all be completed in an apparently automatic manner, with little requirement for conscious effort. Typically, these movements, once

```
rolling over
rising from supine
rising to stand
gait
ascending and descending stairs
running
jumping
hand function and reaching
orofacial movement
balance
```

Figure 1.1 Basic functional movements

established, are not associated with a need for extensive practice or a high level of skill in order to be performed successfully. However, an inability to complete these basic movements effectively may lead to disability and considerable difficulties in the course of everyday life. Although apparently requiring minimal skill, the ability to perform these functional tasks is acquired and refined in the early years of normal human development (Shumway-Cook and Woollacott, 1995).

It is the loss of this apparently effortless activity which is the core of physical rehabilitation and therefore the focus of our measurements.

Purpose of measurement

Measurement is the process of classifying observations that describe phenomena in terms that can be analysed. The measurement process is a natural extension of human curiosity; the need to acquire knowledge and understand phenomena. Links to problem solving are obvious. Data acquired from systematic measurement can shed light on the effects of intervention and the controlled application of external factors. For example, will the use of a walking stick alter stride length, or will the application of high-density rubber insoles reduce the load-bearing characteristics associated with medium-paced running? In the clinical setting, the use of measurement to resolve problems or provide insight into issues where there is uncertainty can lead to improved overall patient care and effective intervention.

Measurement of functional human movement has the potential to inform at different levels, from description to analysis. An ability to provide a detailed general description, the facility to characterize individual functional tasks with reference to specific criteria (such as age) and an understanding of the impact of external factors all provide valuable but differing forms of understanding. The combination of measurement data can also enable analysis, leading to explanations of why motion occurs.

Description
Initially, an ability to form a general description of a functional movement allows us to identify consistent events or phases within a movement. Description therefore has the potential to allow communication based on a common understanding and consistent terminology.

Characterization
At a different level, measurement can identify movement characteristics within a population.

Systematic measurement can reveal important differences in the performance of functional movements due to factors such as age, height, body mass and gender. Knowledge of these characteristic differences can lead to a clearer understanding of an individual's performance, an ability to predict movement patterns of individuals and identification of the life-span changes associated with distinctive movements.

The impact of external factors

On a similar level, but from a different perspective, the measurement process may reveal external factors that have a direct impact on movement performance – for example, the effects of the walking surface on gait pattern and the changes that occur during rising to stand due to seat height. The identification of external factors may lead to ergonomic and therapeutic strategies to facilitate the performance of functional movements.

Analysis

Kinematic data, which describe body motion and kinetic data (i.e. the forces and moments causing motion), can be combined and analysed to explain particular features of movement. This analysis process extends beyond a description of what happens, to the knowledge of why a movement occurs in a particular manner. For example, the analysis of body motion during vertical jumping combined with knowledge of the forces and moments generated has the potential to provide an understanding of the power and muscle behaviour associated with the movement.

Measurement in clinical practice

Measurement of human movement in the clinical setting requires a rigorous and systematic approach. Before clinicians start to gather data, they should have an understanding of the measurement characteristics of the tools to be used. This approach to measurement is not reserved for techniques where complex technology or expensive equipment is required, but should be adopted irrespective of whether the measurement technique is apparently simple or complex.

Clinical measurement tools, where the quality of data has been established, are essential for effective problem solving, decision making and goal setting. These tasks, which form the basis of patient assessment, require measurement tools that can reveal normal and abnormal characteristics of movement. Interpretation of data should form the basis for technique selection and decisions regarding patient management strategies. High-quality measurement data are also required to provide evidence in support of effectiveness of intervention, and therefore must be capable of detecting improvement, deterioration or stasis in the condition of patients. The measurement process is a vital element of the development of evidence-based practice, and is integral to the establishment of clinical effectiveness.

A consideration of the current shortcomings of human movement measurement techniques for use in the clinical setting is useful. The development of measurement tools has not reached the stage where data can be associated directly with diagnosis or ability to predict outcome following disease or trauma. With the development of improved measurement systems, which can reflect essential components of movement, it may be possible to form associations between data, diagnoses and factors predicting outcome. A further requirement is the need to establish both normal subject and patient group data profiles for specific functional human movements. The development of these profiles will include the extent to which population characteristics influence performance. Ultimately, these developments in measurement techniques will lead to higher-quality patient management, with the delivery of more selective and appropriate intervention for individual patients and a greater facility to demonstrate evidence-based practice.

Implications of clinical measurement of human movement

The ethical considerations that apply to individuals receiving medical attention within a health care system, either home- or clinic-based, have implications for the process of measurement of functional human movement.

Measurement should be preceded by an explanation of the processes involved, and agreement should be sought from individual subjects. A number of other factors related to the acceptability of the measurement procedures should be considered. In the development of clinical measurement techniques, it is important to establish the time required to complete the measurement process. Consideration should also be given to practical issues, such as the extent to which subjects are required to undress, techniques for attachment of equipment, and whether the frequency and duration of the proposed measurement procedures are feasible and acceptable.

Technical support may be required to operate and maintain complex measurement systems. Support of this nature may entail assistance with equipment preparation and operation, data analysis and software support and development. The requirement for this level of support is therefore expensive in terms of both time and cost. If funding is not available for these costs, clinicians may have to adopt measurement techniques that are less demanding in terms of technical support. Nevertheless, there is a need to consider the systematic process of enquiry that is appropriate for the development and use of both simple and complex measurement systems.

A scientific approach to measurement of functional human movement

From observations to data

Measurement of functional human movement is the assignment of qualities or quantities to specific characteristics, observations or events. With human movement it is possible to make a single observation, termed a datum. This is a single observable, or potentially observable, phenomenon; a datum is a fact and can be a number (Currier, 1990). Within a scientific approach, which entails the need to incorporate the concept of probability and the natural variations encountered in human subjects, a single datum provides insufficient information. It is therefore necessary to group observations to form data; that is, collections of single observations of units, groups or occurrences.

Variables

In human movement, when a characteristic, observation or event can be measured it is termed a variable. The units attributed to separate variables may differ from one another. For example, in human walking, units of gait speed are expressed as metres per second (ms^{-1}), while units of step length are expressed as metres (m). It follows that the magnitude of a variable can change from one observation to another. Measurement of four consecutive step lengths in a single subject may result in values such as 0.71 m, 0.74 m, 0.81 m and 0.70 m. Variables can be classified as continuous, discrete or derived.

Continuous variables

Measurable observations where the variable can be reported to an unlimited or infinite number of decimal places are termed continuous variables. These variables can be subdivided in an unlimited manner, and can therefore be reported to any level of accuracy required. For example, handgrip strength (force), measured using a grip-strength dynamometer, can theoretically assume infinite numbers of subdivisions. Other examples of continuous variables related to many human movements include acceleration (ms^{-2}), velocity (ms^{-1}), displacement (m) and time(s).

In practice, there are a number of major limitations that constrain the expression of continuous variables in the measurement of human movement. First, the ability to create infinite subdivisions of a continuous variable is limited by the characteristics of the measurement tool. For example, a force plate might be able to measure load under the foot to the nearest Newton, and to report the output of the force plate as a decimal number containing fractions of a Newton would therefore be inappropriate and erroneous.

The second limitation is where a measurement tool is limited in terms of measurement range (the range of values it is capable of expressing). When selecting a measurement tool, it is important to consider the range over which the system is capable of responding and the extent to which the behaviour to be measured alters. For example, it would be inappropriate to use a metre rule to measure the distance walked by a subject in 1 minute; in this case the behaviour (distance covered) is likely to exceed the measurement range of the tool.

A third limitation of a continuous variable is that, in order to express it, we need to record an infinite number of decimal places. Obviously this is impossible, and we must choose to report it to a certain level of accuracy (e.g. 0.14628 N, 0.146 N or 0.1 N).

These limitations mean that, in practice, we cannot have a measuring tool that produces an infinite range of values to an infinite level of accuracy, i.e. a continuous variable. We must therefore choose an appropriate measuring range within which to use the equipment and an appropriate level of accuracy to report the data. This limits the infinite series of values of a continuous variable to a set of discrete but obtainable numbers, i.e. a discrete variable.

Discrete variables

A discrete variable is expressed to a limited number of decimal places. These variables cannot be subdivided in an unlimited manner, and can therefore only be reported to a specific level of accuracy. For example, the number of subjects tested in a gait study (e.g. 20) or the number of repetitions of a movement performed in 10 seconds (e.g. an average of 8.63 repetitions were performed in 10 seconds by the group under study) are both discrete variables where it is inappropriate to further divide the value used to express the variable. The measurement of discrete variables, as values increase or decrease by single increments, leads to an exact value.

Analogue data

A continuous variable that can be recorded at any instant in time is called an analogue signal. An example is when ground reaction force is recorded with a chart recorder, where the force can assume any value within the measuring range and is recorded at all points in time. In order to use such a trace numerically, it is necessary to quantify the force at a given time by measuring the height of the trace at that time. This process is called quantification, and gives rise to a value for the force at a particular instant.

Digital data

If this quantification process is repeated at regular intervals the analogue trace can be turned into a series of numerical values, equally spaced in time, which represent the original analogue signal. This is called a digital signal, and the process is called analogue to digital conversion. In reality, most systems which measure human movements provide data in a digital form with a given measurement range, accuracy and sampling rate, i.e. a discrete digital signal.

Derived variables

Many variables used in the measurement of human movement combine the values from two or more independently measured variables. These derived variables require computation, and express the relationship between two or more separate variables. Data from derived variables can take the form of ratios, proportions, rates or percentages. Examples of derived variables include velocity (ms^{-1}) – a rate expressed by dividing displacement by time; moments (Nm) – a variable expressed by the multiplication of force and perpendicular distance; and statures (stats/s) – a ratio expressed by dividing individuals' walking speed by their height.

Levels of measurement

The measurement and quantification of characteristics, observations or events associated with human movement can produce numbers with different levels of meaning. These differences in level were first proposed by Stevens (1946 and 1951), and are dependent on the logical and mathematical characteristics associated with each number. Classification level also has important implications for analysis and processing of numerical data. While discussion of the statistical implications is beyond the scope of this book, the different levels of numerical data will be considered and related to functional human movement.

Nominal

This is the simplest level of measurement. Data at the nominal level enable classification and the

Characteristic	Level of measurement		Interval	Ratio
	Nominal	Ordinal		
Distinctiveness	*	*	*	*
Ordering in magnitude		*	*	*
Equal intervals			*	*
Absolute zero				*
Distinctiveness	– different numbers assigned to different values of property			
Ordering in magnitude	– larger values represent more of the property			
Equal intervals	– same distance between points on a scale			
Absolute zero	– zero value represents absence of property.			

Figure 1.2 Characteristics of levels of measurement (Polgar and Thomas, 1995)

ability to differentiate classes, observations, persons or traits. The use of numbers at this level is limited, and is only able to identify, classify, differentiate or label members of the category (Currier, 1990). Examples of nominal level data related to human movement would include classification of gender and disease type, and some activities of daily living scales, such as the Nottingham Ten-point ADL Index (Ebrahim *et al.*, 1985). In each case, the data provide knowledge of distinctiveness without attempting to express qualitative differences.

Ordinal

This level of measurement allows traits to be differentiated according to whether there is more than, the same as or less than a particular quality or characteristic. Points on an ordinal scale represent differences, but the extent of the differences can vary. Examples of ordinal data include clinical rating scales such as the Barthel Index (Mahoney and Barthel, 1965), and hierarchical grading systems where it is possible to classify human mobility using a question and a five-point scale (e.g. how far can you walk? – unable, indoors only, 100 m, 500 m, 1 km or more). At the ordinal level it is possible to state that one observation is greater than or less than another, but it is inappropriate to declare the relative sizes of these differences.

Interval

On an interval level measurement scale, the distances between the points are numerically equal and it is therefore possible to use units of measurement. At this level of measurement, the zero point is arbitrary and does not indicate a complete absence of the behaviour. Although most textbooks present temperature as an example of interval data, it is pertinent to consider that joint range of motion values, under certain circumstances, fall into this category.

Ratio

A ratio scale is similar to that of interval but with one additional feature; it is possible to have a total absence of the quantity being measured. For example, it is possible to record a value of 0 N when measuring the force beneath the foot during walking. Other examples of ratio level data that relate to human movement include acceleration and velocity. The existence of an absolute zero enables ratio relationships to be formed – for example, it is possible to claim that the subject

who required 10 s to walk 5 m walked at twice the velocity compared to the subject who covered the same distance in 20 s.

When dealing with human movement, the differentiation between interval and ratio measures can be problematic. When reference is made to the amount of motion from the anatomical position, e.g. degrees of elbow flexion, it is theoretically possible to identify an absolute zero of that quantity and to consider the ratio of measures. In practice, it is difficult to locate the zero position reliably and, consequently, the ability to declare proportional alterations in angular motion (e.g. elbow flexion has doubled or halved) is limited. This would indicate that elbow flexion is interval data. In practice, the differences between interval and ratio measures are minor and both potentially can be subjected to parametric statistical analysis.

The concept of validity

Measurement validity has been defined as 'evidence that a test measures what it is purported to measure' (Anderson, 1994). Validity is a theoretical concept which, if established for a measurement system, would imply that the data recorded were a true reflection of the behaviour being measured under all circumstances.

In reality, measurement systems can only be validated for a particular set of conditions. It is not possible to state that a system is valid without also stating the conditions under which this is true. While it is impossible to establish validity of a measure under all imaginable circumstances, it is possible to conduct a number of validation experiments that demonstrate validity under the conditions envisaged for the study. It is essential then to consider validity when selecting a measurement tool for a given behaviour.

Face validity

During the selection process there is a need to form a judgement regarding the appropriateness of the measurement tool (face validity). This selection process may be straightforward when a measurement tool has been established for a given behaviour, and confirmation in this situation is often achieved by reviewing the literature in the area. Although this approach to determining validity can provide partial evidence based on consensus, there remains a need to examine the theoretical links between observations and potential measures.

Construct validity

When consideration is given to the theoretical associations between the traits or observations to be measured and specific measurement tools, it is possible to form construct validity. This form of validity is related to concepts and hypothetical constructs or arguments. The presence of construct validity in measurement represents a theoretical basis for the measured behaviour. It is particularly important to establish construct validity when measuring a concept that cannot be examined directly, but has to be inferred from indirect observations. An example that exemplifies the difficulties of establishing construct validity is the measurement of muscle strength by the indirect means of limb circumference measurements. Although it has been accepted that cross-sectional muscle area relates directly to muscle strength (Galley and Forster, 1987), circumference measures have been found to seriously underestimate muscle wasting (Young *et al.*, 1982) and growth (Young *et al.*, 1983). This example illustrates the need to address construct validity when selecting a measurement tool for a specific purpose.

Content validity

After defining a construct for a particular behaviour, it is necessary to confirm that all aspects of the behaviour are included in the measurement – this is termed content validity. For example, the content validity of a test inventory designed to measure hand function could be challenged if tests of grip strength were omitted. In human movement studies, batteries of discrete functional tests are often conducted in order to represent generalized ability. When selecting these tests there is a need to ensure that all aspects of the behaviour are included and that, in each case, they are consistent with the arguments supporting construct validity.

Concurrent validity

Where a test or measurement tool has accepted validity, it is possible to establish the validity of a new tool by making direct associations. This process, termed concurrent validity, involves the correlation of outputs from each system, and can establish whether the new system is capable of measuring the same trait or behaviour. The process of establishing concurrent validity is often required when there is a need to replace expensive measurement tools, very often considered the 'gold standard', with simple and inexpensive alternatives.

The validation of movement measurement equipment

The study of functional human movement has made great advances due to the availability of complex and often expensive measurement equipment. Although it is tempting to accept that measurement equipment will inevitably provide the researcher with high quality data, it is important to adopt a sceptical and questioning approach when considering its use. This sceptical approach is exemplified by the need to conduct a series of validation experiments designed to ensure the equipment will provide valid data under all the conditions considered likely to occur during the study. The first issue to be addressed by the researcher before using measurement equipment to study movement should be whether sufficient evidence can be gathered to reject the following null hypothesis:

> the data output from the measurement system lacks both accuracy and precision, and is therefore not fit for its stated purpose.

It follows then that rigorous and systematic testing of the measurement system is required to ensure removal of this doubt.

Accuracy

With instrumentation, the term 'accuracy' is used to indicate differences between 'true' and 'measured' values and, therefore, is a basic consideration in establishing validity. In the context of measurement of human movement, validity or accuracy requires the production of evidence in support of the measurement tool. The gathering of this evidence requires the application of systematic enquiry to establish and confirm the response characteristics of the measurement tool.

Apparently similar systems may vary in performance, and are often used under different conditions. The same models of a commercially available measurement device may have different performance characteristics, and instruments may change with time or become damaged or faulty. Therefore, whether a measurement system is established for a given purpose or not, there is a requirement to test and understand the response characteristics of the system and to determine the extent to which they alter when subjected to internal and external factors. This process, which is characterized by a systematic process of enquiry, is best illustrated by the use of a practical example.

Initially, the first requirement is to know how the output from a device is related to the input. This is established by systematically observing how the measured output values from the instrument relate to reference input values applied to the system; this process is called calibration. Some instruments are pre-calibrated at the time of manufacture and there should be a direct relationship between the input and output such that the measured and reference values are identical. In reality, some error may occur with this response. In addition, it is always worth checking a pre-calibrated instrument as the response may change with time or the device may be damaged or faulty.

To undertake calibration, we need a model of the relationship between input and output values. For most instruments, a linear line model is used; however, some tools may have accurate and predictable non-linear responses (e.g. quadratic, cubic and logarithmic). It should be borne in mind that an instrument with a non-linear response is not necessarily useless, but the errors will also be non-linear and it is therefore usual to seek a tool with a linear response.

To calculate the linear relationship between input and output values, a process of linear regression is used. This statistical technique attempts to fit a straight line through the data in order to account for as much of the difference in the measured data as possible by changes in the reference variable – in other words, the regression tries to minimize the residual errors that exist once the changes in the reference values have been taken into consideration. The calibration of an electrogoniometer is used to illustrate this process (Table 1.1). In this example, reference (input)

values were obtained from a highly accurate engineering protractor and output values from a digital recording system attached to the electrogoniometer. Note that the initial reference value was zero, and that the reference values increased by equal amounts.

A graph of these data would look like Figure 1.3.

The graph illustrates the differences between measured and predicted values. It is necessary to consider techniques for summarizing these differences and expressing the output characteristics of the goniometer and the magnitude of the errors.

The variation in the measured data is modelled by the following expression:

$$Y \text{ (measured)} = mX + c + e$$

where

Y is the output or dependent variable
X is the input or independent variable
m is a constant giving the slope of the regression line
c is a constant giving the offset of the regression line from zero (i.e. the value of Y when X is zero)
e is the random error in the data.

The formula for the systematic relationship between the predicted Y and reference X values is given by:

$$Y \text{ (predicted)} = mX + c$$

In this case, regression calculates the best fitting line through the data so that the sum of squares of the deviation of the measured values from the values predicted by the regression line are minimized.

Table 1.1 Example reference (input) and measured (output) values from an electrogoniometer

Reference X value (units in degrees)	Measured Y value (units in degrees)	Predicted Y value (units in degrees)	Residual error	Absolute residual error
0	1.2	0	−1.2	1.2
10	9.1	10	0.9	0.9
20	21.3	20	−1.3	1.3
30	29.1	30	0.9	0.9
40	41.3	40	−1.3	1.3
50	48.9	50	1.1	1.1
60	60.5	60	−0.5	0.5
70	69.7	70	0.3	0.3
80	79.2	80	0.8	0.8
90	89.9	90	0.1	0.1

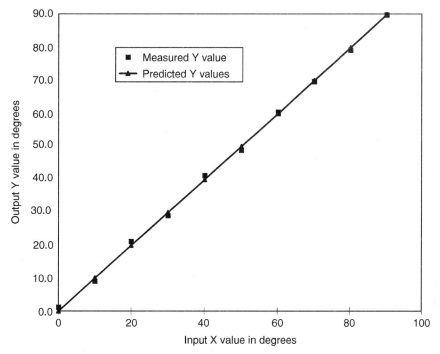

Figure 1.3 Graph of input X values versus output Y values

The regression equation in this case has a value for the slope (m = 0.997) and for the intercept c of zero, i.e.:

$$Y = 0.997X + 0.$$

The result of the regression indicates that the electrogoniometer responds linearly, and that for every degree that was input the system recorded 0.997 of a degree on the output. The input (reference) values are not exactly the same as the output (measured) values; however, they follow the general trend indicated by the straight line with the formula indicated above. In addition, there is a random element to the measured output which means that this relationship is not followed exactly and gives rise to some measured values lying above the line while others are below it. These random differences are indicated by the residual errors. In Figure 1.4, these residual errors are plotted against the measuring range.

If these residual errors are too large for the desired experiment, then it is necessary to find methods to reduce them. These may include redesign of the equipment or improvements in the application. If the errors show a systematic trend then it may be that some other variable is affecting the measured values in a systematic way, and this can be eliminated. This process of reducing the residual errors can be difficult and frustrating.

If the residual errors are small and not likely to affect the outcome of an experiment, then they could be considered random errors that do not require further investigation. It is common to report the accuracy in terms of the distribution of error throughout the range, and by indicating the mean and maximum absolute residual error. In the above example, the mean absolute residual error is 0.8 degrees and the maximum absolute residual error is 1.3 degrees. This means that, on average, the input and measured values varied by 0.8 of a degree and in the worse case by 1.3 degrees. We have therefore established that the electrogoniometer is accurate to within 0.8 degrees under normal circumstances and accurate to within 1.3 degrees in the worst case.

The final measure of accuracy is the percentage linearity. This is calculated by dividing the maximum residual error by the measuring range (the range in the independent X variable), and expressing the ratio as a percentage. In the example we have a maximum residual error of 1.3 and a range of 90 (0 to 90), which gives a percentage linearity of 1.4 per cent.

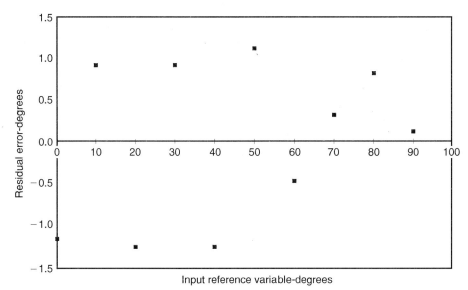

Figure 1.4 Residual error plot

Having established the relationship between the input and output values, it is possible to calculate one from the other using the equation for the straight line derived from the regression, i.e.:

$$Y + mX + c, \quad \text{or} \quad X = \frac{Y - c}{m}$$

If a measurement tool is supplied uncalibrated, there is a need to derive, by means of regression, the relationship between input and output values. If the device is supplied calibrated, then either the equation will be provided or it will be incorporated into the instrument itself so that measured values are 'true'. It is always worth checking that the device supplied is correctly calibrated and that the values are correct.

Frequency response

If the measured dependent variable changes naturally with time, then the instrument must respond sufficiently rapidly to be able to reflect the current value of the measured variable. It must have a frequency response that is sufficiently rapid to allow measurement of the chosen variable. If the measured variable is changing every tenth of a second and the device can only report a value once a second, then the device will not reflect the true changes in the measured variable. In this case the measured variable would appear to adopt the characteristics of a different variable. This process is termed *aliasing*. To prevent a measurement

system from recording data that are aliased, it must be capable of producing precise and accurate samples at a rate that is at least twice that of the changing behaviour.

Reliability

The concept of reliability encompasses repeatability and precision of measures. In the context of measurement of human movement, there is a requirement for measurement tools and the operators of measurement tools to perform reliably under a number of different conditions, otherwise the data collected are meaningless. Reliability can be assessed in a number of different ways; these include intra-rater reliability, inter-rater reliability and test–retest reliability.

Intra-rater reliability refers to the repeatability of a single tester in performing repeated measures. For example, if an individual requires to measure leg length and follows a stipulated protocol for this procedure, repeated measures of each subject should be consistent, with minimal within-subject variation. In this instance, variation is usually attributable to rater error rather than measurement tool error. The consistency of measures between two or more raters is termed inter-rater reliability. In many studies of human movement, tests are conducted by more than one rater. In this situation, it is important to establish consistency within the group of raters when measuring the same phenomenon. If it is possible to use a measurement tool that is immune from error due to tester bias, as in some forms of equipment, then repeated tests are referred to as test–retest reliability.

A common method of testing reliability is to administer the same test on two or more separate occasions. The results of the first test are then compared to those of subsequent tests. Traditionally, correlation coefficients have been calculated to indicate levels of association, with high correlation coefficients of greater than 0.8 taken to indicate good agreement and therefore reliability. More recently, the use of correlation coefficients for expressing reliability has been challenged (Maher, 1993; Shoukri and Edge, 1996) and the use of intraclass correlations (Shrout and Fleiss, 1979; Adams *et al.*, 1995), concordance correlation coefficients (Shoukri and Edge, 1996) or percentage exact agreement and percentage close agreement (Adams *et al.*, 1995) has been advocated.

Precision

The term precision, when applied to measurement tools, refers to the repeatability with which a measured value can be obtained. While this definition could be thought to include all aspects of repeatability, for example repeatability over a number of days or between testers, it is usually taken to refer to the repeatability of a number of samples recorded rapidly over a short period of time. Precision is sometimes also called the 'resolution' or 'stability' of a system.

The precision of a device therefore records how individual samples vary from the mean of a group of samples recorded over a short period of time. If individual samples are very different from the mean, then the device is considered to lack precision. Two almost identical methods of recording precision are reported. One is the standard deviation (s.d.) of the data from the mean, and the other is the root mean square (RMS) value for the data. The s.d. is usually found in clinical publications, while the RMS value is usual in engineering journals and manufacturer's technical sheets. These two formulae differ only in the use of $n - 1$ and n in their respective denominators. When n is large, there is no apparent difference between s.d. and RMS values.

Precision can be calculated by taking a series of measures in quick succession and then reporting their standard deviation. This will gave an indication of the spread of values found in the data. A standard deviation of 2 cm when measuring stride length would imply that 95 per cent of all the recorded values fell within two standard deviations from the mean (i.e. ± 4 cm) and that 99 per cent of values fell within three standard deviations from the mean (i.e. ± 6 cm).

Precision may vary at different points within a measurement range, and it is therefore necessary to measure the precision of the tool throughout the required measurement range. The relative value of the standard deviation with regard to the mean can be expressed as a percentage value using the coefficient of variation (the s.d. divided by the mean, expressed as a percentage). However, caution should be used when interpreting this statistic when the mean value approaches zero, as the coefficient of variation can then rapidly increase or become infinite when the absolute precision of the tool is still very good.

Threats to validity

Hysteresis

Hysteresis is a characteristic of some measurement tools, particularly those that are mechanical and electrical, and means that readings taken when the measurement values are increasing are different to those taken when the measured values are decreasing. Hysteresis therefore represents a systematic error that is dependent upon the direction in which the recording is moving through the measuring range (ascending or descending). Hysteresis is sometimes present in mechanical and electrical systems, due to the storage of mechanical and electrical energy during the ascending phase and its release during the descending phase. Small hysteretic effects may be allowable, but large effects may render the device useless unless the direction in which the data are changing is known. In this case a complicated conversion process is employed. In practice, devices for the measurement of human movement with large hysteretic effects do not make good investigative tools.

Cross-talk

An important factor which can threaten validity is the cross-talk or interference between measuring components when they operate concurrently. A measurement system may comprise a number of separate measuring components where the data from each are channelled to a single recording device. In such a system, the data from each channel may be kept separate or combined to form a derived variable that can reflect performance. An example where the recorded data are kept separate is a multi-channel EMG system, which is designed to record concurrent activity in a number of muscles. Cross-talk can occur in this case when the signal from one muscle is detected in measuring channels allocated to other muscles. With a force platform that can measure forces applied to the upper surface of the device, the measuring components are arranged in three orthogonal axes at right angles to each other. The applied force components can then be resolved into vertical, horizontal and lateral components. With this system, the presence of cross-talk is a major consideration. For example, if the platform is subjected to only vertical forces, then only vertical and not horizontal or lateral forces should be recorded. In many measurement systems with multiple measurement components the potential for cross-talk is revealed by recording the concurrent output from each channel while systematically applying an input to one of the measurement components. The results of this type of test are normally plotted to reveal the extent to which separate measurement components are independent of one another.

Internal factors

With electronic measurement systems, the output characteristics can alter with time. Over a short time period the changes are often due to warm-up effects, and usually occur immediately following power-up. It is important to identify the presence of this effect and, when necessary, include warm-up periods in testing protocols. The operational characteristics of mechanical and electrical components can change over longer periods of time due to wear and the prolonged effects of high temperatures. It is possible to detect these changes with repeated calibration tests, which serve to monitor output characteristics over time.

External factors

The behaviour of measurement instruments can be affected by a wide range of external factors – for example, room temperature, mains voltage fluctuations and fixation methods where measurement components are attached directly to subjects. While some of these external factors lead to systematic changes in measured output and can therefore be modified, many cause random errors which reduce the accuracy of the data. Prior to using a measurement technique, it is necessary to identify both internal and external factors that might cause interference. Systematic development of test protocols, pilot testing and careful examination of initial test data can reveal these factors before extensive testing is carried out.

Conclusion

Within this chapter we have discussed the main theoretical and practical considerations when undertaking measurement of functional human movement. A major concern is to emphasize the need for a sceptical approach to the measurement process, highlighting the requirement for systematic enquiry that can ultimately lead to a clearer understanding of the validity and reliability of measured data. This can be achieved by the careful construction of a series of validation experiments and is an essential prerequisite of a movement measurement study. A few weeks spent exploring the validity of the measurement system can protect the user from a long period of data collection recording flawed and erroneous data.

References

Adams, R. D., Chambers, R. and Maher, C. G. (1995). ICC.EXE. A public domain program for calculating intra-class correlation coefficients and agreement indices. *Proc.12th World Congr. WCPT,* Washington DC, p. 362.

Anderson, K. A. (1994). *Mosby's Medical, Nursing and Allied Health Dictionary.* Mosby Year Books.

Currier, D. (1990). *Elements of Research in Physical Therapy* (3rd edn.). Williams & Wilkins.

Ebrahim, S., Nouri, F. and Barer, D. (1985). Measuring disability after stroke. *J. Epidem. Comm. Health*, **39**, 86–9.

Galley, P. M. and Forster, A. L. (1987). *Human Movement, an Introductory Text for Physiotherapy Students* (2nd edn.). Churchill Livingstone.

Maher, C. (1993). Pitfalls in reliability studies: some suggestions for change. *Aust. J. Physio.*, **39(1)**, 5–7.

Mahoney, F. I. and Barthel, D. W. (1965). Functional evaluation: the Barthel Index. *Md. St. Med. J.*, **14**, 61–5.

Polgar, S. and Thomas, S. A. (1995). *Introduction to Research in the Health Sciences* (3rd edn.). Churchill Livingstone.

Shoukri, M. and Edge, V. (1996). *Statistical Methods for Health Sciences.* CRC Press.

Shrout, P. E. and Fleiss, J. L. (1979). Intraclass correlations: uses in assessing rater reliability. *Psych. Bull.*, **86(2)**, 420–28.

Shumway-Cook, A. and Woollacott, M. H. (1995). Motor control: theory and practical applications. In *A Lifespan Perspective of Mobility*, pp. 269–94. Williams & Wilkins.

Stevens, S. S. (1946). On the theory of scales and measurement. *Science*, **103**, 677–680.

Stevens, S. S. (1951) Mathematics, measurement and psychophysics. In *Handbook of Experimental Psychology* (S. S. Stevens, ed.). John Wiley & Sons.

Young, A., Hughes, I., Round, J. M. *et al.* (1982). The effect of knee injury on the number of muscle fibres in the human quadriceps femoris. *Clin. Sci.*, **62**, 227.

Young, A., Stokes, M., Round, J. M. *et al.* (1983). The effect of high resistance training on the strength and cross-sectional area of the human quadriceps. *Eur. J. Clin. Inv.*, **13**, 411.

2 Measurement parameters

P. J. Rowe

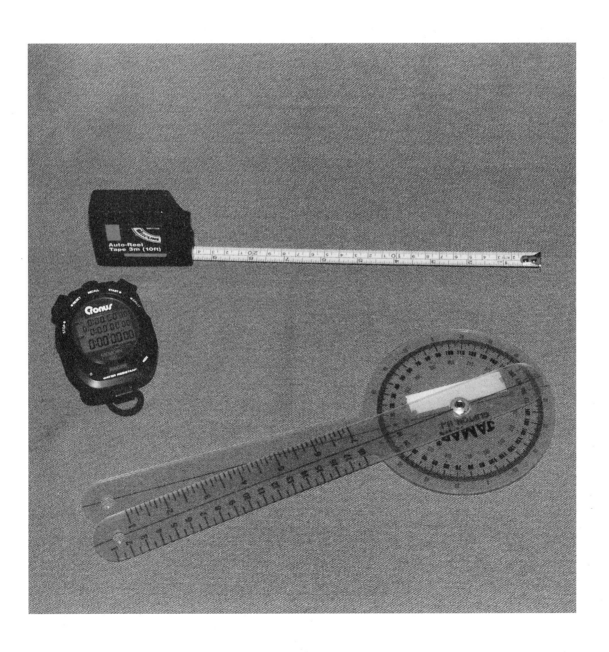

Introduction

When considering a movement analysis study of a functional task we are often faced with what appears to be a bewildering array of measurement techniques and associated equipment. In addition, considerable variation is apparent in the processing, analysis and reporting of data, and in the selection of variables used to combine or summarize the data. A couple of hours spent browsing through the movement analysis literature, or indeed subsequent chapters in this volume, will serve to illustrate the apparent diversity of measurement methodologies and reporting techniques available to the researcher wishing to evaluate a movement activity.

This diversity makes it difficult to begin to plan a measurement study on a particular topic of interest without first embarking on an extensive review of measurement methods and reporting techniques. Questions regarding the choice of equipment often dominate the early stages of the research process, leading to 'equipment driven' project planning.

On first inspecting the movement analysis literature it is not immediately apparent that, while techniques of measurement and reporting vary, the vast majority of these studies record one or more of nine key mechanical variables;

1. Time
2. Linear displacement
3. Linear velocity
4. Linear acceleration
5. Angular displacement
6. Angular velocity
7. Angular acceleration
8. Force
9. Moment of force.

This chapter seeks to explore these nine basic measures, their definitions, meanings and interrelationships, and how they may be combined and transformed to produce derived variables of value in the study of human motion.

General concepts

A defining aspect of animate life and the human race's position in the animal kingdom is the ability to produce motion. This can be illustrated by reference to the definitions of 'animated' (lively, vivacious, having apparent motion) and 'animal' (being endowed with life, sensation and voluntary motion) found in the *Oxford English Dictionary*. Motion is an important element of normal daily life, and restrictions in the quantity or quality of movement can have marked and serious effects on our well-being and, in some circumstances, can be life-threatening. The re-establishment of normal human motion is therefore a common goal of rehabilitation for health professionals.

Conversely, in sporting activities it is often the departure from normal movement that is of interest. Some athletes may seek improvements in the quantity and quality of motion, e.g. sprint runners, while others may seek to reduce movement to a minimum, e.g. archers.

Motion analysis often involves comparison of the subjects under examination with a group of their peers. For this comparison to be valid we require a consistent definition of motion to be employed in all tests, and hence our discussion of the description of motion should begin with a definition of motion itself.

Although we understand the concept of motion and can recognize it when we see it, defining motion actually proves quite a difficult task. Probably the best definition of motion is given by the following:

> Motion is the act or process of changing place or position with respect to some reference point or object.
>
> *Oxford English Dictionary*

This definition contains three important concepts regarding motion.

First, motion is an 'act or process'. This implies that motion, and the movement it produces, take place over a period of time. The laws of physics specifically disallow the science fiction idea that we can be transported instantaneously from one point in space to another. The movement of matter takes time, and has a maximum rate of travel set by the speed of light ($3 \times 10^8 \, \text{ms}^{-1}$). According to Einstein's theory of relativity, movement velocities in excess of this value are impossible and movement will therefore always take time. Hence, time is an important element of movement studies and one of the nine key mechanical variables.

Second, motion involves 'changing place or position'. In order to 'change place', we are required to change location within the universe. Our position within the universe can be fully described using three parameters; this is the concept of three-dimensional space. In most motion analysis situations, the distances (translations) along three axes at right angles to one another (orthogonal) are used to define a point in space. These axes are often labelled X, Y and Z, but conventions vary as to which is defined as which. This method is known as the Cartesian system, and gives three-dimensional Cartesian co-ordinates. However, other co-ordinate systems do exist and are sometimes employed in motion studies.

Changing 'position' can be thought of as involving a change in the orientation of the object (a rotation) rather than a change in the location of the object (a translation). In other words, the object stays where it is but is spinning, and hence changing orientation. An example is given by an ice skater executing a spin at one point on the ice. Again, in three-dimensional space, three parameters are required to fully define the rotational movement of an object. In human motion analysis studies it is normal to define these rotations relative to the three orthogonal axes already defined, i.e. rotations around the X, Y and Z axes.

Thus, the assertion that motion involves 'changing place or position' leads us to the realization that movement can be fully described by reporting the translation of the centre of the object (in three-dimensional space) and the rotation of the object around its centre (in three-dimensional space). Motion in three-dimensional space therefore has six degrees of freedom; three translations and three rotations.

The description of motion using these concepts is known as 'kinematics'. Kinematics is concerned with the geometry of motion, and seeks to describe motion rather than to explain why it occurs. For this reason, it is considered an observational rather than an analytical discipline. The description of translatory motion is known as 'linear kinematics'. Linear kinematics uses three mechanical variables to describe linear motion: linear displacement, linear velocity and linear acceleration (often abbreviated to displacement, velocity and acceleration). The description of rotary motion is known as 'angular kinematics'. Angular kinematics can be described using a similar set of three mechanical variables: angular displacement, angular velocity and angular acceleration. The general motion of an object can thus be fully described by considering the linear and angular kinematics of the object in three-dimensional space. The description of linear and angular kinematics therefore introduces six more of the key mechanical variables used to investigate human movement.

The third and final point of interest in this definition of motion is that motion takes place 'with respect to some reference point or object'. The reference point or object can be any point in the universe, and is very influential in determining what we 'see'. As an example, consider passengers on a train passing a station. They will 'see' the station pass by through the windows while their fellow travellers on the train remain in the same position, and will interpret this as the train moving through the station and leaving it behind. However, it could be that the train is not moving and the station is! The passengers would receive the same visual information in both cases, and would be likely to interpret it in the same way. It is not very often that you see stations on the move and so, in this case, the chances of being wrong are small.

If, however, we take two objects that we know move around, it is not always so clear which is moving and which is stationary. Imagine sitting in a train in a station when the train at an adjoining platform starts to move. Initially we may think that our train has begun to move and the other train is stationary. It is only when we fail to feel the motion of our train or we observe that other objects such as the station have not changed location that we interpret the situation as the other train moving while we are stationary.

Luckily for motion analysis, mechanics recognizes no difference in any of these situations except that the reference point or object from which motion is measured is changing. We would say that if the passengers on the train interpret what they see as the train moving and the station staying still, they have chosen the station as the reference point or object for measuring motion. If they choose to see themselves and the train as stationary and the station passing by the window as moving, they have chosen to name the train as the reference point or object from which to measure motion. All motion must be described relative to some other point or object, and hence the statement that 'all motion is relative'.

Therefore, when describing motion, we must define the origin of motion against which we will measure movement. The choice of reference point or object will affect the data obtained in human motion studies. For example, consider measuring the angle of inclination of the upper body during gait. Some studies have reported the angle of inclination relative to the vertical, while others have reported it relative to the pelvis. Each method gives a characteristic trace for inclination angle against time, but the shapes of the curves and magnitudes of the angles are not the same and it is not possible to convert from one form to the other because the angle of the pelvis to the vertical is not known. The definition of an appropriate reference point or origin is therefore an important aspect of the protocol of any motion analysis study.

While the definition of motion we have used highlights three key points, it is deficient in one aspect – it does not indicate the cause of motion. In the above discussion of relative motion, we often relied on 'feel' to determine whether we were moving or not. Mechanical receptors in our body feel the pushes and pulls applied by gravity, inertia and other objects in contact with the skin. These pushes and pulls are known as forces, and it is the interactions of these forces that determine the motion of our body.

By pushing or pulling, forces attempt to change the motion of objects. Forces can stop objects or make them move faster or slower or in different directions; i.e. they effect the linear kinematics of the object. In addition, forces applied away from with the centre of an object produce an effect that causes the object to spin. This effect is known as a moment of force, and affects the angular kinematics of the object. Forces and moments control the changes in motion of the object. An analysis of the forces and moments acting on an object can be used to predict its subsequent motion. Forces and moments therefore explain the causes of motion rather than simply describing the motion occurring. This branch of mechanics – seeking to explain the causes of motion – is called 'kinetics', and is considered an analytical rather than a purely observational discipline.

This discussion of the causes of motion has introduced the last two of our nine key mechanical variables, namely 'force' and 'moment of force'. A force can be defined as 'that which acts to change (or to try to change) the motion of an object'. If the forces acting on an object are not balanced there will be a net force on the object, and it will begin to move in the direction of the net force, so altering the linear kinematics of the object. If the moments of the forces applied to an object do not balance there will be a net moment on the object, and the object will begin to spin in the direction of the net moment, so altering the angular kinematics of the object. Newton's laws of motion, which will be covered later in this chapter, govern the way in which these interactions affect motion. Forces and moments have an important role in changing the motion of objects and hence they are commonly recorded in human movement studies.

By recording some or all of these nine mechanical variables we are able to describe motion and analyse the causes of motion. The subsequent sections of this chapter will introduce each variable, its definition, and points of note relevant to human movement studies. We will also explore the inter-relationships between these nine variables, and how they can be combined or transformed to produce other measures of use in movement studies. We will begin this process by considering time.

Time

Time is a vital element of motion. Without a change in time, there is no motion. Conversely, motion must take place over time. This relationship between time and motion is often illustrated in popular fiction using statements such as 'time stood still' and 'frozen in time'. It is only in science fiction that we find motion occurring in the absence of time.

The recording of time is therefore an important element of motion analysis. Some studies record the time required to conduct a task, e.g. the time taken to walk 10 m, the time taken to rise from a chair or the time taken to reach and grasp an object. Timings are also used to investigate sub-components of a task (e.g. the stance and swing phase timings in gait) and the timing of specific key actions in a task (e.g. back off the seat, thighs off the seat, and upright stance during rising to stand from a chair).

While much can be gained from these simple and global measures of performance, the data do not indicate how or why the motion occurred to produce these changes over time. We have little information on the quantity or quality of the movement that occurred to produce these overall effects. If we wish to examine the movement more closely we must record one of the other eight variables, and it is here that we encounter the other important issue related to time in motion analysis.

As we have seen, time and motion occur simultaneously. It is usual (though not compulsory) to use time as the independent variable (the variable under our control), and one of the other eight variables as the dependent variable. Put more simply, it is common to record changes in, for example, force against time rather than vice versa. Time has a unique property in that it always advances, and hence no ambiguity can occur when recording variables relative to time. Figure 2.1 shows a force versus time curve generated by a human subject walking over a force plate mounted

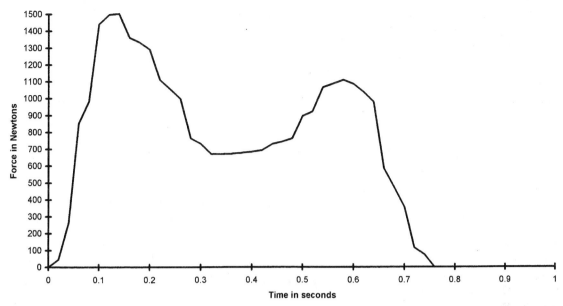

Figure 2.1 Vertical force versus time curve recorded using a floor-mounted Kistler force plate during a single step in a normal human subject

in the floor. For every time point on the X axis, there is one and only one force value recorded on the Y axis.

However, imagine using force as the independent variable and time as the dependent variable

during this same experiment. This would produce the data displayed in Figure 2.2. Now, there are one or more dependent data points for each value of the independent variable, and this will confuse the analysis.

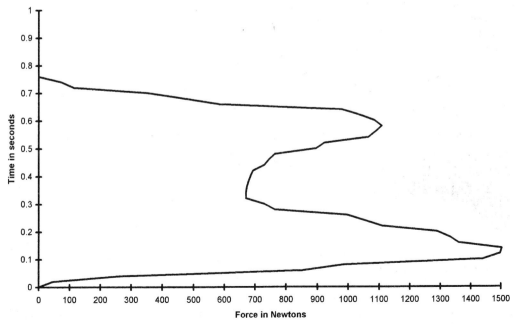

Figure 2.2 Time versus vertical force curve recorded using a floor-mounted Kistler force plate during a single step in a normal human subject

In some limited circumstances we may choose to use time as the dependent variable. For example, we may record lap times during a long distance track running event. In this case, we would record the time for completion of each lap of 400 m and hence time is the dependent variable. Another common example is a 10 m walking test, in which we record the time taken to walk a set distance of 10 m. However, such situations are rare and it is usual to use time as the independent variable against which other variables are recorded.

Having decided to use time as the control variable for recording, we encounter a second issue that requires resolution. Time is a continuum, and progresses in infinitesimally small divisions. Time is therefore a continuous variable otherwise known as an analogue signal. Most transducers designed to record linear or angular kinematics or kinetics produce a continuous output. In days gone by, such signals were fed to analogue recording devices such as chart recorders or oscilloscopes, which also gave out a continuous recording. It was up to the investigator to sample this output and to measure data at key points or regular intervals using, for example, a ruler. This process turns the continuous analogue signal into a series of discrete measures, usually at regular intervals, otherwise known as a digital signal. The decisions about when and where to sample the data stream could be left until the results were available. However, this process of sampling the data, after the event and by hand, was inaccurate and extremely tedious for the investigator.

The advent of high-speed personal computers has transformed the data collection process. The analogue signal produced by the transducer is often fed directly to an 'analogue to digital converter' board mounted internally in the computer. This board, as its name implies, converts the continuous analogue signal into a series of digital samples (numbers) at regular intervals. The sampling interval can be controlled, and can often be made to vary from as many as 20 000 samples per second to as little as one sample per hour.

The use of computers for data recording and analysis has greatly expanded the possibilities for, and the potential of, human motion analysis. However, in order to exploit these gains the researcher must select a frequency for sampling the incoming signal prior to data recording.

At first sight it might appear a good strategy to sample as fast as possible, in order to approximate a continuous signal and delay the choice of ultimate sampling frequency until after the data have been recorded. However, computers have a limited capacity to store data in their memory and, at fast sampling speeds, they do not have time to store the data to disk; hence the storage capacity of the computer is limited. While the memory capacity of computers is expanding, it is unlikely that they will possess sufficient memory in the near future to make this a viable proposition. Even if this were to occur, this strategy is not advisable as it would produce vast quantity of data for storage and processing and would therefore greatly increase the time required to analyse the results of the study being undertaken.

The question, then, is how slowly should we sample in order to properly record the signal and yet store as few data as possible? This is a difficult one to answer. Sampling theory suggests that sampling should occur in excess of twice the highest frequency of interest in the signal you are recording. However, in many motion analysis studies the frequency distribution of the signal is unknown. Even if this knowledge is available, then the significance of different frequency components of the signal is often unknown, and hence it is difficult to decide upon a sampling frequency from theory alone.

A more direct and practical approach is to record some examples of the required signal at a fast sampling speed. Graphs are then drawn of the data, including every data point (i.e. at the chosen sampling frequency), every second data point (i.e. at half the chosen sampling frequency), every fourth data point (i.e. at a quarter of the chosen sampling frequency), etc.

An example of this type of analysis is shown in Figure 2.3. The data displayed here are from the work of Myles *et al.* (1995) and show knee joint flexion angles, recorded using electrogoniometry, during stair climbing in an 88-year-old female subject with a Richard's screw and plate for a fractured neck of femur. In climbing a set of stairs, the subject took three steps involving the knee of the limb shown and three steps with the contra-lateral limb.

Initially, the data recorded and plotted at 100 samples per second (100 Hz) appear smooth (Figure 2.3a). Three peaks of knee flexion can be seen, relating to the swing phase of each stair-climbing step. Smaller features such as those seen at approximately 3 and 5 s and at 4 and 6 s can be seen. These features relate to the activities of weight transference on to the standing limb and swing of the contralateral limb respectively.

When the data are plotted at a sampling frequency of 50 Hz, the graph remains smooth and

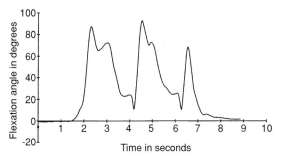

a. Sampling frequency of 100 Hz

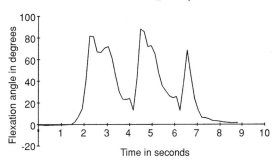

e. Sampling frequency of 6.25 Hz

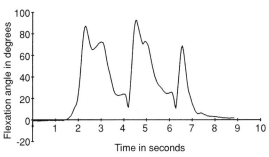

b. Sampling frequency of 50 Hz

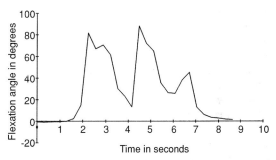

f. Sampling frequency of 3.125 Hz

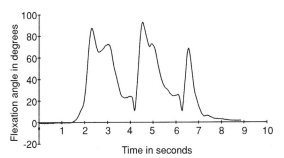

c. Sampling frequency of 25 Hz

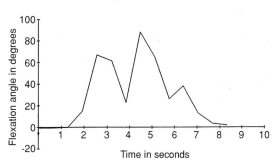

g. Sampling frequency of 1.5 Hz

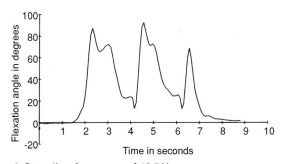

d. Sampling frequency of 12.5 Hz

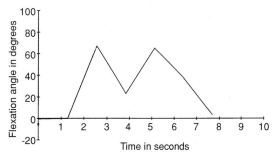

h. Sampling frequency of 0.75 Hz

Figure 2.3 Knee joint flexion angle, recorded using electrogoniometry, during stair climbing in an 88-year-old female subject with a Richard's screw and plate for a fractured neck of femur (Myles *et al.*, 1995)

contains the same salient features (Figure 2.3b). No diminution of the signal appears to occur when the sampling frequency is reduced to half the original. On reducing the sampling frequency further to 25 Hz, the salient feature of the curve remains but some reduction in the smoothness of the curve is observed, particularly at turning points such as peaks and troughs where the signal is changing rapidly (Figure 2.3c). However, the changes are small and might be thought acceptable. Figures 2.3d and 2.3e show the effect of further reducing the sampling frequency to 12.5 Hz and then 6.25 Hz. The increasing roughness of the curve is apparent, but the graphs retain the basic shape and characteristic features of the original. Both these sampling frequencies would appear to be just capable of recording the signal without loss of salient details of pattern. However, sampling at these frequencies would alter the magnitudes of the peak angles recorded in the first two steps by approximately 5°.

Further reductions in sampling rate are shown in Figures 2.3f, 2.3g and 2.3h. In Figure 2.3f, the features at 4, 5 and 6 s have been lost while the larger feature at 3 s has been retained. However, this feature also disappears in Figure 2.3g and, while the curve retains three distinct events, the shape and magnitude of these events (steps) can no longer be considered to represent the original. After a further reduction to a sampling frequency of 0.75 Hz even this similarity is lost, with the curve having a two peak appearance (Figure 2.3h). The signal has been transformed into a different shape – i.e. the signal has been aliased to something else.

This phenomenon of reduced signal quality with reducing sampling frequency ('aliasing') is, to some extent, a feature of all digital sampled signals. It is the task of the experimenter to select a sampling speed that provides sufficient data to examine the aspect of movement under study while not recording data that contain no additional information.

The choice of sampling frequency is context specific. Myles *et al.* (1995) were interested in recording joint angle data from the lower limbs during a short period of stair climbing. They could therefore afford to use a fast sampling frequency for a short period of time without creating vast quantities of data. However, others may wish to examine some other aspect of climbing ability – for example, climbing a series of flights of stairs. This situation would require longer recording periods and may require a reduction in sampling frequency.

While it is not possible to prescribe the sampling frequency required for a particular study, it is hoped that the above example will illustrate a practical way of reaching a decision. In some fields, sufficient work has been undertaken to establish 'normal' sampling frequencies. In gait analysis, a sampling frequency of 50–60 Hz is common; for running, frequencies of 100–200 Hz have been used.

It is interesting to note that the 'gold standard' sampling frequency of 50 Hz used in many gait studies (60 Hz in the USA) can be attributed to the use of television and video cameras, which operate from the electrical mains and hence produce pictures (frames) at the same frequency as the oscillations in the alternating current of the mains (i.e. 50 Hz in the UK and 60 Hz in the USA). It is fortuitous that these electrical mains oscillations occur sufficiently fast for adequate sampling of typical gait signals. However, the analysis of running using these systems was limited until high-speed video and television cameras became widely available. These cameras can produce 100 to 200 frames per second and can therefore suitably quantify fast movements such as running, jumping, vaulting, etc.

In conclusion, for most movement studies time is used as the controlling variable for data collection. The influence of time may subsequently be eliminated either partially (as in gait, where it is common to report measurements relative to the percentage of the gait cycle) or completely (as when plotting angle vs. angle diagrams for a reaching task of the upper limb). However, in order to use modern data recording and sampling methods, a consideration of the time-dependent properties of the variables to be measured is often a vital component of the planning and piloting of a movement measurement study.

Kinematics

Linear kinematics

The linear motion of an object over a period of time can be described fully using three mechanical variables, namely linear displacement, linear velocity and linear acceleration. This section of text will define each variable and explore the relationships between them.

As we have seen, one aspect of movement is the ability to undergo translation. If an object undergoes translation alone, it will move from one location in space to another while maintaining the original orientation of the object (i.e. without rotating). The mechanical variable that describes the location of an object in space is called linear displacement. By definition, linear displacement

indicates the present position of an object relative to a reference point or origin.

It is measured in metres (m).

As we discussed earlier, the object is free to translate in three dimensions (X, Y, and Z axes, or left/right, forwards/backwards and up/down). The linear displacement of an object can therefore be described using three co-ordinates, which indicate the displacement of the object parallel to the three orthogonal axes. The combination of these three co-ordinates indicates how far away the object is from the origin and in what direction. In order to describe the linear displacement of an object we must therefore define both an origin for measurement and a set of three orthogonal axes centred on that origin. We are free to choose any combination of origin and axes orientation, provided we then use this definition throughout the analysis. It is, however, usual to pick axes set with either a geographical significance (vertical, forwards and sideways) or with an anatomical significance (cranial, anterior and lateral).

Linear motion in which the object translates in only one dimension (i.e. a change in only one of the three co-ordinates) will produce movement in a straight line, and this is known as rectilinear motion. If translation occurs in two dimensions, then the object will move within a plane and this is known as two-dimensional curvilinear motion. Finally, if the object exhibits motion relative to all three axes the motion will occur in a three-dimensional volume, and this is known as three-dimensional curvilinear motion.

It is interesting to note that if none of the three co-ordinates of the linear displacement change then the location of the object remains the same, i.e. the object is stationary. Conversely, if any of the three co-ordinates do change, then the object will change location. This change in location will take time, and this leads us on to the second linear kinematic descriptor, linear velocity. Linear velocity is defined as

the rate of change of linear displacement with respect to time.

It is measured in metres per second (ms^{-1}).

Linear velocity can be quantified by considering the change in linear displacement in a given unit of time, i.e. as

Linear velocity =

$$\frac{\text{The change in linear displacement}}{\text{The time taken for the change to occur}}$$

The linear velocity of an object therefore describes how rapidly the object is moving and in what direction the movement is occurring. The linear velocity of an object can again be described using three components of velocity parallel to the three orthogonal axes of the set of axes chosen.

Again it is interesting to note that if all three components are zero the object is stationary, and that if none of the three components of the object's velocity change, it will continue to travel in the same direction at the same speed *ad infinitum*. In this case, the motion of the object would appear the same at any point in time. The object would be undergoing straight-line motion at constant speed. Conversely, if any of the three components of the object's velocity change then the motion of the object will change, and this leads us to our third and final linear kinematic descriptor, linear acceleration, defined as

the rate of change of linear velocity with respect to time.

It is measured in metres per second per second, or in other words metres per second squared (ms^{-2}).

It can be quantified by considering the change in linear velocity in a given unit of time, i.e. as

Linear acceleration =

$$\frac{\text{The change in linear velocity}}{\text{The time taken for the change to occur}}$$

The linear acceleration of an object therefore describes how rapidly the velocity of the object is changing, and in what direction the change is occurring. The linear acceleration of an object can again be described using three components of acceleration parallel to the three orthogonal axes of the axes set chosen.

From these definitions, it is apparent that linear displacement, linear velocity and linear acceleration are inter-related. Linear acceleration is the rate of change of linear velocity with respect to time, and linear velocity is itself the rate of change of linear displacement with respect to time. Changes in displacement can therefore be used to calculate velocity, and changes in velocity can be used to calculate accelerations. Likewise, accelerations can be used to predict changes in velocity, and velocities can be used to predict changes in displacement. These inter-relations can be described using a series of kinematic equations for linear motion, which will now be derived.

Consider an object undergoing linear motion from the origin of measurement to some other location in space with constant acceleration. If:

u is the velocity of the object at the origin
v is the velocity of the object at the final location
s is the final displacement of the object
a is the constant acceleration of the object, and finally
t is the time taken for the change in location to occur

then, from the definition of acceleration

$$\text{Acceleration} = \frac{\text{change in velocity}}{\text{time taken for change}}$$

or $a = \dfrac{v - u}{t}$

hence $a.t = v - u$

or $v = u + a.t$ (equation 1)

In addition, from the definition of velocity

$$\text{Average velocity} = \frac{\text{Change in displacement}}{\text{Time taken for change}}$$

$$= \frac{s}{t}$$

However, the average velocity can also be calculated from the numerical average of the initial and final velocities, i.e.

$$\text{Average velocity} = \frac{u + v}{2}$$

hence $\dfrac{s}{t} = \dfrac{u + v}{2}$

or $s = \dfrac{t(u + v)}{2}$

However, from equation 1 we have that

$v = u + a.t,$

and hence

$$s = \frac{t(u + (u + a.t))}{2}$$

and multiplying out we have

$s = u.t + \frac{1}{2}\, a.t^2$ (equation 2)

Alternatively, if we return to

$$s = \frac{t(u + v)}{2}$$

and rearrange equation 1 to give

$$t = \frac{(v - u)}{a}$$

then $s = \dfrac{(v - u)}{a} . \dfrac{(u + v)}{2}$

hence $2.a.s = (v.u + v^2 - u^2 - u.v)$

or $2.a.s = (v^2 - u^2)$

and finally $v^2 = u^2 + 2.a.s$ (equation 3)

In summary, we have developed three equations which relate linear displacement, linear velocity, linear acceleration and time.

$v = u + a.t$ (equation 1)

$s = u.t + \frac{1}{2}a.t^2$ (equation 2)

$v^2 = u^2 + 2.a.s$ (equation 3)

These equations are valid for all linear motion in which the acceleration is constant. They predict that the linear velocity developed by a constant acceleration is directly proportional to the time over which the acceleration is applied (equation 1), while the linear displacement changes as a square of that time (equation 2). While these equations are useful for calculating overall aspects of a movement, such as the average acceleration or the final velocity, most human movements involve fluctuating accelerations. In order to evaluate these situations we must return to the basic definitions of linear velocity and linear acceleration.

Figure 2.4 shows the displacement of a normal subject during a 6 m walking test recorded using rotary encoder-based movement measuring (see Chapter 3). If we wished to calculate the normal walking velocity of the subject, we could select a portion of this curve which excluded initiation or termination of gait (in this case from 3–5 s) and determine the change in displacement that has occurred (2.8 m, from 2.2–5.0 m). By dividing the change in displacement by the change in time we could calculate the velocity of the subject during gait (in this case, 1.4 ms^{-1}). In this process we have divided a change in displacement (on the vertical axis) by a change in time (on the horizontal axis). We have therefore calculated the average slope (or gradient) of the curve between these two points in order to determine the average velocity during this

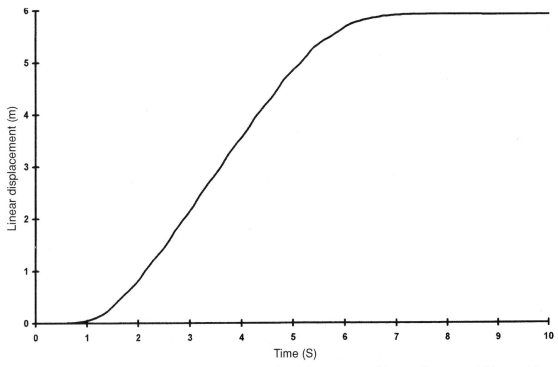

Figure 2.4 Linear displacement recorded during a 6 m, level, free speed walking test in a normal 34-year-old male subject (Rowe, 1997)

period. The slope of the displacement time curve therefore indicates the velocity of the object.

A closer inspection of the curve will reveal that the gradient of the curve fluctuates over this period of time. If we wish to characterize the velocity more closely, we will need to choose shorter and shorter intervals of time. Eventually, if we make the periods of time very small, we will be able to calculate the velocity of the object at any point in time. The process of calculating slopes, i.e. rate of change, is known as differentiation, and hence velocity is also defined as the first differential of displacement.

The use of high-speed computer-controlled sampling and data processing has meant that this process can now be implemented relatively easily using spreadsheets. Two important restrictions, however, are that the sampling frequency must be sufficiently fast to characterize the signal, and that the signal must be sufficiently smooth to allow sensible estimation of the slopes.

Figure 2.5 shows the linear velocity of a human subject during a 6 m walking test calculated from the data in Figure 2.4 using this process. The build up of velocity during the earlier portion of the activity can clearly be seen, as can the drop off in

velocity as the activity terminates. During the free speed walking section of the activity (the middle section of the trace), the velocity is seen to fluctuate rhythmically with each step between 1.2 and $1.6\,\mathrm{ms^{-1}}$, with an average of approximately $1.4\,\mathrm{ms^{-1}}$. These fluctuations indicate that walking velocity is not a constant but varies continuously during each step.

Turning our attention now to linear acceleration, it is apparent that similar rules apply. Linear acceleration is defined as the rate of change of linear velocity with respect to time, and is therefore indicated by the slope of the velocity – time curve. Acceleration is the first differential of velocity and therefore the second differential of displacement. We can use the same numerical process to estimate accelerations from velocities as we used to estimate velocities from displacement. Figure 2.6 shows the accelerations generated during a 6 m walking test of a normal subject estimated from the data in Figure 2.5.

During the initial phase of the movement, positive accelerations dominate as the subject begins to build up speed. During the middle period, positive and negative periods of acceleration occur as the subject speeds up and then slows down, and

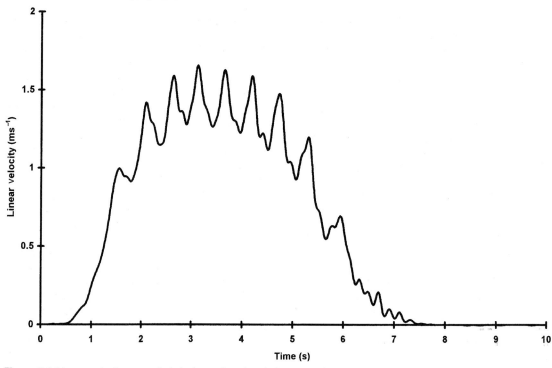

Figure 2.5 Linear velocity recorded during a 6 m, level, free speed walking test in a normal 34-year-old male subject (Rowe, 1997)

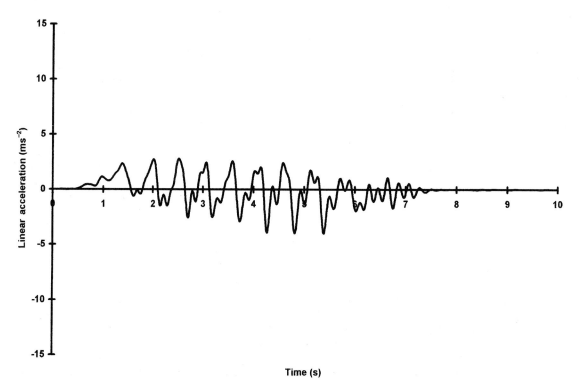

Figure 2.6 Linear acceleration recorded during a 6 m, level, free speed walking test in a normal 34-year-old male subject (Rowe, 1997)

during the later stages of the activity negative accelerations dominate as the subject slows down and comes to rest. Again, care must be taken to sample at a sufficiently high frequency and that the signal is sufficiently smooth for valid estimation of the accelerations.

From this discussion it is possible to see that by measuring displacement it is possible to estimate velocities and accelerations. These three variables are 'chained together'. It may also be apparent that the process can be operated in the opposite direction, i.e. using accelerations to predict velocities and velocities to predict displacements. In our discussion of linear kinematic equations, the first equation developed was from the definition of linear acceleration and stated that

$$v = u + a.t$$

Inspection of this equation indicates that the final velocity of an object is dependent on its initial velocity and the product of acceleration and time. Returning to the graph of acceleration versus time (Figure 2.6), it can be seen that between two points in time the product of acceleration and time is given by the area of the acceleration versus time curve between the two time points. If this area is positive, then the object will accelerate and its velocity will increase. If the area is negative, then the object will decelerate (a negative acceleration) and its velocity will decrease.

The velocity of the object can therefore be determined by calculating the area under the curve from the beginning of the movement, provided we know the initial velocity of the subject on commencement of activity. This can be estimated by multiplying the acceleration for each period of time by the time between samples, and then summating these values over the entire activity. This process of area calculation is called integration and, therefore, velocity is the first integral of acceleration.

This process of integration assumes that the acceleration can be considered constant for the short periods of time between samples without producing significant error. In effect, the area under the acceleration time curve is calculated using a series of rectangular strips (a histogram). This process will only be valid if the acceleration is near constant for each strip and hence the area can be estimated appropriately using this approximation. The sampling frequency is of key importance in this respect, and we must ensure that the samples are sufficiently frequent that little change in acceleration occurs between them.

Finally, as we have seen, a similar relationship is evident between velocity and displacement to that illustrated between acceleration and velocity. The final displacement of an object is therefore directly related to its initial displacement and the product of its velocity and the time over which the velocity acts. Again, provided we know the initial displacement of the object (usually we define this point as the origin), we can estimate the displacement of the object at any point in time after that by calculating the cumulative area under the velocity versus time curve. Positive areas will cause the displacement to increase and negative areas will cause the displacement to decrease. Displacement is therefore the first integral of velocity and the second integral of acceleration.

These inter-relationships between the kinematic variables aid our understanding of motion and can be used by the movement scientist to predict variables which are not directly measurable with the available instrumentation. It is therefore possible for movement analysis systems to measure displacements, but to infer velocity and acceleration data. Likewise, it maybe possible in some situations to use acceleration data to predict the velocities and displacements of a subject.

Angular kinematics

The angular motion of an object over a period of time can also be fully described using three mechanical variables, namely angular displacement, angular velocity and angular acceleration. This section of text will define each variable and then explore the relationships between them.

If an object undergoes angular motion (rotation) alone it will change orientation with respect to one or more of the three axes used to define motion, although its centre will remain at the same location. The mechanical variable that describes the orientation of an object in space is known as angular displacement and, by definition,

indicates the present orientation of an object relative to a reference point or origin and a line.

It is measured in radians or degrees.

As we discussed earlier, the object is free to rotate around any of the three axes (X, Y, and Z axes, or left/right, forwards/backwards and up/down). The angular displacement of an object can therefore be described using three angles, which indicate the orientation of the object relative to each orthogonal axis. The combination of these three angles indicates the orientation of the object.

It is interesting to note that, if none of the three angles of the angular displacement change, then the orientation of the object remains the same (i.e. the object is stationary). Conversely, if any of the three angles do change, then the object will change orientation. This change in orientation will take time, and this leads us on to the second angular kinematic descriptor; angular velocity, defined as

the rate of change of angular displacement with respect to time.

It is measured in radians per second or degrees per second.

It can be quantified by considering the change in angular displacement in a given unit of time, i.e.

$$\frac{\text{Angular}}{\text{velocity}} = \frac{\text{The change in angular displacement}}{\text{The time taken for the change to occur}}$$

The angular velocity of an object therefore describes how rapidly the object is spinning and in which direction the movement is occurring. The angular velocity of an object can again be described using three components of angular velocity related to the three orthogonal axes of the axes set chosen.

It is interesting to note that if all three components are zero the object is stationary, and that if none of the three components of the object's angular velocity change the object will continue to spin in the same direction at the same rate *ad infinitum*. In this case, the motion of the object would appear the same at any point in time. Conversely, if any of the three components of the object's angular velocity change, then the motion of the object will change. This leads us to our third and final angular kinematic descriptor; angular acceleration, defined as

the rate of change of angular velocity with respect to time.

It is measured in radians per second squared or degrees per second squared.

Angular acceleration can be quantified by considering the change in angular velocity in a given unit of time, i.e.

$$\frac{\text{Angular}}{\text{acceleration}} = \frac{\text{The change in angular velocity}}{\text{The time taken for the change to occur}}$$

The angular acceleration of an object therefore describes how rapidly the angular velocity of the object is changing, and in which direction the change is occurring. It can again be described

using three components of angular acceleration related to the three orthogonal axes of the axes set chosen.

From these definitions, it is apparent that angular displacement, angular velocity and angular acceleration are of a similar form and are inter-related in a similar manner to their linear equivalents. Angular acceleration is the rate of change of angular velocity with respect to time, and angular velocity is itself the rate of change of angular displacement with respect to time. Changes in angular displacement can therefore be used to calculate angular velocity and changes in angular velocity can be used to calculate angular accelerations. Likewise, angular accelerations can be used to predict changes in angular velocity and angular velocities can be used to predict changes in angular displacement. These inter-relations can again be described using a series of kinematic equations for angular motion, which are directly parallel to those for linear motion.

Consider an object undergoing angular motion from the origin of measurement to some other orientation in space with constant angular acceleration. If

ω_i is the initial angular velocity of the object
ω_f is the final angular velocity of the object
θ is the final angular displacement of the object
α is the constant angular acceleration of the object, and finally
t is the time taken for the change in orientation to occur

then, from the definition of angular acceleration

$$\frac{\text{Angular}}{\text{acceleration}} = \frac{\text{Change in angular velocity}}{\text{Time taken for change}}$$

or $\alpha = \dfrac{\omega_f - \omega_i}{t}$

hence $\alpha.t = \omega_f - \omega_i$

or $\boldsymbol{\omega_f = \omega_i + \alpha.t}$ (equation 4)

In addition, from the definition of angular velocity

$$\frac{\text{Average}}{\text{angular}}_{\text{velocity}} = \frac{\text{Change in angular displacement}}{\text{Time taken for change}}$$

$$= \frac{\theta}{t}$$

However, the average angular velocity can also be calculated from the numerical average of the initial and final angular velocities, i.e.

$$\text{Average angular velocity} = \frac{\omega_i + \omega_f}{2}$$

hence

$$\frac{\theta}{t} = \frac{\omega_i + \omega_f}{2}$$

or

$$\theta = \frac{t(\omega_i + \omega_f)}{2}$$

However, from equation 4 we have that

$$\omega_f = \omega_i + \alpha.t$$

and hence

$$\theta = \frac{t(\omega_i + (\omega_i + \alpha.t))}{2}$$

and, multiplying out, we have

$$\boldsymbol{\theta = \omega_i.t + \tfrac{1}{2}\alpha.t^2} \qquad \text{(equation 5)}$$

Alternatively, if we return to

$$\theta = \frac{t(\omega_i + \omega_f)}{2}$$

and rearrange equation 4 to give

$$t = \frac{(\omega_f - \omega_i)}{\alpha}$$

then

$$\theta = \frac{(\omega_f - \omega_i)}{\alpha} . \frac{(\omega_i + \omega_f)}{2}$$

hence

$$2.\alpha.\theta = (\omega_f.\omega_i + \omega_f^2 - \omega_i^2 - \omega_i.\omega_f)$$

or

$$2.\alpha.\theta = (\omega_f^2 - \omega_i^2)$$

and finally

$$\boldsymbol{\omega_f^2 = \omega_i^2 + 2.\alpha.\theta} \qquad \text{(equation 6)}$$

In summary, we have developed three equations which relate angular displacement, angular velocity, angular acceleration and time:

$$\boldsymbol{\omega_f = \omega_i + \alpha.t} \qquad \text{(equation 4)}$$

$$\boldsymbol{\theta = \omega_i.t + \tfrac{1}{2}\alpha.t^2} \qquad \text{(equation 5)}$$

$$\boldsymbol{\omega_f^2 = \omega_i^2 + 2.\alpha.\theta} \qquad \text{(equation 6)}$$

These equations are valid for all angular motion in which the angular acceleration is constant. They predict that the angular velocity produced by a constant angular acceleration will be directly proportional to the time for which the angular acceleration is applied (equation 4), and that the angular displacement will change as a square of this time (equation 5). As with the equations for

linear kinematics, these angular equations are useful for calculating overall aspects of a movement such as the average angular acceleration and the final angular velocity of a movement when the angular acceleration can be assumed to be constant. However, most human movements involve fluctuating angular accelerations and in these circumstances we must, as with linear kinematics, resort to the basic definitions and apply these for very short periods of time.

As we have seen, the situation for angular kinematics is a direct parallel of that for linear kinematics. We can therefore use the same numerical methods for differentiation and integration in angular motion as those developed for linear motion earlier in this chapter. In addition, the inter-relationships between the variables are parallel and we can therefore conclude that angular velocity is the first differential of angular displacement and angular acceleration is the second differential of angular displacement. Likewise, angular velocity is the first integral of angular acceleration and angular displacement is the second integral of angular acceleration. We have the same 'chain' between the variables as is apparent for the linear kinematic variables.

An example of the inter-relationships between the three angular kinematic variables is shown in Figures 2.7, 2.8 and 2.9. Figure 2.7 shows the angular displacement of the knee in the flexion/extension direction, recorded using electrogoniometry, during a single gait cycle of level, free speed walking by a female child aged 10 years (Hazlewood *et al.*, 1994). This trace shows the classic two-peak appearance of normal knee flexion during gait.

Figure 2.8 shows the first differential of this data, i.e. the angular velocity. Initially, on heel contact, the knee has a large angular velocity causing flexion. This rapidly diminishes and during the majority of the stance phase the knee shows a slight negative angular velocity, indicating the knee is slowly straightening. At toe off and during early swing, the angular velocity reverts to rapid flexion as the body is propelled forward and the knee starts to swing. Finally, an equally rapid negative angular velocity is produced in late swing to return the limb to the near neutral position ready for the next heel strike.

The angular acceleration curve shown in Figure 2.9 indicates that four periods of angular acceleration (or deceleration) are required to produce this motion. An initial negative acceleration from heel strike to mid stance is required to slow the rate of

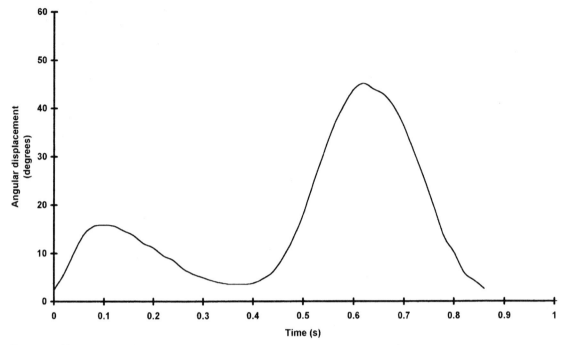

Figure 2.7 Knee angular displacement recorded using electrogoniometry during a single gait cycle of level, free speed walking in a female child aged 10 years (Hazlewood *et al.*, 1994)

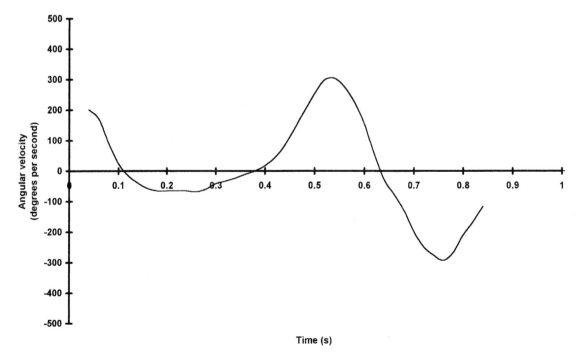

Figure 2.8 Knee angular velocity recorded using electrogoniometry during a single gait cycle of level, free speed walking in a female child aged 10 years (Hazlewood *et al.*, 1994)

flexion of the knee and to start to produce extension. A second period of positive angular acceleration occurs in late stance and early swing, causing rapid flexion of the knee and push off. A third period of negative angular acceleration follows, which has the effect of slowing down the rate of flexion and then starting to produce an extending velocity which causes the knee to come to a maximum flexed position and start to extend. Finally, at the very end of the cycle, just prior to heel strike, a short period of positive angular acceleration occurs in order to slow down the rate at which the knee is extending so that it comes to heel strike in a straight but not hyper-extended position.

The linear and angular kinematic variables and their inter-relationships provide much of interest to the motion scientist. They can be used to describe normal, pathological and excellent performance. They can be used to compare and contrast subjects and groups of subjects, and may indicate in what aspect the motion is abnormal, allowing the clinician to focus in on problem areas.

However, a more careful consideration of this issue will indicate that, even if we can fully describe the accelerations of the object and hence predict its subsequent motion, we have no knowledge of the cause of the motion. For example, a cyclist coming down a hill may have a given acceleration due to:

1. the effects of gravity alone
2. the effects of gravity and propulsion from the legs
3. the effects of gravity and resistance from the brakes or
4. gravity, propulsion from the legs and resistance from the brakes together.

Similarly, the lower leg during the later stages of swing phase in gait may descend and straighten due to:

1. the effects of gravity alone
2. the effects of gravity and propulsion from the quadriceps group of muscles
3. the effects of gravity and the resistance of the hamstrings muscle group or (most likely)
4. the effects of gravity and the quadriceps and hamstrings muscle groups.

Therefore, if we wish to analyse the causes of motion, we need to consider the forces acting on the object. It is the combined effect of these forces which determines the acceleration of the object, and hence its subsequent motion. If we remove

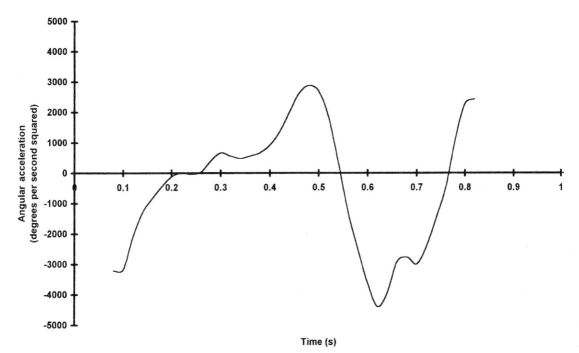

Figure 2.9 Knee angular acceleration recorded using electrogoniometry during a single gait cycle of level, free speed walking in a female child aged 10 years (Hazlewood *et al.*, 1994)

these forces from the object, as for example in space, then the motion of the object will remain unaltered for infinity.

Kinetics

Forces and moments

Much of the credit for our current understanding of mechanics and, in particular, the relationship between forces and motion can be ascribed to Sir Isaac Newton (1642–1727). His book *Principia* (1687), or *Principles*, revolutionized the study of mechanics and was one of the outstanding scientific contributions of the age. Newton, who was self-educated, can be said to have to have established the field of mechanics by setting out the rules that govern the relationship between forces and motion.

Newton carried out many meticulous observations of experimental situations, and reduced what he saw to three basic principles, or 'laws'. Initially these were regarded as absolute laws, governing all motion in the universe. However, around the turn of the 20th century, the 'laws' were brought into question when physicists tried to apply them to motion at very high speeds (close to the speed of light, $3 \times 10^8 \, \text{ms}^{-1}$). Einstein showed that, at these very high velocities, Newton's 'laws' needed correction. However, for human motion the correction factors are minute and can be ignored without any loss of accuracy. Newton's laws are now regarded as 'rules of thumb' for all movements except those at very high speeds.

Newton observed the motion of objects on the earth in a highly meticulous way. If he did (as legend would have it) think up his laws sitting under an apple tree with a bruise on his head, then his thoughts were clearly affected by long hours of experimentation in his laboratory. These are the three principles he proposed.

Newton's first law of motion

A body which is at rest will remain at rest unless some external force is applied to it, and a body which is moving at a constant speed in a straight line (a constant velocity) will continue to do so unless some external force is applied to it.

Newton's first law implies that matter has a built-in reluctance to change its state of motion. If it is stationary it will stay stationary, or if it is moving at a certain speed in a certain direction it will continue to do so unless a force is applied to it

from outside. We are all quite familiar with this finding. We know it is often difficult to make things move. We also know it is often difficult, and sometimes painful, to make things stop. The property of objects by which they resist changing their motion is known as 'inertia'.

All objects possess inertia to some degree or another. Inertia can occur in two forms; a reluctance to undergo linear motion, which is known as mass, and a reluctance to undergo angular motion, which is called moment of inertia. Because the first law is associated with the property of inertia, it is sometimes referred to as the law of inertia.

During his experiments, Newton also observed that the rate of change of velocity with respect to time (or the acceleration) of an object was:

1. directly proportional to the force applied and
2. inversely proportional to the inertia (mass) of the object.

From this he proposed his second law.

Newton's second law

When an unbalanced force acts on a body it produces an acceleration which is proportional to the force and inversely proportional to the inertia of the body, and is in the direction of the force.

This is often simplified to

force = mass × acceleration

or

f = m.a

(where the force and acceleration are in the same direction).

Finally, Newton observed the interactions between objects and developed a third law.

Newton's third law

If a body exerts a force on a second body, then the second body will exert an equal and opposite force on the first body; or, for every action there is an equal and opposite reaction.

For obvious reasons, this is sometimes referred to as the law of reaction.

The crux of the relationship between force and linear acceleration is given in the numerical summary of Newton's second law (i.e. F = m.a). This equation indicates that the acceleration produced by a force will be in the direction of the force, and will be directly proportional to the size of the force and indirectly proportional to the mass of the object. Larger forces will cause larger accelerations and subsequent changes from straight-line motion at constant speed (i.e. changes in velocity). The greater the mass of the object, the less it will accelerate under the influence of a given force. If multiple forces act on an object, then it is the net or resultant force produced when all the forces have been added together that will determine the movement of the object.

If we are able to measure the force(s) on an object and we know its mass, we can determine the acceleration that the force or group of forces will produce, and we will be able to predict the subsequent velocities and displacements of the object over time. Therefore, our chain of mechanical variables should really begin with force, which can be related to acceleration and thence to velocity and displacement. Force is the cause of linear motion and it is therefore common in movement studies to record the forces used in an activity.

Exploiting the chain in the opposite direction (i.e. using accelerations to predict forces) is more problematic. We can use Newton's second law to predict the net force required to produce this acceleration. However, the human body can often produce this net force in a variety of ways, using the musculature of the body. For example, there are 22 muscles which cross the hip joint and, because many of these muscles have similar actions, considerable redundancy exists in the system. We may predict a certain net force is required to produce the desired acceleration, but this can be achieved by one muscle alone, a group of muscles with similar actions working in combination, an agonist and antagonist pair or even by a combination of an agonist group and an antagonist group. If we then add the influence of pathology and possible spasticity, the problem becomes a complex one with many solutions. We therefore require some method to predict the actual behaviour of the body.

Electromyography (EMG) studies of certain key muscles are often used to determine which muscles are active at which point in the movement, and hence to determine the solution the body has selected. It is also usual to assume that the body will pick a solution that minimizes the amount of force produced or the energy consumed in contraction. However, such analyses are rare and complex and have therefore remained primarily a laboratory-based research interest.

Turning to angular motion, the factor that determines changes in the angular kinematics is not the magnitude of the force but the moment it produces about the centre of the object. Large moments will cause the object to have a large angular acceleration. In addition, objects with a lot of mass distributed away from their centre (i.e. a large moment of inertia) will be difficult to spin (i.e. a large inertia to angular motion). These observations for angular motion parallel those for linear motion, and can be expressed using a version of Newton's second law for angular motion:

$$T = I \cdot \alpha$$

where

T is the moment (or torque) applied to the object
I is the moment of inertia of the object around the axis of rotation and
α is the angular acceleration of the object.

Larger moments will produce greater angular accelerations, and objects with large moments of inertia will be reluctant to move and hence produce low angular acceleration. Moment (or torque) is therefore the causal factor for angular motion. If we can measure the moments applied to an object and we know its moment of inertia relative to the centre of the rotation, then we can calculate its angular acceleration and hence predict the angular velocities and angular displacements it will undergo. Likewise, if we can determine the angular acceleration of an object, we can predict the net moment required to produce that movement. Again, this moment can be produced in a variety of ways by the body, and EMG can be used to help determine the solution it chooses. Moment is therefore a key factor in determining angular motion and for this reason it is commonly recorded in movement studies.

Derived variables

In our discussion we have covered the nine key mechanical variables used to record movement. However, mechanics makes use of certain combinations of these to produce derived variables, which can provide a different viewpoint for analysis. Of particular interest to the movement scientist are impulse, momentum, work and energy. It is often not understood that these variables are simply re-expressions of Newton's second law using the inter-relationships between kinematic variables. To illustrate this, we can transform Newton's second law using the kinetic equations we developed earlier in the chapter to arrive at the definitions of impulse and momentum.

$$f = m.a$$

But $$v = u + a.t$$

or $$a = \frac{(v-u)}{t}$$

hence $$f = m.\frac{(v-u)}{t}$$

or $$\mathbf{f.t = m.v - m.u} \qquad \text{(equation 7)}$$

In this equation, the variable on the left-hand side (i.e. the product of the force and time) is called the impulse of the force. The variables on the right-hand side consist of a mass multiplied by a velocity, giving the momentum of the object, so on the right-hand side we have the final momentum minus the initial momentum, which is the change in momentum. This equation therefore indicates that the impulse of the force is equal to the change in momentum of the object. This redefinition of Newton's second law is useful in that the momentum before and after an event can be calculated and, provided the time between the two points is known, we can predict the average force generated. The impulse/momentum equation can be used to give a slightly different perspective on the cause of motion.

An angular version of the impulse/momentum equation can be derived in a similar fashion.

$$T = I.\alpha$$

but $$\omega_f = \omega_i + \alpha.t$$

or $$\alpha = \frac{(\omega_f - \omega_i)}{t}$$

hence $$T = I.\frac{(\omega_f - \omega_i)}{t}$$

or $$\mathbf{T.t = I.\omega_f - I.\omega_i} \qquad \textbf{(equation 8)}$$

The variable on the left-hand side of the equation, which is the product of the moment and time, is known as the angular impulse of the force. On the right-hand side we have two variables that combine the moment of inertia of the object with its angular velocity, and this variable is known as the angular momentum of the object. The equation therefore indicates that the angular impulse is equal to the change in angular momentum of the object.

Similarly, we can redefine Newton's second law using equation 3 from the kinematics section:

$$f = m.a$$

but $$v^2 = u^2 + 2.a.s$$

or $$a = \frac{(v^2 - u^2)}{2.s}$$

hence $$f = m.\frac{(v^2 - u^2)}{2.s}$$

or $$\mathbf{f.s = \tfrac{1}{2}m.v^2 - \tfrac{1}{2}m.u^2}$$

In this equation, the variable on the left-hand side (the product of the force times the displacement in the direction of the force) is known as the work done by the force. On the right-hand side we have variables of the form, half the mass times the velocity of the object squared. This is known as the kinetic energy of the object, and so the right-hand side of the equation represents the change in kinetic energy. The work/energy equation therefore indicates that the work done by a force is equal to the change in energy of the object (in this case a change in kinetic energy). Many forms of energy exist but, from a mechanical point of view only, three are important: the kinetic energy due to the object's linear velocity, the potential energy due to the object's position in a gravitational field (which gives it the potential to move and hence do work), and finally the rotational kinetic energy of the object due to its angular velocity.

The potential energy of an object is given by the formula

Potential energy $= m.g.h$

where

m is the mass of the object
g is the gravitational constant at that point in space and
h is the height above a chosen datum (sea level, floor level, etc.)

The rotary kinetic energy is given as follows:

$$\tfrac{1}{2}I.\omega^2$$

where

I is the moment of inertia of the object and
ω is the angular velocity of the object.

The work/energy equation therefore indicates that the work done on the object is equal to the change in the total mechanical energy (the sum of the kinetic, potential and rotary kinetic energies) of the object, i.e.

$$\mathbf{f.s} = (\tfrac{1}{2}\mathbf{mv}^2 - \tfrac{1}{2}\mathbf{mu}^2) + (\mathbf{mgh_2} - \mathbf{mgh_1})$$
$$+ (\tfrac{1}{2}\mathbf{I}\omega_f^2 - \tfrac{1}{2}\mathbf{I}\omega_i^2) \qquad \text{(equation 9)}.$$

By recording the linear and angular kinematics of a body segment and using a knowledge of the mass and moment of inertia of that segment, it is possible to calculate the fluctuations in kinetic, potential, rotary kinetic and total mechanical energy of the segment and hence to make inferences about the work done on that segment by the muscles that cross its boundaries. This technique has been used in complex pathologies such as cerebral palsy to shed light on which muscles are being used to provide energy to segments of the body. Attempts have also been made to model the effects of surgery on specific muscles or muscle groups, and hence predict the likely effect of this type of surgery on the subject's subsequent function. These studies are sometimes supplemented by respiratory gas analysis during movement, which can be used to assess the rate of energy consumption for the body as a whole. Again, these analyses are complex and time-consuming, and remain the priority of a few specialist research centres.

Impulse, momentum, work and energy are derived variables that aid our understanding and discussion of human movement. Like Newton's original laws, they help to explain the causes of motion and are therefore grouped alongside forces and moments as kinetic variables.

Summary

In conclusion, a full mechanical analysis of motion can be achieved by describing nine key variables related to motion. These variables can be recorded directly using a variety of equipment or, in some circumstances, they can be inferred from one another. In addition, the variables can be combined in a variety of ways to provide further insight into the mechanics of motion. Finally these variables can be presented and processed using a variety of different methods. These methods are often specific to the human functional movement that is being evaluated.

This chapter has attempted to report the basic mechanical variables used in motion analysis, their definitions, inter-actions and combinations. The following chapter will present the equipment choices available to the movement scientist. Subsequent chapters will illustrate the processing and presentation issues related to specific functional activities in humans.

All the equipment systems and functional studies reported in this volume, however, will have one thing in common; the data they present will be based solely on the recording of one or more of these nine key mechanical variables. Therefore, in planning a movement study, the researcher should think primarily about the aspect or aspects of movement which reflect the desired outcome of the study. Subsequently, consideration can be given to the method of processing and presenting data and to the most appropriate equipment with which to record it. In this way it is hoped that we can develop outcome-specific, rather than equipment-driven, research projects, thereby producing research work of greater relevance to the patient, health professional, scientific community and general public.

References

Baer, G. D., Rowe, P. J., Crosbie, J., Fowler, V. E. and Durward, B. R. (1995). Measurement of body segment displacement during functional activities. *Physiotherapy*, **81 (10)** 643.

Hazlewood, M. E., Brown, J. K., Rowe, P. J. and Salter P. M. (1994). The use of therapeutic electrical stimulation in the treatment of hemiplegic cerebral palsy. *Dev. Med. Child Neur.*, **36**, 661–73.

Myles, C., Rowe, P. J., Salter, P. M. *et al.* (1995). An electrogoniometry system used to investigate the ability of the elderly to ascend and descend stairs. *Physiotherapy*, **81**, 639.

Rowe, P. J. (1997). An inexpensive method of measuring one, two or three dimensional displacement of the human body during a range of human movement studies. In *Proc. XVIth Cong. Int. Soc. Biomech.* August 25–29, Tokyo, Japan, p. 5.

3 Measurement systems

P. J. Rowe

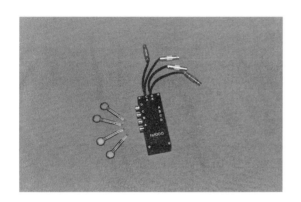

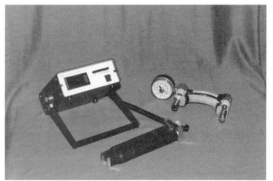

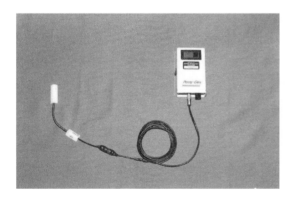

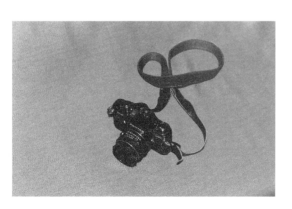

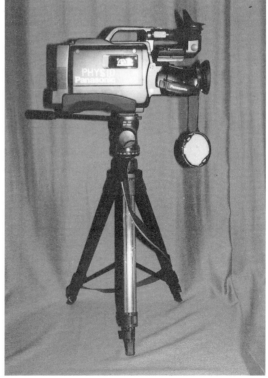

Introduction

A study of the literature relating to a particular functional task will reveal a plethora of measurement systems used to record and process the data presented in these studies. These systems range from commercially available equipment to hand-built, one-off prototype systems. The current drive for scientific research designed to support evidence-based rehabilitation, as well as the widespread availability of computer technology and the increasing involvement of the engineering community in clinical measurement, is likely to encourage this diversity.

A chapter such as this, which attempts to review the measurement systems currently available for analysing human movement, therefore requires a method of grouping together systems in some logical order so as not to become a long list of distinct and separate reviews of individual systems. One method which is often used to review measurement systems is to subdivide them into 'clinical analysis' and 'scientific or research' systems. This division is neither helpful nor appropriate, implying that clinical measurement and scientific research are mutually exclusive. By inference it suggests that clinical measurement must be unscientific and unrelated to research, and that scientific research must by its nature be of no relevance to clinical practice. Clearly clinical measurement and scientific research are mutually inclusive, and rehabilitation involves scientific clinical measurements that facilitate the forming and testing of research hypotheses and hence lead to evidence-based practice.

Alternatively, systems are often categorized based on the cost and complexity of purchasing the system, operating the equipment and interpreting the data produced. These are obviously important considerations that can affect the availability of systems in the clinical environment and also their usefulness to the clinical researcher. However, focusing on the cost and complexity of the system alone does not provide an appropriate assessment of its potential to contribute to the clinical sciences.

Many systems classed as complex and costly tools a decade ago are now commonplace in clinical measurement, while nuclear magnetic resonance imaging, computerized tomography scanning and 24-hour monitoring of ECGs are all relatively expensive procedures that have been introduced to patient care protocols within the last decade. The benefits that these clinical measure-ments bring to diagnosis, treatment and outcome are thought to outweigh the costs involved in obtaining and operating the systems and training staff in their use and interpretation.

In addition, the cost, complexity and user-friendliness of a tool are often functions of the numbers being produced. Initially personal computers were expensive, complex and capable of only a very limited range of applications. Widespread acceptance of personal computers and their mass production means that they are now widely available, relatively inexpensive, user-friendly and capable of a wide variety of tasks. The widespread acceptance of a particular clinical measurement system by practising therapists as part of their normal patient treatment protocols is likely to result in similar changes in the state of development of that clinical measurement system. Mass production is likely to reduce the cost and apparent complexity of the device and to increase its functionality.

The 'value' of a particular system is therefore a multifaceted issue, and involves the following factors:

cost
complexity
availability
transportability
robustness
speed of testing
patient comfort and acceptability
patient coverage
operator training
data processing requirements
accuracy of the data
reliability of the test
usefulness of the results in diagnosis, treatment
   and assessment and
staffing costs, etc.

The clinical measurement of human movement is a relatively young and undeveloped scientific discipline and hence the advantages and disadvantages of different measurement systems are only gradually beginning to emerge. Many of these systems have not received sufficient exploration by clinical researchers to allow a mature assessment of their value to be made. It is hoped that the drive towards evidence-based practice will add impetus to both the development of these systems and their evaluation as tools for clinical measurement.

In the light of this discussion it would be unwise arbitrarily to divide the systems into groups based on single pairs of descriptors, such as 'clinical' and 'research' or 'inexpensive' and 'expensive'. However, a full analysis of the strengths and weaknesses of all the different measurement systems currently available or indeed those presented in this book is beyond the scope of this chapter and would be of limited value. Such an analysis would quickly require revision to keep pace with technological changes, be based on the sole opinion of the author and require to be altered for different clinical and functional scenarios. An understanding of the systems can only fully be developed by studying the literature and through discourse between researchers. The later chapters in this book are designed to indicate the most common selections made for different functional activities, and some of their strengths and weaknesses.

This chapter will therefore attempt to give an introduction to this debate by providing a broad outline of the types of measurement systems currently available for the analysis of human motion. The systems will be classified and presented in relation to the types of data they can produce, and not in terms of their cost, complexity, availability or perceived worth. This review will therefore concentrate on the primary kinematic parameters that are recorded and reported by each system.

Motion analysis systems

Motion analysis systems can be divided into two main measurement approaches:

1. Those that attempt to record or predict all nine kinematic parameters accurately in three dimensions, and hence provide a full biomechanical analysis of the movement being analysed.
2. Those that attempt to record or predict only a subset of these nine parameters that can be used to evaluate human movement but which do not provide sufficient data to conduct a full biomechanical analysis of motion.

For the purposes of this chapter, we will refer to the former as full biomechanical analysis systems and to the latter as movement evaluation systems.

Full biomechanical analysis systems provide expansive and accurate data but tend to be complex and costly. They have tended to be used in situations where a precise and detailed knowledge of the forces and moments developed in the body is needed; for example, to calculate the required strength of joint implants or to evaluate patients with complex pathologies such as cerebral palsy.

In contrast, movement evaluation systems often provide sufficient data to characterize the patients and their clinical rehabilitation but cannot analyse the cause of the deficit. However, they are often less expensive to purchase and simpler to operate. Examples of the use of these types of systems include electrogoniometry to record outcome following joint replacement, instrumented walkways to evaluate stroke patients, and grip strength dynamometers to evaluate hand-strengthening exercises.

Both approaches offer considerable benefit and potential to the research-minded clinician, and it is important that they continue to develop alongside one another. Many examples of both types of approach can be found in the subsequent chapters of this volume.

This chapter starts with a review of the development of full biomechanical analysis systems, their current state of development and the type of data produced, then continues by reviewing the types of other movement evaluation techniques and systems available. It is hoped that this will expose readers to the broad spectrum of measurement systems available and allow them to take the first steps towards selecting a measurement method that fulfils their requirements.

Finally, it should be noted that many studies reported in the literature have used a combination of these simpler movement evaluation systems to analyse movement and that often the combined system is of greater value than either of the systems alone. For example, it is common practice in gait analysis to record both angular displacement of the joints and the timing of footfalls and, in this way, report the angular displacement of a joint at different stages of the gait cycle. It is impossible here to report all the possible or even the reported combinations of systems, but it is hoped that, by examining the spectrum of systems available, the reader will come to appreciate the combinations of systems that can be commissioned and the types of data they can produce. Further illustrations of these hybrid combinations will be apparent in each of the function-specific chapters that follow.

Full biomechanical analysis of movement

Attempts have been made to evaluate human movement scientifically since the times of Ancient Greece (Steindler, 1953). However, movement is often a rapid and complex activity that is therefore difficult to record visually and, as a result, movement studies are heavily dependent on the available technology. This continues to be the case, and the advent of new computer technologies has greatly expanded the range and scope of current systems and their potential to contribute to the establishment of evidence-based practice. Many advances in human movement studies were first developed for the study of human walking or gait. This trend continues today, although other functional activities are now receiving significant attention.

Technologically assisted observation of motion can be thought to have originated in the nineteenth century, with the introduction of the photographic camera. The advent of the camera allowed the measurement of linear and angular displacement of various parts of the body during movement to be recorded accurately for the first time. The work of Marey (1895), using a camera and stroboscope to take multiple exposure single plate photographs, and of Muybridge (1902), using a bank of cameras to take a sequence of single exposure plates, helped to identify key aspects of human movement and, in particular, gait.

Murray and associates used a system of interrupted light photography to assess the gait of normal subjects and patients with hip pain, hip fusion, hip replacement and knee replacement (Collopy *et al.*, 1977; Gore *et al.*, 1975, 1985, 1986; Murray *et al.*, 1964, 1971, 1972, 1975, 1976, 1979, 1981a, 1981b, 1984; Murray and Gore, 1981). In their technique, the patients wore appropriately positioned reflective targets while walking along a walkway in semidarkness. Images of the markers were recorded on single photographic plates using an interrupted light source that flashed 20 times a second. The photographs obtained were enlarged and the position of the markers measured by hand, providing data on the sagittal, frontal and transverse rotations and displacement of all major body segments and joints. However, the technique demanded that the subjects walk in semidarkness and be illuminated by a bright and rapidly flashing light and, despite considerable attempts to familiarize the subjects with the system, it must be doubtful whether they functioned normally under such circumstances.

In an attempt to remove the irritating light source, Soderberg *et al.* (1975) replaced the passive markers used by Murray with active markers made from light emitting diodes (LEDs) of various colours. These markers were flashed at a rate of 25 Hz as the subject walked in front of a 35 mm colour camera. Normand *et al.* (1985) developed a similar three-dimensional system. The use of LEDs removed the irritating light source, but patients were still required to walk in semidarkness and were now encumbered with several LEDs and associated wires, electronics and power supply. Furthermore, the development and enlargement of the photographic plates and the manual analysis of the data obtained required a considerable period of time and led to a delay before the results were available.

The development of cinefilm in the early part of the twentieth century offered an alternative method of taking serial photographs. Cinefilm techniques such as those developed by Elftman (1939), the University of California (1947), Paul (1967) and Grieve (1968) have been used widely in gait analysis. Most modern systems are similar to the method described by Paul (1967), in which two cine cameras positioned in front of and to the side of the subject were driven at 50 frames per second by synchronous electric motors. Markers placed on appropriate landmarks were used to track body segments. The film was developed, projected on to a screen and the position of the markers measured manually.

Cinefilm techniques provide a non-invasive and unobtrusive method of analysis. Apart from the bright lights necessary, the sound of the cameras and the attachment of small skin markers, the patient is left to function in an otherwise normal environment. However, cinefilm is expensive to purchase and develop, and the technique remains slow and laborious despite considerable attempts to automate the analysis.

Interrupted light photography and cinematography are essentially 'off-line' systems, in that a delay is required after data collection in order to process the data and produce the results. In order to produce results more rapidly, 'on-line' or 'real time' systems are required, which can automatically detect anatomical markers and require little operator involvement in the data processing. Most recent developments in these optical systems have been targeted at this issue.

One of the first automatic motion measurement systems was developed by Winter *et al.* (1972). In this system, a television camera and video recorder were used to record the gait of a subject wearing large passive retroreflective markers while walking across a normally lit room. The video recording was then played back through a special TV–computer interface, which determined the position of each marker in a grid of 96 vertical and 96 horizontal lines. Due to the coarseness of the grid it was necessary that the field of view of the camera covered the smallest possible area, but all the markers needed to remain in view during the movement. To achieve this, the camera was mounted on a trolley and pushed alongside the subject. The position of the markers was related to static markers on the background wall.

Cheng *et al.* (1975) interfaced a TV camera directly to a minicomputer, so eliminating the video recorder and producing a real time, on-line system. The system had a vertical and horizontal resolution of 1 part in 240, but was unable to detect more than one marker per TV camera line. This was a serious drawback in cases where different markers appeared at the same height.

Jarrett (1976), working at the University of Strathclyde, Glasgow, developed an automatic three-dimensional television system. The system used three synchronized cameras linked to a PDP12 computer to record the three-dimensional displacement of a number of small markers. The markers were illuminated by bright halogen lights, and placed on key anatomical landmarks from which the position of body segments could subsequently be reconstructed. The system had an accuracy of approximately 1 part in 300 for the three-dimensional analysis and allowed markers at equal heights. More recently, the system has been improved to reduce data processing time (Jarrett *et al.*, 1980; Andrews, 1982) by using a series of routines that enable the markers to be tracked automatically from one frame to the next and by

replacing the bright halogen lights with invisible infrared lights. A similarly constructed system is available commercially (*Vicon®*, by Oxford Metrics Ltd).

With this type of system, a typical movement analysis involves placing sets of three markers on each individual limb segment. The position of these markers relative to the proximal and distal joint of the segment is recorded in three dimensions. This is then used to determine the location and orientation of that limb segment in three dimensions, and hence to calculate the location of both the proximal and distal joints. A typical analysis of the lower limb during gait involves three markers on the shank (used to calculate the position of the knee and ankle) and three markers placed on the pelvis (used to calculate the location of the hip).

The subject, wearing suitably positioned markers, is asked to walk in front of the cameras and data are recorded at 50 Hz (50 frames per second). Following the test, the pictures from each camera are examined in turn. For each camera, the first frame in which all the markers are visible is found and the markers are then numbered manually by the operator. The computer program then looks at the next frame from that camera and attempts to

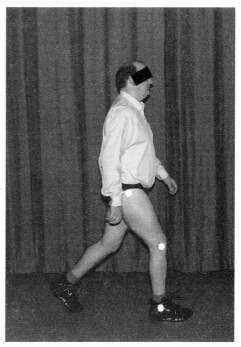

Figure 3.2 Retroreflective markers in use from the Mac Reflex® system

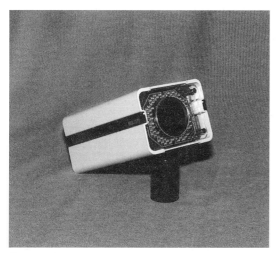

Figure 3.1 A typical motion analysis camera from the Mac Reflex® system

'track' the markers from the first frame to this second frame. Having identified the markers in the second frame, the software moves on to the third frame and so on. This process is repeated until all frames have been processed for all cameras.

However, in some frames individual markers can be obscured from the view of the camera by various body parts. During gait the arms swing backwards and forwards and, in so doing, obscure the markers attached to the pelvis. In addition, the lower leg shows marked rotation during swing and this rotation may cause the markers to be rotated to the 'dark side' of the lower leg when viewed from some of the cameras. Both these issues can lead to 'missing' markers. A further problem occurs if two markers appear at the same point of view of the camera, i.e. their trajectories appear to converge. The camera cannot separate the two markers, and when they move apart again the system does not know which one is which. Missing markers and trajectory conflicts therefore pose a challenge to automatic marker tracking and data analysis. Despite advances in tracking routines and the use of multiple cameras to try to prevent missing markers, tracking of the markers remains problematic and often requires the intervention of the operator. This makes it a time-consuming and expensive process.

Once the data from each camera have been processed, they can be combined to calculate the three-dimensional location of each marker. Theoretically, a marker need only appear in the view of two cameras to enable its three-dimensional co-ordinates to be calculated. However, data from three or more cameras have been shown to improve the accuracy of the calculations and to limit the problems associated with missing markers, and hence it is usual to use three or more

cameras. If both sides of the body need investigation simultaneously, this can lead to a requirement for six cameras.

Once the location of each marker is known for each frame, the data can be used to calculate the locations of the joint centres in three-dimensional space. From these, a host of displays can be produced, including the translation and rotation of each joint in three dimensions, the angle of one joint with respect to another, and stickman drawings showing the spatial and angular configuration of the lower limb (Figure 3.3). Finally, by using the data from successive frames, it is possible to draw time graphs of the various kinematic parameters and to animate the action using stickmen or other graphical procedures. Ultimately these systems provide a comprehensive three-dimensional description of the linear and angular kinematics of the body during the activity. This type of analysis was pioneered using the lower limb during gait (Crowninshield *et al.*, 1978), but recently other activities and body segments have begun to be analysed and there has been particularly wide use of these techniques for the analysis of sporting excellence.

Taylor *et al.* (1982) modified a similar system to use larger markers. By calculating the centre of these large markers (rather than the edge of the small ones, as had been done previously) Taylor was able to increase the accuracy to 1 part in 500. Taylor and colleagues also used sophisticated pattern recognition and tracking routines in order to reduce the amount of time needed to analyse the results. Shape recognition techniques and generalized models of locomotion have been used to facilitate automatic marker recognition and tracking by the *Elite®* motion analyser (1987), marketed by Bioengineering Technology and Systems.

There are now a number of commercially available multiple-camera, light-reflecting marker systems currently on the market in addition to the *Vicon®* and *Elite®* systems already mentioned. These include the *Ortho Trak® II* and its derivatives (*Gait Trak, Foot Trak, Spine Trak* and *Lift Trak*) produced by the Motion Analysis Corporation; the *Mac Reflex Motion Analysis System®* produced by Qualisys AB, and the *Primas®* system produced by HCS Vision Technology BV.

Due to the problems associated with tracking passive light-reflecting markers, some workers have attempted to produce markers that can be differentiated from one another in some way. Woltring (1974), Woltring and Marsolais (1980),

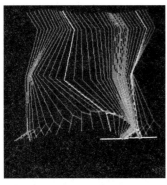

Figure 3.3 A typical stickman figure

Soderberg and Gabel (1978), Andriacchi *et al.* (1979) Andriacchi and Galante (1980) used 'active' infrared light emitting diode (LED) markers to replace the light source and passive reflecting markers used in previous systems. The markers were flashed one at a time in sequence, and could therefore be identified individually without the need for operator interference. Up to 30 markers could be used simultaneously, with a maximum sampling frequency in excess of 300 Hz. The ability to track markers and reconstruct motion automatically represented a considerable advantage. However, the system required the subject to wear the active LED markers and power supply, and either an umbilical cord or telemetric receiver for synchronization. This represented a considerable encumbrance. In addition, Andriacchi's system proved vulnerable to stray reflections from the walls of the laboratory, and in order to overcome this problem the walls and floor had to be covered in non-reflective material at considerable expense. A commercial version of this system, *Selspot*, is available from Selspot AB. Other active marker systems are also commercially available, including *Costel* from Log.in SRL and *Watsmat* and *Optotrak*® from Northern Digital Inc.

An alternative system was developed by Mitchelson (1974) called *Coda*. The system used markers made up of retroreflective coloured glass prisms. Three detectors were used to locate the markers, each consisting of a revolving mirror used to scan the field of view using infrared light supplied by a powerful arc lamp. Light falling on a marker was reflected back to the detector and the angle from the marker to detector was recorded. The markers were located in three-dimensional space using two detectors separated by 1 m that scanned the field of view from side to side, and a third detector which scanned from top to bottom. Twelve coloured markers could be used, and were automatically identified from the colour of the reflected light. The system could track all twelve markers automatically at up to 300 Hz for 6 s with an accuracy of 1 part in 500. The use of revolving components makes this system vulnerable to mechanical failure. The mounting of the detectors in a single metre-long box limits the system's field of view, and hence the applications which can be studied. Activities involving rotation are a particular problem. However, the speed and accuracy of the system are high and it can produce 'real time' results. An updated version of this system is currently available as the *Coda-3*, from Movement Technologies Ltd.

Finally, video technology has been used to record the output of the cameras and then play back the action from each camera in turn to a video digitizer, which is either hand operated or semi-automatic. These systems require less complex camera–computer interfaces, and also less computing power to run; they therefore offer a less expensive alternative to the television systems mentioned previously. However, the video digitization process is often slower and less accurate than that for television systems. Video systems currently available include the *Peak Performance System*® (Peak Performance Technologies Ltd), *Ariel Performance Analysis System*® (Ariel Performance Analysis Systems Ltd), the *Biomechanics Workstation*® (Salford College of Technology) and the *SP2000*® (Eastman Kodak Company).

In summary, all the aforementioned imaging systems are able to locate markers in three-dimensional space. By using a number of markers to identify body segments of interest, these systems are able to determine the linear and angular displacements of body segments and joints in three dimensions during dynamic activities. If a force-measuring device such as a force plate or hand dynamometer is included in the system, it is possible to estimate the forces and moments generated at the joints by these external loads. The inclusion of anatomical data from X-rays and other sources, and the use of a theoretical model of likely muscle activity, allow an estimate of the muscle and soft tissue forces required from the body to counter the externally generated moments. By considering the combined effects of the external and internal loads, an estimate of the force exerted on the joint during the activity can be made (Paul, 1976). In this way it is possible not only to describe the kinematics of motion, but also to carry out a full biomechanical analysis of the movement. This indicates the muscles controlling motion, the likely loading placed on structures within the body, and the transfers of energy from one segment to another (Ishai, 1975; Kelley *et al.*, 1978; Kelly, 1984; Winter, 1983, 1985).

When dealing with patients with chronic disabilities, such as children with cerebral palsy or patients with muscular dystrophy, full biomechanical analysis provides a powerful technique for the scientific assessment of the functional and neurological impairment of the patient. This can then be used to determine the success of a treatment regime. In addition, full biomechanical analysis of normal and pathological function is vital in order to determine the loads on joints and therefore influence the design and strength of joint replacements. Full biomechanical analysis is considered essential to provide a fundamental understanding of human movement, to provide normative data for comparison, and in the clinical assessment of patients with complex disabilities or undergoing complex operations.

Limitations

Full biomechanical analysis has some limitations. The initial capital costs incurred in setting up a gait analysis laboratory are considerable, and may include expenditure on buildings, decor, testing equipment and computer systems. Running costs such as staff wages, staff education, consumables, equipment maintenance and patient transport may be considerable. Quanbury, writing as long ago as 1985, stated that a fully equipped biomechanical analysis laboratory required a capital outlay of £150 000 on testing equipment alone and that running costs were likely to exceed £50 000 per annum. A fully equipped biomechanical analysis laboratory therefore represents a large monetary investment, which few clinical departments (apart from specialist centres) can afford.

The testing procedure can also be long and arduous for the patient, particularly if pain is present. Few systems are capable of providing immediate results, and data processing times may lead to considerable delays before the results can be studied. The results themselves are complex, and a considerable amount of education and training is required before they can be interpreted. The use of force plates places spatial restrictions on the testing procedure and may make testing difficult. In order to improve accuracy, the fields of view of the optoelectronic sensing devices are often concentrated on a small volume, making it difficult to follow the action during, for example, a number of steps, vaulting or stair climbing.

Despite these limitations, full biomechanical analysis systems remain a powerful and impressive analysis tools with which to study issues in human movement and clinical rehabilitation. The capital costs, running costs and complexity of these systems are likely to limit their use to the most complex analytical situations, in which the initial outlay is offset by the insight gained from data produced. In other circumstances, the evaluation needs of clinical practice can often be met in simpler, less expensive and more direct ways.

Movement evaluation systems

Visual movement evaluation

Perhaps the most common and complex evaluation of human movement is made by the unaided human eye. Our ability to detect abnormal patterns of movement is remarkable. The brain's ability to process the data from our binocular vision system is highly tuned, complex and versatile. Despite this ability to recognize abnormality, visual movement evaluation has some serious limitations.

First, it is dependent on the 'skill' of the individual observer. Even with considerable training and formalized methods of recording the movement (Brunnstrom, 1964; Koerner, 1984; Olney *et al.*, 1979; Tracy *et al.*, 1979), it is often difficult to get agreement between observers. Krebs *et al.* (1985) found visual gait analysis to be 'only moderately reliable', while Saleh and Murdoch (1985) indicated that visual gait analysis missed many gait abnormalities that could be detected by full biomechanical analysis systems.

Visual movement analysis is a 'real time', one-off activity. It is not possible to repeat the observation or to provide a permanent record of the activity. In addition, many human functions and activities take place at relatively high speed and this cannot be observed in detail by the human eye. For instance, it is often difficult to observe heel strike in gait. This leads to problems when evaluating, for example, children with cerebral palsy, where it may appear that they produce an acceptable heel strike but on subsequent analysis it can often be shown that they strike the ground with the metatarsals alone. Finally, visual observation only allows estimates of linear and angular displacement to be made. Velocities may sometimes be construed, but accelerations, forces and moments cannot be observed and therefore the causes of motion remain unrecorded.

In order to overcome these limitations, the clinical researcher has attempted to produce more scientific and objective measures of movement.

Timing

Arguably the most basic objective measure available is the time taken to perform some or all of a task. Timing can be achieved using clocks, wristwatches, stopwatches, and switches connected to computers. Considerable clinical information can be obtained from such simple measures. Simply recording the time taken to rise from a chair, walk 10 m or reach for a cup can provide objective information regarding the extent of functional impairment in a patient group. Patients' performance can be compared to matched normal subjects, and used to chart their recovery or deterioration.

Additionally, it is often possible to break down functional tasks into separate phases of activity and to time these phases individually. For example, a gait cycle can be split into stance and swing, and stance itself can be split into double support and single support phases (Perry *et al*., 1979). Climbing stairs can also be split into periods of stance and swing, while rising from a chair can be split into phases of leaning forward, ascent and establishing stability in standing.

In many situations the timing of activities and phases of activities can be greatly facilitated by the use of a video camera and recorder. The video allows repeated observation of the function, and it is therefore possible to time different phases or activities on different showings of the video. Repeated estimates can be made, allowing both inter- and intra-observer variability to be measured, and the video tape provides a permanent record of the activity for future reference and further analysis.

Video recorders with slow motion playback are particularly valuable, as they allow the phases to be timed at a reduced speed. Events therefore take longer to occur, and this allows transitory events such as double support in gait to be measured. The resulting values can then be converted to real time values, provided the playback speed of the recorder is known or can be calculated. Many modern video recorders are ideally suited to this task in that they can play back in slow motion at fixed speeds and without loss in picture quality.

A quick and sophisticated gait analysis system has been produced using a camcorder mounted on a tripod, a video recorder, and a multi-memory stopwatch (Wall and Crosbie, 1997). A video recording is made of the subject walking. The operator attempts to focus in on the feet while keeping both feet in the field of view of the camera. This can easily be done by panning the camera to follow the subject across the floor. The video is played back in slow motion, and the time between successive heel strikes and toe offs is recorded using the multi-memory stopwatch. In this way it is possible to record all the temporal parameters of gait, quickly and efficiently, for a number of consecutive gait cycles. This technique lends itself to the analysis of other functional activities.

Timing can also be facilitated using beams placed across the path of the movement. As the body or a body part passes through the beam, the continuity of the beam is interrupted. Using two such beams it is possible to time the passage of the body part from one location to the other. Timing can also be facilitated by switches attached to anatomical landmarks (for example, footswitches during gait, running or stair climbing) or to objects which the body contacts (for example, the back rest and seat of a chair during rising to stand). Arrays of switches built into a flat surface as, for example, seen in walkmats or pressure distribution plates can be used to identify the timing and pattern of contact between the switches and various parts of the body.

Linear displacement

Linear displacement in one-, two- or three-dimensional space is probably the next most commonly reported kinematic variable. Most of the systems used to measure linear displacement have been developed for applications in gait analysis. More recently, these techniques have been adapted to record other functional activities.

Since man first left footprints in the primeval mud, the effect of human weight bearing on the earth's surface has been used to study the spatial patterns of gait. By coating a subject's feet with water-soluble paint or talcum powder, it is possible to produce a record of the footfalls used during gait. However, the technique is rather messy and quite laborious to analyse. Recognizing this, Boenig (1977) used markers attached to the soles of the shoes and soaked in coloured ink to record the spatial positioning of the feet during locomotion along a 0.5 m wide strip of white paper. The positions of the resultant ink marks were then measured by hand using a ruler. A similar system using felt-tip marker pens was reported by Cerny (1983). This testing method, although simple and quick to conduct, had three main disadvantages. The results were analysed manually, requiring 20 minutes of data processing time per traverse of the paper; considerable quantities of paper were used; and the system gave no information on the temporal asymmetries of gait.

A similar but more efficient technique has been developed for recording the spatial parameters of gait (Wall and Crosbie, 1997). The subject walks along a 10 m walkway, which is marked with a regular grid. A video recording of the subject is made simultaneously from the side and from behind, using two camcorders mounted on tripods. Each camera is panned by an operator to follow the subject. By playing back the video and freezing it at points where the foot is flat on the floor it is possible to measure, from the grid, the forward and mediolateral displacement of the feet and, hence, to calculate step, stride length and step width. In addition the video can be used to calculate the temporal parameters of gait, leading to a comprehensive analysis of the footfalls during gait.

Various authors have attempted to automate this type of analysis using a walkmat capable of measuring the contact between the feet and the floor. Wall *et al.* (1976) used an instrumented walkway that consisted of two sets of parallel conducting rods set into groves in a corrugated walking surface at right angles to the direction of forward progression. The rods were connected by a series of electrical resistances to a power supply. Conductive strips placed on the soles of the subject's shoes linked two adjacent rods, so completing the electrical circuit. The current flowing through the circuit could be used to calculate the position of the foot relative to the beginning of the mat, and gave the temporal parameters of gait as well as step and stride length. It has been used to investigate normal subjects, total hip replacement patients and subjects with neurological problems (Wall *et al.*, 1978, 1981).

Similar systems have been reported using pressure-sensitive rod switches (Gabel *et al.*, 1979), photochemically etched boards (Durie and Farley, 1980; Gifford and Hutton 1980) and longitudinal resistive wires (Arenson *et al.*, 1983). Two-dimensional walkmats capable of measuring step width and foot angle as well as step and stride length have been developed by Gabell and Nayak (1984) and Hirokawa and Matsumara (1987). Recently, Al-Mijalli *et al.* (1993) have reported the design of a portable two-dimensional walkmat suitable for use in the clinical environment.

Walkmats, while providing information on the contact between the feet and the floor, are essentially intermittent devices. Nothing is known about the displacement of the foot while in the air. Various authors have attempted to develop systems that can give a continuous recording of one-, two- or three-dimensional linear displacement.

A simple continuous displacement recording system was reported by Mukherjee and Ganguli (1977). In this system, a tachogenerator (a wheel which gives an electrical signal as it is turned) and continuous loop string were used to record the forward progression of the pelvis during gait. Law (1987) used two tapes and two recorders to monitor the forward progression of the left and right feet during gait. This system allowed the temporal and

spatial patterns of the feet to be recorded, and also gave information regarding the velocity of the feet during swing (Law and Minns, 1989).

More recently, Crosbie and Eisenhuth (1993) have reported a similar device which uses an optical encoder attached to a wheel to record movement of a weighted string wrapped round the wheel. The encoder is made up of a small, lightweight disc with 500 slots cut in it, and the slots pass between the source and sensor of a light emitting diode as the disc rotates. Each slot causes the output of the device to produce a pulse of electricity and, by counting these pulses and the direction of spin of the disc, it is possible to record the movement of the encoder and hence the string. Crosbie *et al.* (1996) have used this device to record upper and lower trunk translations associated with stepping. The device has since been modified by Baer *et al.* (1995) to allow direct connection to a computer. By using two of these devices attached to the same anatomical landmark it is possible to record planar motion, and by using three devices it is possible to record three-dimensional displacements in a hemispherical volume. Baer and co-workers have used this device to measure a range of functional activities, including gait, sitting, rising to stand, standing, sitting down, reaching and pointing (Baer *et al.*, 1995). While this technique is still in its infancy, it is simple to use and inexpensive, costing a few hundred pounds. The data produced is accurate and three-dimensional, and as such this system has much to commend it as an alternative to camera systems when undertaking three-dimensional analysis of motion in a limited volume of space and where information is required on only one or two anatomical landmarks.

Angular displacement

Angular displacement is also of considerable interest to the researcher and clinician. Mobility in the human is produced by a series of angular displacements at adjacent joints, and it is often the function of these joints which is the focus of rehabilitation. It is not surprising, therefore, that a number of attempts have been made to record angular displacement directly. Perhaps the simplest and most common clinical measurement made in a rehabilitation setting is that of joint range, using a manual goniometer. While of interest, these passive measures of joint motion do little to reveal the function of a joint during dynamic activities. Fluid-filled and gravity goniometers attached to the subject can be used to record the range of motion of the subject during quasi-static movements, and may be assisted by video recordings. However, these devices have poor dynamic characteristics because they take time to 'settle' before a reading can be taken, and this makes them impractical for functional analysis. Researchers have therefore looked for devices that respond more rapidly to angular displacement changes.

Electric goniometers (or electrogoniometers) that record angular displacement as a changing electrical voltage have been widely reported in the literature. Finley and Karpovich (1964) reported an electrogoniometer that consisted of a rotary potentiometer wired to a battery as a variable resistor (or potential divider) and attached to the subject using two lever arms. They used this device to investigate normal and pathological gaits. Finley and Karpovich's device was uni-dimensional, in that it used one potentiometer placed on the lateral side of the joint at the level of the joint centre to measure the flexion–extension angle of the joint. Electrogoniometers were developed for both the knee and ankle, and were held in position using a metal chassis strapped to the limb. The output was recorded using a chart recorder. A similar method was reported by Trnkoczy and Badj (1975).

However, human joints are complex structures and often allow motion (both rotational and translational) in more than one plane. The centre of rotation often alters during the joint range, giving rise to a polycentric joint. The use of this type of uni-dimensional electrogoniometer with a single fixed axis of rotation to measure polycentric joints inevitably leads to restriction in the motion of the joint under observation or to unwanted movement of the instrument relative to the joint.

Tala *et al.* (1978) attempted to provide a polycentric uni-dimensional electrogoniometer using a three bar linkage with a potentiometer at each of the two hinges. The joint angle was determined using a trigonometric combination of the outputs of the two potentiometers. However, this device was essentially planar and did not allow abduction, adduction or rotation of the joint.

Lamoreux (1971) introduced a 'self-aligning' electrogoniometer, which used an exoskeleton of metal bars and straps attached to the leg. The various sections of the device were connected using parallelogram linkages that allowed abduction, adduction and translation, but not rotation. Johnston and Smidt (1969) developed a three-dimensional potentiometer goniometer with linkage bars, and

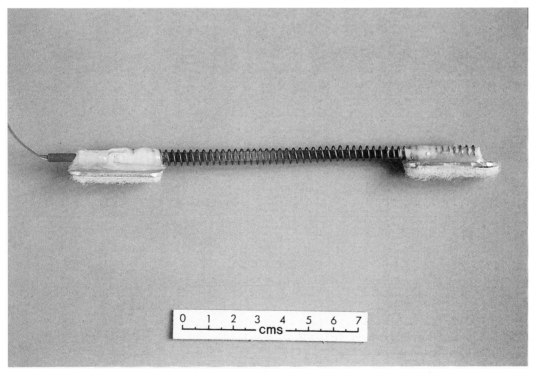

Figure 3.4 A Strathclyde electrogoniometer (Rowe *et al.*, 1987)

this has been used by Smidt and Johnston (1972), Wadsworth *et al.* (1972), Stauffer *et al.* (1974) and Kettlekamp *et al.* (1979) to study gait. Similar devices have been developed and extensively used to study motion by Townsend *et al.* (1977), Gore *et al.* (1979), Chao (1980) and Perry (1981). Potentiometer goniometers are commercially available from Biokinetics, Chattex and MIE Medical Research. These potentiometer devices with their single fixed axis of motion have found widespread use; however, they remain limited due to the restrictions of the exoskeleton needed to allow for the polycentric and three-dimensional nature of joints.

Nicol (1988) developed a new form of 'flexible' electrogoniometer, which used a long strain-gauged shim as the measuring device and could accommodate for the polycentric and three-dimensional nature of joints. Rowe *et al.* (1987, 1989) adapted this device (Figure 3.4) for clinical use, recording flexion/extension of the hips and knees of both legs during gait (Figure 3.5), rising from and sitting in a chair and ascending and descending stairs, both in a group of normal subjects and in a group of patients undergoing total hip replacement (Paul and Hamblen, 1986; Rowe, 1990). Using the

same device, Macmillan (1989) investigated elbow function in rheumatoid arthritis and elbow replacement.

The device is now commercially available from Penny and Giles Biometrics Ltd, and comes in one- and two-dimensional versions. Hazlewood *et al.* (1994) used these devices to investigate the effect of electrical stimulation on the function of children with cerebral palsy (Figure 3.6), and Myles *et al.* (1995) used the devices to study hip, knee and ankle movement during stair climbing in the elderly and in subjects following a fractured neck of femur.

These flexible electrogoniometers have found widespread applications in human movement analysis and, when care is taken to look after them and mount them on the body in an appropriate manner, they can provide accurate, valid and reliable results. Recently a number of alternative flexible electrogoniometers have been introduced, including the *Greenleaf Wristsystem* from Greenleaf Medical Systems and the *Bioback* system from Proteo Service. However, the mode of operation and accuracy of these devices has not as yet been reported in the literature.

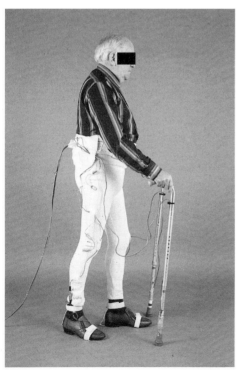

Figure 3.5 A clinical gait analysis system using flexible electrogoniometers (Rowe *et al.*, 1987)

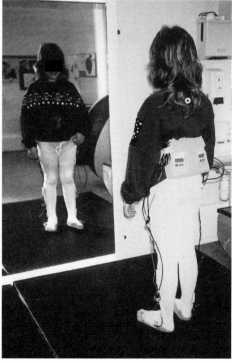

Figure 3.6 A portable gait analysis system using Penny and Giles electrogoniometer (Hazlewood *et al.*, 1994)

An alternative to electrogoniometry was introduced by An *et al.* (1988), who used a magnetic tracking device called a *3-Space Isotrak®* from Polhemus Navigation Sciences Division, McDonald Douglas Electronics Company. The Isotrak consists of a source that develops a three-dimensional electromagnetic field and a small sensor that is able to record its position and orientation relative to the source (Figure 3.7). By attaching the source

and sensor to the proximal and distal limb segments of a joint the experimenter is able to record linear and angular displacement of the joint in all three dimensions. The six degrees of freedom of the joint can therefore be examined simultaneously without a direct physical connection across the joint. The system has been used by, amongst others, Pearcy and Hindle (1989) and Hindle *et al.* (1990) to measure the range of motion of the lower back, and by Rowe and White (1996) to measure the three-dimensional kinematics of the lumbar spine during gait in patients with back pain (Figures 3.8 and 3.9).

Subsequent versions of the device are now available, and include a version with one source but four independent sensors and a version with two sources and up to six sensors.

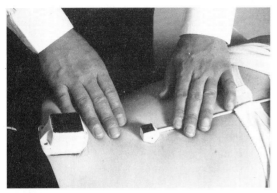

Figure 3.7 Isotrak source and sensor mounted on the back (Rowe and White, 1996)

Accelerometers

As was mentioned in the previous chapter, if the displacement of an object is recorded carefully and rapidly it is possible to process the data so as to estimate the velocity and acceleration of the body. Acceleration is particularly useful, as it is directly related to motive force by Newton's second law of

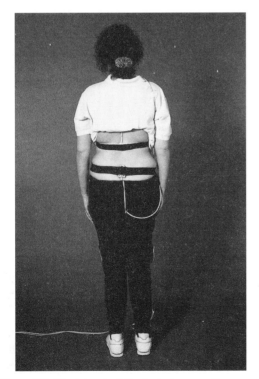

Figure 3.8 Attachment of the Isotrak measuring lumbar spinal motion in standing (Rowe and White, 1996)

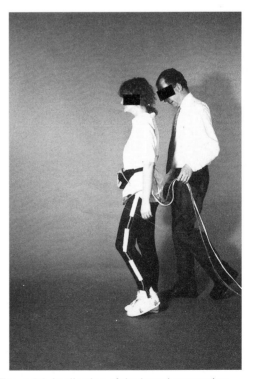

Figure 3.9 Application of the Isotrak measuring lumbar spinal motion during gait (Rowe and White, 1996)

motion (F = ma). Accelerations can, in some circumstances, be measured directly using accelerometers (Vivoda, 1986). These devices contain a small mass connected to a spring or flexing beam, and an electronic device that can measure the deflection of the mass when the device is accelerated. This deflection is proportional to the acceleration experienced by the small mass. Commercially available accelerometers include those produced by Radio Spares Components and J. P. Biomechanics.

Accelerometers have been used to measure accelerations directly, and can theoretically be used to predict velocity and displacement; however, this procedure is more problematic than when using displacement to predict velocity and acceleration, as it is affected severely by any form of drift or system inaccuracy. These errors are integrated and therefore continue to affect the data even when the noise and drift have abated; as a result, accelerometers have not found widespread use in motion analysis.

Force transducers

A number of force-measuring devices have been used to evaluate human motion. Most popular has been the force plate, a three-dimensional force-measuring device mounted in a floor or other surface. Force plates have been extensively used to investigate abnormalities and asymmetries in the loading patterns of the lower limbs in various pathologies during gait (Andriacchi *et al.*, 1977; Charnley and Pusso, 1968; Jacobs *et al.*, 1972; Jansen *et al.*, 1982; Pedotti, 1977). In these studies, the three-dimensional components of the ground reaction force and the moments generated about the three principal axes of the plate are recorded. These systems require that the foot of the limb under investigation be placed wholly upon the upper surface of the plate and that the contralateral limb remains clear of the plate. This, along with the need to conceal the plate to avoid targeting, means that it is often necessary to conduct a series of walks before a successful recording is made, and for patients with pain and severe functional limitation this represents a substantial problem. Despite these issues, force plates are now widespread and commonly form part of a gait analysis system. Commercial force plates are available from Kistler Instruments Ltd, The Bertec Corporation and AMTI Inc.

Force plates have also been used to assess balance while both sitting and standing. Sackley and Baguley (1993) used a force plate mounted in the seat of a chair to measure balance in patients who have suffered a stroke. Durward and Rowe (1995) have developed a system which uses eight force plates, four mounted in the seat of a chair and four mounted under the feet, to examine the load distribution during sitting, rising to stand, standing and sitting down in normal and stroke subjects. Various commercial balance assessment systems are available which incorporate one or more force plates, including the *Nottingham Balance Platform* from Nottingham Rehabilitation Services and the *Balance Master* from Neurocom International Inc. A system for superimposing the output of a force plate, as a force vector, on top of a video image of the subject was reported by Tait and Rose (1979), and subsequently by Cook (1981). This device, called a video vector, is commercially available from MIE Medical Research Ltd as the *Video Vector Generator*. A similar but inexpensive device has recently been reported by Rowe (1996).

Other force transducers have been used to study functional activities. Most notable is the use of instrumented force measuring walking aids to record the supportive forces generated during gait (Bennett *et al.*, 1979; Bergmann *et al.*, 1978; Opila *et al.*, 1986, 1988; Rowe 1990).

Attempts have been made to record the pressure distribution under the feet, which gives rise to the ground reaction force, using a matrix array of force transducers. These systems have tended to be less accurate than their force plate counterparts, but are useful in that they indicate not only the force being generated but the points of high pressure between the foot and floor. This is of particular benefit for those interested in foot problems such as bunions, excessive pronation or diabetes. Commercial systems include the *Musgrave Footprint* from W. M. Automation, the *Computer Dyno Graphy (CDG) System* from Infotronic, the *Emed Pressure Plate* from Novel Gmbh and the *Pedobaragraph* from Baltimore Therapeutic Equipment.

Both Infotronic and Novel also make flexible in-shoe devices that can record the pressure distribution between the sole of the foot and the shoe during activity (the *CDG In-shoe Pressure Device* and the *Emed In-shoe Pressure Device*, respectively). However, the sole of the foot is a curved surface and there is little room in normal shoes for a transducer and wiring. For these reasons the sensors are usually clustered at key anatomical points such as the heel and metatarsals, and do not cover the whole of the sole of the foot.

Moments

Moments generated at the joints by concentric, eccentric and isometric muscle activity can be measured during non-weight bearing prescribed activities using 'isokinetic' measuring devices such as the *Akron*, *KinCom* and *Cybex*. The moments exerted by a subject on a number of different manual tools can be measured during a number of work-related activities using the *BTE Work Simulator* produced by the Baltimore Therapeutic Equipment Company; however, no direct measurement system exists to measure joint moments during functional activities.

Other scientific measures of human movement

Electromyography (EMG), which is the measurement of the electrical activity of muscles caused by contraction of the muscle, has been widely used in studies of human movement. Various methods of detecting the electrical noise produced by muscles are available, including surface electrodes, fine wire electrodes and needle electrodes. EMG recordings are very difficult, if not impossible, to equate with the force developed by the muscle. While EMG can be used to indicate the activity of a muscle, morphological differences, muscle length–tension relationships and fatigue all complicate the relationship between the electrical activity of the muscle and the force generated by the muscle. Even if an EMG could indicate the force generated by the muscle, the anatomical position of the muscle would also need to be recorded before the data could be used to calculate the muscle moment produced and, hence, determine the nature of the motion likely to be produced. EMG is therefore useful as an adjunct to movement studies, but cannot be thought to evaluate movement itself. There is an excellent exposé of the issues related to EMG in *Muscles Alive: Their Functions Revealed by Electomyography* by Basmaijan (1974).

Energy expenditure has also been used to evaluate functional activity (Arborelius *et al.*, 1976; McBeath *et al.*, 1980; McNicol *et al.*, 1980; Pugh, 1973; Waters *et al.*, 1987). The amount of energy expended can be calculated by recording oxygen consumption or, in certain instances, by recording heart rate. Such physiological measures are beyond the scope of this chapter. However, extreme caution must be taken when trying to equate changes in energy expenditure with the mechanical cost of a functional activity. While there may be a causal relationship for activities where the muscle activity and mechanical work done are very simply related (for example, repeated concentric contraction of the biceps to lift a weight), this is often not the case. The situation is usually a complex one, involving many muscles in three dimensions and with varying forms of contraction and co-contraction. If this were not sufficient reason for care, the energy used can be altered by a variety of clinical factors such as obesity, circulatory problems and drug therapy. Energy studies therefore provide little analytical information regarding the mechanics of functional movement in subjects with an underlying pathology.

In summary, a number of movement assessment systems are available to the clinical researcher. These systems are able to record one or more kinematic variables for one or more joints or limb segments, but comprehensive coverage of all nine aspects of movement for a number of joints or body segments would not be practical with such equipment. These systems are therefore useful for characterizing motion and movement deficits, but are usually unable to identify the cause. To do this, a full biomechanical assessment is often required. However, movement assessment systems can usefully be employed to produce outcome measures for a number of clinical movement measurement purposes. In comparison to full biomechanical analysis, such systems are inexpensive, relatively simple to use and portable, and hence may offer a valuable alternative for clinical measurement of motion.

Summary

At the present time there exists a considerable spectrum of motion measurement systems available to the clinical researcher. In presenting these tools and systems the author has attempted to indicate that, for a particular research topic, a number of outcome measures are available, and that these measures can often be recorded in a number of ways. Therefore, when initiating a clinical research project, the investigator must select an appropriate outcome measure (for example, angular displacement of the knee during gait in knee replacement surgery) and a system by which this measure can be recorded (such as cameras, electrogoniometer, Isotrak, etc.).

The measure and the system will be affected by the nature of the research question being asked. For example, 'does the patient use the knee replacement normally?' may be more efficiently investigated by kinematic systems such as electro-goniometers or the Isotrak, which are simple to use and inexpensive. However, the question 'why is the motion of the knee different in patients with knee replacements?' may require a full bio-mechanical analysis using cameras, force plates and EMG, and the calculation of kinetic para-meters such as energy transfers between segments and the muscle work done.

While it is impossible to predict the exact nature or cost of motion measurement systems that will be available in the near future, it seems likely that the human movement scientist will continue to need to commission a system which addresses the measure-ment issues of specific interest to a particular project. It would be overkill indeed (but not unheard of) for a £200 000 full biomechanical analysis system to be used to record the walking speed or stance time of a group of subjects, when a stopwatch and video recorder would achieve the same ends with a considerable saving in time and money.

The author encourages those who read this chapter to plan their investigations based on the nature of the research question posed, the type of data needed, the level of accuracy considered appropriate and the detail required from the results. Having established these requirements, the inves-tigator can then seek a method that can determine the required data with the maximum efficiency and minimum expenditure of time and money. In other words, the question should precede the measure-ment system and not *vice versa*.

By presenting some of the historical develop-ments in this chapter, it is hoped to encourage readers to create systems and solutions that are appropriate to their situation. Most of the current analysis systems have been developed by medical engineers with an eye to clinical assessment needs. Some have included input from orthopaedic sur-geons, sports scientists and physiotherapists. How-ever, the field of human movement analysis is in a developmental stage, and direct involvement of clinicians in the design, operation and reporting of these measurement systems is vital if the recording of human movement is to become a regular activity in the clinical environment.

References

Al-Mijalli, M., Solomonides, S., Spence, W. *et al.* (1993). Design specification of a walkmat system for the measure-ment of temporal and distance parameters of gait. *Gait and Posture*, **1,** 119–120.

An, K. N., Jacobsen, M. C., Berglund, L. J. and Chao, E. Y. S. (1988). Application of a magnetic tracking device to kinesiologic studies. *J. Biomech.*, **21(7),** 613–20.

Andrews, B. (1982). *On-line Locomotion Analysis using Television Techniques*. PhD thesis, University of Strathclyde, Glasgow, UK.

Andriacchi, T. and Galante, J. (1980). The influence of total hip and knee replacement on gait. *Proc. Int. Conf. Rehabil. Eng.*, Toronto, pp. 71–4.

Andriacchi, T., Ogle, J. and Galante, J. (1977). Walking speed as a basis for normal and abnormal gait measurements. *J. Biomech.*, **10,** 261–8.

Andriacchi, T., Hampton, S., Schultz, A. and Galante, J. (1979). Three-dimensional co-ordinate data processing in human motion analysis. *J. Biomech. Eng.*, **101,** 279–83.

Arborelius, M., Carlsson, A. and Nilsson, B. (1976). Oxygen intake and walking speed before and after total hip replace-ment. *Clin. Orthop.*, **12,** 113–15.

Arenson, J., Ishai, G. and Bar, A. (1983). A system for monitoring the position and time of feet contact during walking. *J. Med. Eng. Tech.*, **7(6),** 280–4

Baer, G. D., Rowe, P. J., Crosbie, J., Fowler, V. E. and Durward, B. R. (1995). Measurement of body segment displacement during functional activities. *Physiotherapy*, **81 (10)** 643.

Basmaijan, J. V. (1974). *Muscles Alive: Their Functions Revealed by Electromyography*. Williams & Wilkins.

Bennett, L., Murray, P., Murphy, E. and Sowell, T. (1979). Locomotion through cane impulse. *Bull. Prosth. Res.*, **10(31),** 38–47.

Bergmann, G., Kolbel, R. and Rohlmann, A. (1978). Walking aids – their effect on forces transmitted at the hip joint and proximal end of the femur. *Biomechanics*, **VI(B),** 264–9.

Boenig, D. (1977). Evaluation of a clinical method of gait analysis. *Phys. Ther.*, **57(7),** 795–8.

Brunnstrom, S. (1964). Recording gait patterns of adult hemiplegic patients. *Phys. Ther.*, **44,** 11.

Cerny, K. (1983). A clinical method of quantitative gait analysis. *Phys. Ther.*, **63(7),** 1125–6.

Chao, E. (1980). Justification of a triaxial goniometer for the measurement of joint rotation. *J. Biomech.*, **13,** 989–1006.

Charnley, J. and Pusso, R. (1968). The recording and analysis of gait in relation to surgery of the hip joint. *Clin. Orthop.*, **58,** 153–64.

Cheng, I., Koozekanini, S. and Fatehi, M. (1975). A simple computer–television interface system for gait analysis. *IEEE Trans. Biomed. Eng.*, **22,** 259–60.

Collopy, M., Murray, M., Gardener, G. *et al.* (1977). Kinesiologic measurements of functional performance before and after geometric total knee replacement. *Clin. Orthop.*, **126,** 196–202.

Cook, T. (1981). Vector visualization in gait analysis. *Bull. Pros. Res. (Conf. Rep.)*, **10–35(18/1),** 308–9.

Crosbie, J. and Eisenhuth, J. (1993). Transducer for the measurement of linear displacement of body segments. *Med. Biol. Eng. Comput.*, **31,** 430–2.

Crosbie, J., Durward, B. D. and Rowe, P. J. (1996). Upper and lower trunk translations associated with stepping. *Gait and Posture*, **4(1),** 26–33.

Crowninshield, R., Johnston, R., Andrews, J. and Brand, R.

(1978). A biomechanical investigation of the human hip. *J. Biomech.*, **11**, 75–85.

Durie, N. and Farley, R. (1980). An apparatus for step length measurement. *J. Biomed. Eng.*, **2**, 38–40.

Durward, B. R. and Rowe, P. J. (1995). Measurement of total vertical force and time during rising to stand in normal and hemiplegic subjects. *Physiotherapy*, **81**, 640.

Elftman, H. (1939). Forces and energy changes in the leg during walking. *Am. J. Physiol.*, **125**, 339–56.

Finley, F. and Karpovich, P. (1964). Electrogoniometric analysis of normal and pathological gaits. *Res. Q.*, **35(3)** (supp.), 379–84.

Gabel, R., Johnston, R. and Crowninshield, R. (1979). A gait analyzer/trainer instrumentation system. *J. Biomech.*, **12**, 543–9.

Gabell, A. and Nayak, U. (1984). The effect of age on variability in gait. *J. Geront.*, **39**, 662–6.

Gifford, G. and Hutton, W. (1980). A microprocessor-controlled system for evaluating treatments for disabilities affecting the lower limb. *J. Biomed. Eng.*, **2**, 46–8.

Gore, T., Flynn, M. and Stevens, J. (1979). Measurement and analysis of hip joint movements. *Eng. Med. (ImechE)*, **8**, 21–5.

Gore, D., Murray, M., Sepic, S. and Gardner, G. (1975). Walking patterns of men with unilateral surgical hip fusion. *J. Bone Jt. Surg.*, **57(A)**, 759–65.

Gore, D., Murray, M., Gardner, G. and Sepic, S. (1985). Hip function after total vs. surface replacement. *Acta Orthop. Scand.*, **56**, 386–90.

Gore, D., Murray, M., Gardner, G. and Mollinger, L. (1986). Comparison of function two years after revision of failed total hip arthroplasty and primary hip arthroplasty. *Clin. Orthop.*, **208**, 168–73.

Grieve, D. (1968). Gait patterns and speed of walking. *Biomed. Eng.*, **March**, 119–22.

Hazlewood, M. E., Brown, J. K., Rowe, P. J. and Salter P. M. (1994). The use of therapeutic electrical stimulation in the treatment of hemiplegic cerebral palsy. *Dev. Med. Child Neur.*, **36**, 661–73.

Hindle, R. J., Pearcy, M. J., Cross, A. T. and Miller, D. H. (1990). Three-dimensional kinematics of the human back. *Clin. Biomech.*, **5**, 218–28.

Hirokawa, S. and Matsumara, K. (1987). Gait analysis using a measuring walkway for temporal and distance factors. *Med. Biol. Eng. Comput.*, **25**, 62–74.

Ishai, G. (1975). *Whole Body Gait Kinetics*. PhD thesis, University of Strathclyde, Glasgow.

Jacobs, N., Skorecki, J. and Charnley, J. (1972). Analysis of the vertical components of force in normal and pathological gait. *J. Biomech.*, **5**, 11–34.

Jansen, E., Vittas, D., Hellberg, S. and Hansen, J. (1982). Normal gait of young and old men and women. *Acta Orthop. Scand.*, **53**, 193–6.

Jarrett, M. (1976). *A Television/Computer System for Human Locomotion Analysis*. PhD thesis, University of Strathclyde, Glasgow.

Jarrett, M., Moore, P. and Swanson, A. (1980). Assessment of gait using components of the ground reaction vector. *Med. Biol. Eng. Comput.*, **18**, 685–8.

Johnston, R. and Smidt, G. (1969). Measurement of hip joint motion during walking, an evaluation of an electrogoniometric method. *J. Bone Jt. Surg.*, **51(A)**, 1083–94.

Kelley, D., Dainis, A. and Wood, G. (1978). Mechanics and muscular dynamics of rising from a seated position. *Biomechanics*, **VB**, 127–34.

Kelly, I. (1984). *Forces in the Joints of the Lower Limb before and after Hip Arthroplasty*. MD thesis, University of Edinburgh.

Kettlekamp, D., Johnston, R., Smidt, G. *et al.* (1979). An electrogoniometric study of knee motion in normal gait. *J. Bone Jt. Surg.*, **52(A)**, 775–90.

Koerner, I. (1984). *Observation of Human Gait* (a study guide to accompany videocassettes). Health Sciences Audiovisual Education, Univeristy of Alberta.

Krebs, D. E., Edelstein, J. E. and Fishman, S. (1985). Reliability of observational kinematic gait analysis. *Phys. Ther.*, **65**, 1027–33.

Lamoreux, L. (1971). Kinematic measurements in the study of human walking. *Bull. Prosth. Res.*, **10(15)**, 3–84.

Law, H. T. (1987). Microcomputer-based, low-cost method for measurement of spatial and temporal parameters of gait. *J. Biomed. Eng.*, **9**, 115–20.

Law, H. T. and Minns, R. A. (1989). Measurement of spatial and temporal parameters of gait. *Physiotherapy*, **75**, 81–4.

Marey, E. (1895). *Movement*. Heinemann.

Macmillan, F. S. (1989). *Performance of the Rheumatoid Elbow following Elbow Arthroplasty*. PhD thesis, University of Strathclyde, Glasgow.

McBeath, A., Bahrke, M. and Balke, B. (1980). Walking efficiency before and after total hip replacements as determined by oxygen consumption. *J. Bone Jt. Surg.*, **65(A)**, 807–10.

McNicol, M., McHardy, R. and Chalmers, J. (1980). Exercise testing before and after hip arthroplasty. *J. Bone Jt. Surg.*, **62(B)**, 326–31.

Mitchelson, D. (1974). *CODA instrument for 3D Movement Recording*. Report Number 145, Loughborough University of Technology.

Mukherjee, P. and Ganguli, S. (1977). Detection of gait abnormality from tachographic data. *J. Med. Eng. Tech.*, **1(2)**, 106–7.

Murray, M. and Gore, D. (1981). Gait of patients with hip pain or loss of hip joint motion. In *Clinical Biomechanics*. Black & Dumbleton, Churchill Livingstone.

Murray, M., Drought, B. and Kory, M. (1964). Walking patterns of normal men. *J. Bone Jt. Surg.*, **46(A)**, 335–60.

Murray, M., Gore, D. and Clarkson, B. (1971). Walking patterns of patients with unilateral hip pain due to osteoarthritis and avascular necrosis. *J. Bone Jt. Surg.*, **53(A)**, 259–74.

Murray, M., Brewer, B. and Zuege, R. (1972). Kinesiologic measurement of functional performance before and after McKee–Farrar total hip replacement. *J. Bone Jt. Surg.*, **54(A)**, 237–56.

Murray, M., Brewer, B., Gore, D. and Zuege, R. (1975). Kinesiology after McKee–Farrar total hip replacement. *J. Bone Jt. Surg.*, **57(A)**, 337–42.

Murray, M., Gore, D., Sepic, S. and Gardner, G. (1984). Function after revision of failed total hip arthroplasty. *Acta*

Orthop. Scand., **55**, 59–62.

Murray, M., Gore, D., Brewer, B. *et al.* (1976). Comparison of functional performance after McKee–Farrar, Charnley and Muller total hip replacement. *Clin. Orthop.*, **121**, 33–43.

Murray, M., Gore, D., Brewer, B. *et al.* (1979). A comparison of the functional performance of patients with Charnley and Muller total hip replacements. *Acta Orthop. Scand.*, **50**, 563–9.

Murray, M., Gore, D., Brewer, B. *et al.* (1981a). Comparison of Muller total hip replacement with and without trochanteric osteotomy. *Acta Orthop. Scand.*, **52**, 345–52.

Murray, M., Gore, D., Brewer, B. *et al.* (1981b). Joint function after total hip arthroplasty. *Clin. Orthop.*, **157**, 119–24.

Muybridge, E. (1902). *The Human Figure in Motion*. New York – Dover Publications.

Myles, C., Rowe, P. J., Salter, P. M. *et al.* (1995). An electrogoniometry system used to investigate the ability of the elderly to ascend and descend stairs. *Physiotherapy*, **81**, 639.

Nicol, A. (1988). A new flexible electrogoniometer with widespread applications. *Biomechanics*, **X**, 1029–33.

Normand, M., Richards, C., Filton, M. *et al.* (1985). A simplified method of tridimensional analysis of gait movements. *Biomechanics*, **IX(A)**, 255–59.

Olney, S. J., Elkin, N. D. Lowe P. J. *et al.* (1979). An ambulation profile for clinical gait evaluation. *Physiother. Can.*, **31**, 31–85.

Opila, K., Nicol, A. and Paul, J. (1986). Biomechanical analysis of limb loads in aided gait using elbow crutches. In *Biomechanics and Current Interdisciplinary Research* (S. Perren and E. Schneider, eds.), pp. 567–72. Martinus Nijhoff.

Opila, K., Nicol, A. and Paul, J. (1988). Quantification of the function of walking aids. *Biomechanics*, **XA**, 147–72.

Paul, J. (1967). *Forces at the Human Hip Joint*. PhD thesis, University of Glasgow.

Paul, J. (1976). Loading on normal hip and knee joints and on joint replacements. In *Engineering in Medicine, Vol. 2: Advances in Artificial Hip and Knee Joint Technology* (Schaldach and Wohmann, eds.). Springer-Verlag.

Paul, J. and Hamblen, D. (1986). *Clinical and Biomechanical Investigation of the Lower Limb Function in Patients with Polyarthritis following Single Joint Replacement*. Report to the Scottish Home and Health Department. Contract Number K/RED/4/C42. University of Strathclyde, Glasgow.

Pearcy, M. J. and Hindle, R. J. (1989). New method for the non-invasive three-dimensional measurement of human back movement. *Clin. Biomech.*, **4**, 73–9.

Pedotti, A. (1977). Simple equipment used in clinical practice for evaluation of locomotion. *IEEE Trans. Biomed. Eng.*, **24(5)**, 456–65.

Perry, J. (1981). The techniques and concepts of gait analysis. *Bull. Prosth. Res.* , **18(1)** (Conf. Rep.), 279–81.

Perry, J., Bontgranger, E. and Antonelli, D. (1979). Footswitch definition of basic gait characteristics. In *Disability. Proceedings of a Seminar on Rehabilitation of the Disabled, August 1978* (Kennedi, Paul and Hughes, eds.). Macmillan.

Pugh, L. (1973). Oxygen uptake and energy cost of walking before and after unilateral hip replacement, with some observations on the use of crutches. *J. Bone Jt. Surg.*, **55(B)**, 720–45.

Quanbury, A. (1985). The clinical gait lab: form and function. *Biomechanics*, **IX(A)**, 509–72.

Rowe, P. J. (1990). *The Evaluation of the Functional Ability of Total Hip Replacement Patients*. Thesis, University of Strathclyde, Glasgow.

Rowe, P. J. (1996). Development of a low-cost video vector for the display of ground reaction forces during gait. *Med. Eng. Phys.*, **18(7)**, 591–5.

Rowe, P. J. and White, M. (1996). Three-dimensional lumbar spinal kinematics during gait following mild musculoskeletal low back pain in nurses. *Gait and Posture*, **4**, 242–51.

Rowe, P. J., Nicol, A. and Kelly, I. (1987). A microcomputer based system for the assessment of hip function. In *Proc. Conf. Gait Anal.Med. Photogrammetry*, pp. 42–4. Oxford Orthopaedic Engineering Centre.

Rowe, P .J., Nicol, A. and Kelly, I. (1989). Flexible goniometer computer system for the assessment of hip function. *Clin. Biomech.*, **4**, 68–72.

Sackley, C. M. and Baguley, B. I. (1993). Visual feedback after stroke with the balance performance monitor. *Clin. Rehab.*, **7**, 189–95.

Saleh, M. and Murdoch, G. (1985). In defence of gait analysis. *J. Bone Jt. Surg.*, **67B**, 237–41.

Soderberg, G. and Gabel, R. (1978). A light-emitting diode system for the analysis of gait. *Phys. Ther.*, **58**, 426–32.

Soderberg, G., Reiss, R., Johnston, R. and Gabel, R. (1975). Kinematic and kinetic changes during gait as a result of hip disease. *Biomechanics*, **V(2)**, 437–43.

Stauffer, R., Smidt, G. and Wadsworth, J. (1974). Clinical and biomechanical analysis of gait following Charnley total hip replacement. *Clin. Orthop.*, **99**, 70–77.

Steindler, A. (1953). A historical review of the studies and investigations made in relation to human gait. *J. Bone Jt. Surg.*, **35(A)**, 540–42 and 728.

Tait, J. and Rose, G. (1979). The real time video vector display of ground reaction forces during ambulation. *J. Med. Eng. Tech.*, **3(5)**, 252–5.

Tala, J., Quanbury, A., Steinke, T. and Grahame, R. (1978). A variable axis electrogoniometer for the measurement of single plane movement. *J. Biomech.*, **11**, 421–5.

Taylor, K., Mottier, F., Simmons, D. *et al.* (1982). An automated motion measurement system for clinical gait analysis. *J. Biomech.*, **15(7)**, 505–16.

Townsend, M., Izak, M. and Jackson, R. (1977). Total motion knee goniometry. *J. Biomech.*, **10**, 183–93.

Tracy, K. B., Montague, E. C., Gabriel, R. P. *et al.* (1979). Computer assisted diagnosis of orthopaedic gait disorders. *Phys. Ther.*, **59**, 268.

Trnkoczy, A. and Badj, T. (1975). A simple electrogoniometric system and its testing. *IEEE Trans. Biomed. Eng.*, **22(3)**, 257–9.

University of California (1947). Fundamental studies of human locomotion and other information relating to the design of artificial limbs. In *Subcontractors Report to the Committee on Artificial Limbs, National Research Council Prosthetic Devices Research Project* (2 volumes). College of Engineering, Serial Number CAL 5, The Project, Berkeley, California.

Vivoda, E., Jenkins, S., Stanish, W. and Putnam, C. (1986). Gait patterns of accelerometry. *Orthop. Trans. (IEEE)*, **10(1)** (abstract)**,** 93.

Wadsworth, J., Smidt, G. and Johnston, R. (1972). Gait characteristics of subjects with hip disease. *Phys. Ther.*, **52(8)**, 829–39.

Wall, J. C. and Crosbie, J. (1997). Accuracy and reliability of temporal gait measurement. *Gait and Posture*, **4**, 293–6.

Wall, J., Dhanendran, M. and Klenerman, L. (1976). A method of measuring the temporal/distance factors of gait. *Biomed. Eng.*, **December,** 409–12.

Wall, J., Charteris, J. and Hoare, J. (1978). An automated on-line system for measuring the temporal patterns of foot/floor contact. *J. Med. Eng. Tech.*, **2**, 187–90.

Wall, J., Ashburn, A. and Klenerman, L. (1981). Gait analysis in the assessment of functional performance before and after total hip replacement. *J. Biomech. Eng.*, **3**, 121–7.

Waters, R., Perry, J., Conaty, P. *et al.* (1987). The energy cost of walking with arthritis of the hip and knee. *Clin. Orthop.*, **214**, 278–84.

Winter, D. (1983). Energy generation and absorption at the ankle and knee during fast, natural and slow cadences. *Clin. Orthop.*, **175**, 147–54.

Winter, D. (1985). Use of normalized profiles in the assessment of the kinetics of pathological gait. *Biomechanics*, **IX(A)**, 520–24.

Winter, D., Greenlaw, R. and Hobson, D. (1972). Television – computer analysis of kinematics of human gait. *Comput. Biomed. Res.*, **5**, 498–504.

Woltring, H. (1974). New possibilities for human studies of real time light spot position measurement. *Biotelemetry*, **1**, 136–46.

Woltring, H. and Marsolais, E. (1980). Optoelectronic (Selspot) gait measurement in two- and three-dimensional space: a preliminary report. *Bull. Prosth. Res.*, **17(2)**, 46–52.

Systems and suppliers

Vicon Motion Analysis System
Oxford Metrics Ltd
Unit 14, 7 West Way
Botley
Oxford OX2 0JB
UK
Telephone +44 1865 244656

Elite Motion Analyser
Bioengineering Technology and Systems
Vai Capecelatro, 66-I 20148
Milano
Italy
Telephone +39 2 4047896

Ortho Trak Motion Analysis System (including Gait Trak, Foot Trak, Spine Trak and Lift Trak).
Motion Analysis Corporation
3650 North Laughlin Road
Santa Rosa
California
USA
Telephone +1 707 579 6500

MacReflex Motion Analysis System
Qualisys AB
Ogardesvagen 2
433 30 Partille
Sweden
Telephone +31 363010

Primas Motion Analysis System
HCS Vision Technology BV
Hurksestraat 18d
5652 AK Eindhoven
Netherlands
Telephone +31 40 521637

Selspot Motion Analysis System
Selspot AB
Sallarangsgatan 3
S-431 37 Molndal
Sweden
Telephone +46 31 278992

Costel Motion Analysis System
Log.In SRL
Via Aurelia 714
00165 Roma
Italy
Telephone +39 6 6807044

Watsmart and Optotrak Motion Analysis Systems
Northern Digital Inc.
403 Albert Street
Waterloo
Ontario N2L 3V2
Canada
Telephone +1 519 884 5142

Coda-3 Motion Analysis System
Movement Technologies Ltd
Unit 5
The Technology Centre
Epinal Way
Loughborough
Leicestershire LE11 0QE
UK
Telephone +44 1509 267637

Peak Performance Motion Analysis System
Peak Performance Technologies Inc.
7388 S Revere Parkway
Suite 801
Englewood
Colorado 80112
USA
Telephone +1 303 799 8686

Ariel Motion Analysis System
Ariel Performance Analysis Systems Inc.
6 Alicante
Trabuco Canyon
California 92679
USA
Telephone +1 617 964 2042

*Biomechanics Workstation, Video Motion
Analysis System*
Salford College of Technology
Adelphi Campus
Fredrick Road
Salford M6 6PU
Telephone +44 161 736 6541

SP2000 High-speed Video Motion Analysis System
Eastman Kodak Company
11633 Sorrento Valley Road
San Diego
California 92121
USA
Telephone +1 516 667 1200

*Biokinetics Potentiometer Electrogoniometer
System*
Biokinetics Inc.
1710 Westminster Way
Annapolis
Maryland 21401
USA
Telephone +1 301 849 3401

Chattex Potentiometer Electrogoniometer System
Chattex Corporation
101 Memorial Drive
P.O. Box 4287
Chattanooga
Tennessee 37405
USA
Telephone +1 615 870 2281

MIE Potentiometer Electrogoniometer System
MIE Medical Research Ltd
6 Wortley Moor Road
Leeds LS12 4JF
UK
Telephone +44 1532 793710

*Penny and Giles Flexible Electrogoniometer
System*
Penny and Giles Biometrics Ltd
Blackwood
Gwent NP2 2YD
UK
Telephone +44 1495 228000

Greenleaf Wristsystem Electrogoniometer System
Greenleaf Medical Systems
2248 Park Boulevard
Paolo Alto
California 94306
USA
Telephone +1 415 3216135

Bioback Electrogoniometer System
Proteo Service
11, Rue des Buttes
21000 Dijon
France
Telephone +41 80715078

Isotrak Electromagnetic Tracking System
Polhemus Ltd
c/o TDS Digitizers Ltd
Lower Phillips Road
Blackburn BB1 5TH
UK
Telephone +44 1254 667 921

Accelerometer System
R.S. Components Ltd
P.O. Box 99
Corby
Northants NN17 9RS
UK
Telephone +44 1536 201201

Shock Meter Accelerometer System
J. P. Biomechanics
J. C. Peacock & Sons Ltd
Clavering Place
Newcastle-upon-Tyne
UK
Telephone +44 91 2329917

Kistler Force Plate
Kistler Instruments Ltd
Whiteoaks
The Grove
GB-Hartley Wintney
Hants RG27 8RN
UK
Telephone +44 1716 691 5100

Bertec Force Plate
Bertec Corporation
819 Loch Lomond Lane
Worthington
Ohio 43085
USA
Telephone +1 614 436 9966

AMTI Force Plate
Advanced Medical Technology Inc. (AMTI)
151 California Street
Newton
Massachusetts 02158
USA
Telephone +1 617 964 2042

Nottingham Balance Platform
Nottingham Rehab. Ltd
Ludlow Hill Road
West Bridgeford
Nottingham NG2 6HD
UK
Telephone +44 1159 452345

Balance Master
NeuroCom International Inc.
9570 SE Lawnfield Road
Clackamas
Oregon 97015–9943
USA
Telephone +1 503 653 2144

Video Vector Generator
MIE Medical Research Ltd
6 Wortley Moor Road
Leeds LS12 4JF
UK
Telephone +44 1532 793710

Musgrave Footprint Pressure Plate
W. M. Automation
Unit 18
Kilroot Park
Larne Road
Carrickfergus
Co. Antrim
N. Ireland
UK
Telephone +44 19603 51955

CDG Pressure Plate
Infotronic Gait Analysis Systems
P.O. Box 73
7650 AA Tubbergen
Netherlands
Telephone +31 6 52919720

Emed Pressure Plate
Novel Electronics Inc.
Suite 266 Box 82
11th Avenue South 511
Minneapolis
Minnesota 55415
USA
Telephone +1 612 332 8605

Pedobaragraph Pressure Plate
Baltimore Therapeutic Equipment Co.
7455 L New Ridge Road
Hanover
Maryland 21076
USA
Telephone +1 301 850 0333

CDG In-Shoe Pressure Device
Infotronic Gait Analysis Systems
PO Box 73
7650 AA Tubbergen
Netherlands
Telephone +31 6 52919720

Emed In- Shoe Pressure Device
Novel Electronics Inc.
Suite 266 Box 82
11th Avenue South 511
Minneapolis
Minnesota 55415
USA
Telephone +1 612 332 8605

Akron Isokinetic Machine
HNE Akron
1 Farthing Road
Ipswich
Suffolk IP1 5AP
UK
Telephone +44 1473 463096

Cybex Isokinetic Machine
Nomeq Healthcare and Rehabilitation Equipment
c/o Pharma Plast Ltd
23/24 Thornhill Road
North Moons Moat
Redditch
Worcestershire B98 9NL
UK
Telephone +44 1527 64222

Kincom Isokinetic Machine
Chattanooga Group Ltd
Talisman Road
Bicester
Oxfordshire OX6 0JX
UK
Telephone +44 1869 322555

BTE Work Simulator
Baltimore Therapeutic Equipment Co.
7455 L New Ridge Road
Hanover
Maryland 21076
USA
Telephone +1 301 850 0333

4 Rolling over and rising from supine

A. F. VanSant

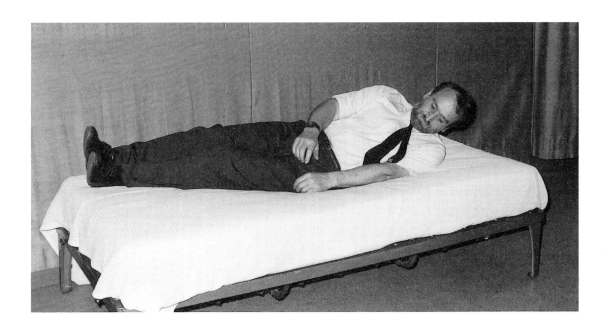

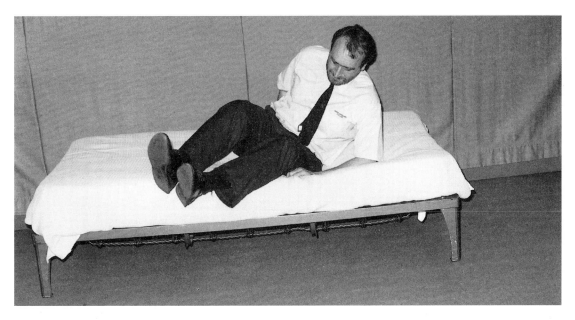

Introduction

The actions of rolling from the supine position to the prone position and rising from the supine position to standing are important elements in the functional skills of daily life, and physical therapists routinely teach these tasks to individuals whose physical impairments interfere with the ability to perform them. In addition to their practical importance in assuring physical independence, these actions are also of significance in theories of motor development and motor control. Although the focus of this chapter is on the methods and results of a programme of research of these functional skills, theoretical perspectives will be included to allow appropriate interpretation of the information regarding human performance in these tasks.

Theoretical and practical considerations in the study of rolling and rising

The tasks of rolling and rising fall within the general concept of 'righting' movements, which were brought to the attention of physical therapists by Bobath (1965). Originally described in the early part of this century, righting movements were initially considered to be reflexive actions that assured proper body alignment and attainment of the upright posture. According to the hierarchical theory of central nervous system (CNS) function, righting movements were mediated in the midbrain of the CNS and were an integral part of what Bobath (1965) termed the 'normal postural reflex mechanism'. To right oneself was to assume erect bipedal stance, the normal posture of the human species. From a developmental perspective, rising from a recumbent position on the floor has been considered the ultimate righting task, an important milestone in maturation reflecting independence from others in the performance of fundamental physical tasks.

During infancy, rising from the floor is accomplished by the action of rolling from the supine position into prone and then erecting the body through a series of transitional postures which may include quadruped, plantigrade, squatting, kneeling, and half-kneeling (McGraw, 1945; Schaltenbrand, 1928). As righting abilities develop across infancy and early childhood, the individual acquires the ability to move from one body posture to another more advanced posture while combating the force of gravity in the process. Each new posture represents an elevation of the centre of mass of the body over a diminishing base of support, and thus skills such as rising from supine to sit, or assuming the quadruped position from a prone position, are also righting actions. In large measure, the motor milestones of infancy represent the acquisition of righting abilities; however, although the ability to perform righting movements is typically accomplished during the first 15 months of life, developmental change within righting tasks continues beyond infancy (VanSant, 1990).

According to Schaltenbrand (1928), mature form in rising from the recumbent position is characterized by symmetry of trunk and limb action. Adults were said to rise by flexing the head, trunk and lower limbs from a supine position to assume a sitting position, and then moving forward to squat and stand. Schaltenbrand further claimed that this adult form of rising could be observed in children of about 4–5 years of age.

Bobath (1965) can be noted for her recognition of the fact that individuals with motor impairments due to cerebral palsy, cerebrovascular accident or traumatic brain injury present with disorders of righting. As a result of the work of the Bobaths (1972), therapists became increasingly interested in the 'quality' of motor performance in righting movements used to perform functional skills.

Although righting actions had been purported to be fully developed in early childhood, I routinely observed healthy young adults using more primitive forms of righting when asked to rise from the floor. My theoretical perspective at that time suggested that healthy individuals who showed less than mature form in rising were demonstrating either developmental delay or the behaviour expected after the peak of maturity (and thus were on a downward course of developmental regression characteristic of aging). Neither alternative was a particularly appealing interpretation of these observations of healthy young adults. Yet the hierarchical theory of development from which initial studies of righting were conceived (Schaltenbrand, 1928; McGraw, 1945) offered no alternative explanation, and thus my interest in righting behaviours led to intriguing theoretical questions.

Methods of studying righting movements: the problems of technology – a personal perspective

Righting behaviours, unlike walking, are not easily studied as single plane movements. Because of their rotational nature, I quickly realized that to pursue a kinematic investigation of these actions a three-dimensional cinematographical method would be needed. I had undertaken a three-dimensional analysis of the standing posture of children with cerebral palsy during my Master's thesis work (VanSant, 1976). That study was filled with difficulties emanating from the limitations of technology. I needed the services of civil engineers to locate the cameras accurately with respect to the filming field, used a graphic plotter to generate co-ordinate readings of body landmarks, and faced the challenge of trying to interface a data terminal in the laboratory with the main university computer. It was also necessary at that time to write a data reduction program in FORTRAN language, and each of these steps took several weeks to accomplish.

The struggle with technology seemed endless. The university computer would default at certain points when running my FORTRAN program but, after weeks of reducing the program to small steps and printing out intermediate values that would then be re-entered into smaller programs, I accomplished my goal – a postural configuration for each of 30 children with spastic cerebral palsy. Although I was able to answer my research question, the angles portraying postural alignment were not analogous to clinical goniometric measures. This greatly limited the applicability of my findings to clinical practice, and I learned an important lesson: technology often lags behind our desire to understand more about human posture and movement.

I was still interested in describing righting behaviours. The lessons learned from my experience with three-dimensional kinematics suggested that, if I were to pursue a kinematic approach, I would be spending a great deal of time in the laboratory solving technical problems; also that it was quite expensive to maintain and upgrade my data collection and analysis system. I therefore began a search for a more expedient approach to the problem of describing righting behaviours, looking for a method that would be less dependent on technology and less expensive, yet would yield clinically useful information regarding righting behaviours.

The component approach to movement description

In the late 1970s, Roberton (1977, 1978), a physical educator, described the development of overarm throwing in young children, and created the 'component approach' to movement analysis in order to describe throwing movements in greater detail than was available in earlier reports. Classic portraits of developmental stages in throwing (Wild, 1938) described body action as a whole, portraying the general features of the body movement. However, Roberton experienced difficulty classifying children's throwing movements when using Wild's descriptions; for example, the child's trunk movements might correspond to one of Wild's descriptions while the limb movements did not, or leg action might be classified at one developmental level while arm action corresponded to another.

Roberton therefore divided body action into 'component parts' to achieve reliable categorization of the children's movements. A component is a part of a body action, typically describing the movements of a region of the body. For example, action of the axial region (comprised of head and trunk movements) may be one component of body action, while upper and lower limb movements may represent two separate components. Researchers select these components for a variety of practical and theoretical reasons. To characterize action of the entire body, however, a sufficient number of components must be identified to describe comprehensively the movements of all body regions.

Roberton described the throwing action within components she selected. In the process of a more refined description, she discovered aspects of the developmental process that had been hidden from previous investigators. Specifically, she discovered that the development of movement patterns in the throwing task does not occur across all components of the body in a locked step fashion; rather, one component may advance to a new stage of behaviour while another remains stable (Roberton, 1978).

In a similar way to Roberton's (1977) experience with throwing movements, I found that descriptions of righting movements (McGraw, 1945; Schaltenbrand, 1928) lacked detail and were often not comprehensive of all body regions. Seeing promise in Roberton's method I decided to learn it, and have subsequently used the component approach to provide more refined descriptions of righting actions.

The component method applied to righting tasks

Application of the component approach to the description of rising from the floor required delineation of components for study. I selected three components of body action: the upper limbs, the axial region, and the lower limbs. I was influenced in this selection by reports of neuro-anatomical studies of descending motor control systems of the brain, which were conducted in the laboratories of Lawrence and Kuypers (1968a and 1968b). I decided to define components of action that allow investigation of the developmental progression and interaction between axial and limb movements and which are grounded to some degree in neuroanatomical structure.

To gather data, two video cameras are used to record the subject's movements when performing 10 sequential trials of the righting task. Typically, one camera is placed facing the foot of an exercise mat or the bed and another is placed facing one side of the mat or bed. Although in some of our initial studies only one camera was used, we currently use two cameras for all studies. All subjects are asked to lie in the supine position on an exercise mat or on the bed and, on the command 'Go', to rise or roll as quickly as possible. The task is repeated 10 times, and all trials are videotaped. Subjects are allowed to rest between trials and to stop participation at any time for any reason.

It should be noted that form (not speed) is the primary concern in all studies. However, after discovering that young adults who are being videotaped while performing a movement task are concerned about 'correct performance', I now ask for 'quick movement' to prevent subjects from focusing on the form of their movements and possibly deliberately altering their movement patterns. This request allows comparison across many different subject groups, but it can also be considered a limitation of the studies because speed generally affects motor performance. As my theoretical interest lies predominantly in the realm of life-span change in motor behaviour, the ability to compare across age groups is of greater

importance than any limitation produced by this admonition.[1]

The remainder of this chapter focuses on the results of our studies of the tasks of rising from the supine position and rolling from the supine position to the prone position. The studies reported below include those conducted on individuals of varying ages without known impairments or disabilities. In addition, some reports of our studies of individuals with known disabling conditions, such as low back pain and brain injury, are included. Our knowledge of performance within these righting tasks is broadening over the years, and recently we have begun investigations of the influence of various 'control parameters' on the emergence of movement patterns within these tasks. Areas appropriate for further investigation will be pointed out to the reader.

Rising from the supine position

Two tasks have been studied that involve rising from the supine position: rising from the floor and rising from bed. Each is discussed separately below. A summary then follows at the end of this section.

Rising from the floor

The prototypical task of righting is rising from a supine position on the floor to erect stance. Early researchers (McGraw, 1945; Schaltenbrand, 1928) described the circuitous route that infants took in accomplishing this action. They first roll from supine into the prone position and push up with their hands to assume the quadruped posture, then elevate the buttocks by extending the knees until the weight is born on hands and feet. Next they flex the knees, lowering the buttocks into a squatting position, and then lift the hands from the surface and extend the legs and trunk to reach the erect posture.

Over time, this round-about approach to the vertical is replaced with a more direct route that proceeds with flexion of the trunk and legs from the supine position to assume a sitting, then squatting, posture, followed by extension to bring the body to erect stance. The gradual development of the more direct and symmetrical form of rising was reported to be accomplished over the period of

---

[1] Detailed discussion of the method can be found in the Proceedings of the Eugene Michels Research Forum (VanSant, 1993) available through the American Physical Therapy Association, 1111 North Fairfax Street, Alexandria, VA22314, USA

Table 4.1 Rising from a supine position on the floor: movement patterns of the Upper Limbs

Movement pattern	Description
Push and Reach to Bilateral Push with Thigh Push	One or both hands are placed on the supporting surface beside the pelvis. After an initial push, one arm reaches across the body and the hand is placed on the surface. Both hands are placed on the knee and then the arms are lifted and used for balance.
Push and Reach to Bilateral Push	One hand is placed on the supporting surface beside the pelvis. The other arm reaches across the body and the hand is placed on the surface. Both hands push against the surface to an extended elbow position. The arms are then lifted and used for balance.
Push and Reach with Thigh Push	One or both arms are used to push against the support surface, or to reach forward. Pushing and reaching movements give way to a single arm push against the support surface. One or both hands are placed on the knee, and then the arms are lifted and used for balance.
Push and Reach	One or both arms are used to push against the support surface. If both arms are used, there is an asymmetry or asynchrony in the pushing action, or a symmetrical push gives way to a single push pattern.
Symmetrical Push	Both hands are placed on the surface. Both hands push symmetrically against the surface prior to the point when the arms are lifted synchronously and used to assist with balance.
Symmetrical Reach	The arms reach forward, leading the trunk, and are used as balance assists throughout the movement.

early childhood, with so-called 'mature form' appearing at about the age of 4–5 years (McGraw, 1945; Schaltenbrand, 1928).

My first study of righting involved a group of healthy young adult subjects. After gathering the data in the manner described above, the movement patterns of each component were described by reviewing the videotaped performances. A set of descriptive categories of upper limb (UL), axial region (AR) and lower limb (LL) patterns were identified. Descriptions were then used to classify movement across all trials of all subjects. An external rater then used the categorical descriptions to classify movements for a random sample of 30 trials, and percentages of exact agreement were calculated. These percentages of exact agreement were all greater than 90 per cent, indicating good objectivity of the written descriptions. Four UL patterns, four AR patterns and five LL patterns

were identified in that original study. The UL and AR pattern descriptions remain virtually unchanged since that original study, although additional UL and AR patterns have been added that were identified in subsequent studies of older (Luehring, 1989) and younger individuals (VanSant, 1988a; Marsala and VanSant, 1998). The movement pattern descriptions described in Tables 4.1, 4.2 and 4.3 are those used in our most recent studies of rising from the floor, and represent all patterns that have been described up to 1997.

In addition to the identification and description of component actions, the first study of 32 young adults confirmed the reports of McGraw (1945) and Schaltenbrand (1928) that the most common form of rising in young adults involved a symmetrical action (Figure 4.1). This initial study also began to provide an understanding of the great variability in rising action among individuals of

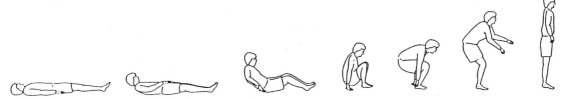

Figure 4.1 Symmetrical rising in young adults (VanSant, 1988b)

Table 4.2 Rising from a supine position on the floor: movement patterns of the Axial Region

Movement pattern	Description
Full Rotation Abdomen Down	The head and trunk flex and rotate until the ventral surface of the trunk contacts the support surface. The pelvis is then elevated to or above the level of the shoulder girdle. The back extends up to the vertical, with or without accompanying rotation of the trunk.
Full Rotation Abdomen Up	The head and trunk flex and/or rotate until the ventral surface of the trunk faces, but does not contact, the support surface. The pelvis is then elevated to or above the level of the shoulder girdle. The back extends from this position up to the vertical, with or without accompanying rotation.
Partial Rotation	Flexion and rotation bring the body to a side-facing position or beyond, with the shoulders remaining above the level of the pelvis. The back extends up to the vertical, with or without accompanying rotation.
Forward with Rotation	The head and trunk flex forward, with or without a slight degree of rotation. Symmetrical flexion is then interrupted by rotation or extension with rotation. Flexion with slight rotation is corrected by counter-rotation. One or more changes in the direction of rotation occur. A front or slightly diagonal facing is achieved before the back extends to the vertical.
Symmetrical	The head and trunk move symmetrically forward past the vertical. The back then extends symmetrically to the upright position.

Table 4.3 Rising from a supine position on the floor: movement patterns of the lower limbs

Movement pattern	Description
Pike	The legs are flexed toward the trunk and may be rotated to one side with knees or a knee and foot in contact with the ground. Both feet then contact the support surface. The legs are fully extended to a pike position. Slight flexion of the legs is followed by full extension during the rise.
Jump to Pike	The legs are flexed toward the trunk and rotated until both knees contact the support surface, while the legs remain flexed. Next the legs are fully extended to a pike position. Both feet are then lifted simultaneously off the support surface. The feet land back on the support surface in closer proximity to the hands, with the hips and knees flexing to a squat position. The legs are then extended during the rise.
Kneel	The legs are flexed toward the trunk and rotated to one side, allowing both knees to contact the support surface. Half-kneeling may then be assumed, or a squat pattern. When the legs extend one or more balance steps may be taken.
Jump to Squat	The legs are flexed and/or rotated to one side. Both legs are then lifted simultaneously off the support surface and may be derotated. The feet land back on the support surface, with the hips and knees flexing to a squat or semi-squat position.
Half-kneel	Both legs are flexed toward the trunk as one or both legs are rotated to one side. A half-kneeling pattern is assumed, with one foot and one knee contacting the surface. The forward leg pushes into extension as the opposite legt moves forward and extends.
Asymmetrical/Wide-Based Squat	One or both legs are flexed toward the trunk, assuming an asymmetrical, crossed-leg or wide-based squat. The legs push into an extended position. Crossing or asymmetries may be corrected during extension by stepping action.
Narrow-Based Symmetrical Squat	The legs are brought into flexion with the heels approximating the buttocks in a narrow-based squat, or balance steps (or hops) may follow the symmetrical rise.

this age. The component approach proved to be a parsimonious method to capture and characterize this variability. The relatively small number of UL, AR and LL patterns were being used in many different combinations by the subjects, and 33 of 80 possible combinations of AR and limb movement patterns were observed. However, most subjects were quite consistent in performing the same combination of UL, AR and LL patterns across 10 trials of rising. Thus, in adult subjects, inter-individual variability was high and intra-individual variability was low.

In subsequent studies of young children it became clear that young adults demonstrate the majority, but not all, of the patterns of movement that can be used to perform the rising task. I identified an AR pattern Full Rotation Abdomen Down, and a LL pattern Jump to Squat when studying young children (VanSant, 1988a) (Figure 4.2). Two additional LL limb patterns were described in a recent study of infants and toddlers: Pike, and Pike Jump to Squat. Younger children also demonstrate greater variation across trials of the task, but demonstrate a fewer number of

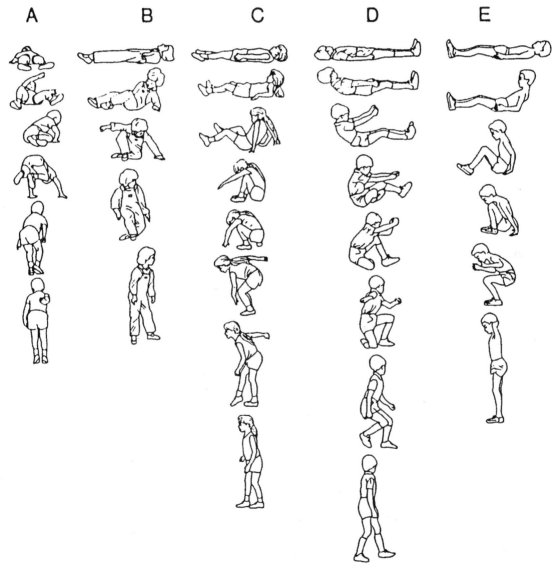

Figure 4.2 Variability in children's rising movements (VanSant, 1988a)

different combinations of action in rising. Thus, while they appear to try several different strategies across their trials, they use strategies similar to other young children and show less inter-individual variability than adult subjects.

Luehring's (1989) work with older adults led to the identification of two new UL patterns: Push and Reach to Bilateral Push with Thigh Push, and Push and Reach with Thigh Push. These two latter patterns involve pushing with the ULs on the thighs, seemingly to assist with LL and AR extension to the upright posture. In our subsequent study of young children (Marsala and VanSant, 1998), these two Thigh Push patterns were observed in the youngest subjects. In younger subjects it also appears that this strategy is being used to assist with knee and trunk extension.

Over a series of years we have outlined developmental sequences for this task (VanSant, 1991a; VanSant 1991b). The sequences are a series of movement patterns within each of the three components of body action, and the incidence of each pattern varies with age in each component (VanSant, 1989a). The form of that age-related variation is such that patterns common in early childhood are often observed later in the life span, although close inspection of these recurring patterns reveals subtle differences that separate the performance of children and adults (VanSant, 1991c). Thus we have documented that movement patterns vary with age across the human life span in this rising task (VanSant, 1997).

Our studies of rising in special populations began with a study of adults who had sustained a traumatic brain injury. Individuals with moderate and severe head injury were studied across a period of 3–12 months following injury (VanSant, 1991d). The same methods were used to gather data as reported above for our studies of those without disabling conditions. Those with moderate injury typically used rotation patterns that represented 'developmental regression' at 3 months following their injury. These individuals recovered age-appropriate patterns with less rotation by 6 months post-injury, but demonstrated some 'regression' to the use of rotational patterns again at 9 months post-injury. I interpret this somewhat disturbing trend in the data as an indication that following rehabilitation, individuals did not have sufficient opportunity to remain physically active. They demonstrated 'regression' following a period of active rehabilitation. Such a finding points to the need for continued physical activity beyond the period of rehabilitation for those with traumatic brain injury.

The relationship between physical activity and performance in this rising task has been documented by both Luehring (1989), in her study of active and less active older adults, and by Green and Williams (1992), who studied the movement patterns of young adults reporting varying levels of participation in physical activity. In both instances the less active individuals demonstrated a greater proportion of trials employing a rotational approach to the upright posture.

More recently, we have begun to investigate the stability of movement patterns when external constraints are applied. These constraints include weights applied to the trunk (Dhawan and VanSant, 1995) and ankle orthotics (King and VanSant, 1996). Dhawan and VanSant (1995) demonstrated that movement patterns change form when 10–15 per cent of an individual's body weight is added to the body. Trunk patterns appear to be differentially sensitive to this additional weight. Those young adults who demonstrated symmetrical patterns without wearing additional weight changed to asymmetrical patterns when weights were added. Those demonstrating asymmetrical patterns when not wearing additional weight did not change patterns as often. Dhawan used dynamic pattern theory (Scholtz, 1990) to interpret her findings, and suggested that asymmetrical patterns are more stable than symmetrical ones and may be considered 'attractor' patterns.

King and VanSant (1996) asked healthy young adults to rise while wearing unilateral and bilateral solid ankle foot orthotics (SAFO) on their lower limbs. Without the orthotics, this group of subjects most commonly demonstrated a combination of upper limb action involving a push and reach pattern of the UL, forward with rotation pattern of the trunk, and an asymmetrical squat pattern when rising without the SAFO. When subjects wore the SAFO on the right limb or on both limbs, the pattern seen most commonly in the trunk was a partial rotation pattern. We found the SAFOs' influence to be most apparent when individuals were transferring weight from their buttocks onto the feet when assuming a squat position. The orthotics prevented ankle motion, and the subjects adopted a compensatory strategy that involved rotation of the trunk to allow weight to be transferred onto the feet.

We continue to study the influence of physical constraints on the rising task, and are particularly interested in determining how physical dimensions of the body influence performance of it. It appears that this work may lead to an answer to my original question regarding why healthy young adults do not all demonstrate symmetrical form in rising. The answer to that question probably revolves not around issues related to the maturation of the nervous system but rather around issues related to physical activity and body dimensions, two inter-related factors that are increasingly being shown to affect performance in this task.

Rising from a supine position in bed

Sarnacki (1985) completed the first in a series of studies describing the movement patterns used to rise from a supine position on a bed. Her goal was to identify component movement patterns for this task and to propose a developmental sequence for each action component. Four body action components were studied. The need for four components arose because she was unable to view simultaneously both upper limbs from either of the two cameras used to videotape the subjects' performances. Thus the actions of the upper limbs were described as two separate components, termed the 'near upper limb' (NUL) and 'far upper limb' (FUL), referring to their proximity to the camera

Table 4.4 Rising from bed: Far Upper Limb movement pattern categories

Movement pattern	Description
Lateral Lift and Push	The upper limb lifts or slides on the supporting surface toward the head of the bed. The entire upper limb, or some portion of it, is placed on the bed and pushes. The upper limb extends until the hand is the only part of the limb remaining on the bed. The hand lifts and the limb may be used as a balance assist.
Push	The entire upper limb, or some part of it, pushes into the bed. The upper limb extends until the hand or elbow is the only part of the upper limb remaining on the bed. The hand or elbow lifts and the limb may be used as a balance assist.
Double Push	The entire upper limb lifts toward the head of the bed and pushes, or pushes into the bed without lifting. The extremity extends until the hand or elbow is the only part of the upper limb remaining on the bed. The hand or elbow lifts and the hand is placed on the bed, usually near the edge, and pushes. The hand lifts and the extremity may be used as a balance assist.
Lift and Push	The upper extremity lifts off the bed and may reach across the body. The hand is placed on the bed or on the ipsilateral lower limb at some point before reaching the edge of the bed. The hand lifts and the extremity may be used as a balance assist.
Lift or Lift and Reach	The upper extremity lifts off the bed and may reach across the body. The extremity may be used as a balance assist.

Table 4.5 Rising from bed: Near Upper Limb movement pattern categories

Movement pattern	Description
Lateral Lift and Push	The upper limb lifts or slides on the supporting surface toward the head of the bed. The entire upper extremity is in the extended or nearly extended position, and the hand is the only part of the extremity remaining on the bed. The hand lifts, and the extremity may be used as a balance assist.
Grasp and Push	The upper limb slides or lifts, positioning the hand to grasp the edge of the bed. The entire upper extremity, or some part of it, pushes down on the bed while the hand grips on the edge. The upper extremity lifts and may be used as a balance assist.
Push	The entire upper extremity, or some part of it, pushes into the bed. The extremity lifts from the bed and may be used as a balance assist.
Lift and Reach*	The leading upper extremity is lifted off the bed without pushing. The extremity may be used to reach forward or as a balance assist.

* Identified in McCoy's study of adolescents (McCoy and VanSant, 1993)

positioned to obtain a side view of the subject when lying supine in bed.

Sarnacki, after videotaping 35 young adult subjects each performing 10 trials of rising from bed, described movement patterns for each of the four action components. She identified five FUL patterns (Table 4.4), three NUL patterns (Table 4.5), four movement patterns of AR (Table 4.6), and four patterns of the LL (Table 4.7). The most common combination of movement patterns used by young

adults to rise from bed involved pushing with the FUL, grasping the edge of the bed and then pushing with the NUL, a roll-off pattern in the AR, and asynchronous lifting with synchronous placement of the LL on the floor. This 'profile' of rising from bed, although the most common across the trials of the 35 subjects, was observed in only 10 per cent of the trials (Figure 4.3).

Fifty-seven different combinations of rising were seen, representing nearly 24 per cent of

Table 4.6 Rising from bed: Axial Region movement pattern categories

Movement pattern	Description
Pelvis Leading	The lower trunk rotates to the side. At side lying, the upper side of the pelvis drops to the bed, and the trunk lifts and turns toward side facing. The subject may be in a symmetrical sitting position posture before standing.
Lateral Roll	The head and trunk turn toward the side-facing position, with minimal flexion toward the foot of the bed. In the side-facing position, one buttock is off the bed, and the shoulders and pelvis are aligned and displaced toward the head of the bed. When the buttocks come off the bed, the head and trunk are displaced toward the head of the bed or a symmetrical sitting posture is observed.
Roll-off	The head and trunk flex and turn toward side facing with the weight shifted to one buttock. Just before both buttocks come off the bed, the head and trunk are displaced toward the head of the bed through lateral flexion or rotation of the trunk.
Come to Sit	The head and trunk flex symmetrically or flex and turn toward side facing by pivoting on one or both buttocks. Just before both buttocks come off the bed, the trunk is in a symmetrical sitting posture, though it may be flexed forward.

* As revised by McCoy and VanSant (1993).

Table 4.7 Rising from bed: Lower Limb movement pattern categories

Movement pattern	Description
Step Off	The lower extremities are lifted asynchronously off the bed. The far extremity may push on the bed before lifting. The far extremity flexes toward the chest such that the thigh is above the near extremity thigh. The feet are usually placed on the floor asynchronously, and the near extremity may begin to extend before the far extremity foot is placed on the floor.
Asynchronous with Leg Extension	The lower extremities are lifted asynchronously off the bed. The far lower extremity may push on the bed prior to lifting. The thighs remain parallel as they move across the bed. The far lower extremity may be extended as it moves across and over the edge of the bed. The far lower extremity foot is in front of the near lower extremity leg as the legs descend toward the floor. The feet are placed on the floor, and the lower extremities extend to the upright position.
Asynchronous	The lower extremities are lifted asynchronously off the bed. The far lower extremity may push on the bed before lifting and is usually medially rotated. The thighs are parallel as they move across the bed, and the legs are parallel as they descend toward the floor. The feet are placed on the floor simultaneously, and the lower extremities extend to the upright position.
Synchronous	The lower extremities are lifted or slid simultaneously off the bed. A brief push on the bed may proceed the lifting. The lower extremities move together over the edge of the bed. The feet are placed on the floor simultaneously. The lower extremities extend to the upright position.

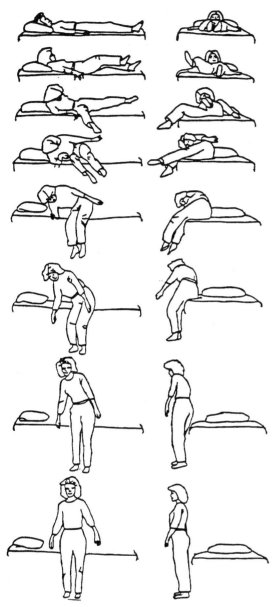

Figure 4.3 Most common form of rising from bed in young adults (from Sarnacki, 1985)

movement patterns observed but, interestingly, the percentage of possible combinations observed was similar across the two tasks.

Since Sarnacki's original study, additional investigations have added to our knowledge of performance in the task of rising from bed. The first focused on older children and adolescents performing this task (McCoy and VanSant, 1993). Sixty adolescents were studied: 20 aged 11 years, 20 aged 14 years, and 20 aged 17 years. We found the movement pattern descriptions developed by Sarnacki for both upper limbs and lower limbs to be accurate descriptors of movements used by adolescents to rise from bed. The axial region movement patterns, however, were re-written to be more reflective of the actions observed in adolescents and to make it easier to generalize these pattern descriptions.

Although the limb pattern descriptions were accurate, one new near upper extremity pattern was identified that had not been reported by Sarnacki (1985). This pattern was termed Lift and Reach (McCoy and VanSant, 1993), and is reported in Table 4.5. Adolescents demonstrated a comparable degree of inter-individual variation in rising actions. Eighty-nine different combinations of component action were seen in performances of the 60 subjects (28 per cent of the 320 possible combinations). Age differences in variability were found such that the 11-year-old subjects demonstrated 67 different profiles of rising, whereas the 14- and 17-year-old subjects demonstrated 40 and 44 different combinations, respectively. Thus, inter-individual variability appeared to decrease with age. No subject used the same combination of movement patterns across all 10 trials of rising.

We were able to identify one combination of movement patterns that was relatively common across age groups (Figure 4.4). That form of rising involved grasping and pushing with the NUL, a double push with the FUL, a come to sit pattern of the AR, and asynchronous lifting of the LL with one leg extended in front of the other as the feet descended from the bed to the floor. This form of rising was seen on approximately 6 per cent of the trials of the 11-year-old subjects, 12 per cent of the trials of 14-year-olds and 15 per cent of the trials of the 17-year-old subjects. Two other action profiles were seen with equal frequency in the 11-year-old subjects. These two profiles included similar lower extremity and far upper extremity action, differing only in axial region or near upper limb movements. Thus 11-year-old children are much more variable than young adults in their performance of the task

the 240 mathematically possible combinations of component actions. This degree of variability is comparable to the 21 different combinations of movement observed among 32 subjects performing the task of rising from the floor (VanSant, 1988b), representing approximately 26 per cent of a possible 80 combinations. In the task of rising from bed, adding a fourth component contributed to the increased number of combinations of

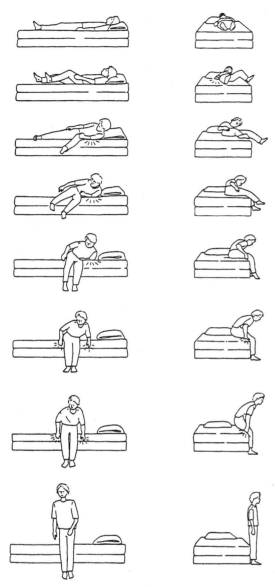

Figure 4.4 A common form of rising from bed across later childhood and adolescence (from McCoy and VanSant, 1993)

of rising from bed, and 14- and 17-year-old teens are slightly less variable than young adults.

Ford Smith and VanSant (1993) reported the patterns used by individuals between the ages of 30 and 60 years when rising from bed, and investigated age differences in the performance of this task across middle adulthood. Ninety-three individuals participated, with at least 30 subjects 30–39 years old, 30 subjects 40–49 years old, and 30 subjects 50–60 years of age. As in previous studies, each performed 10 self-paced trials of rising from a supine position in bed. We were able to use the categories developed by Sarnacki without modification. No new patterns were discovered in this age group. The most common form of rising differed between the youngest group of subjects (30–39 years old) when compared to the older two groups (40–49 and 50–60 years old). Subjects in their thirties rose using a Double-Push pattern with the FUL while first grasping the edge of the bed and then pushing with the NUL. These subjects demonstrated a Come to Sit pattern of the AR, and the LLs were lifted asynchronously off the bed and carried to the side with the limbs aligned as the feet were lowered to the floor. This pattern was demonstrated in 12 per cent of the trials of this younger age group. The two older groups varied from the younger group only in LL action. In the older subjects, the LLs were lifted synchronously off the bed and carried to the side, and lowered to the floor simultaneously. This latter pattern, although the most common profile for these two age groups, was seen in only 8 per cent and 14 per cent of the trials of those in their forties and fifties, respectively.

Subjects in their thirties as a group demonstrated 57 movement pattern combinations out of a possible 248 combinations (28 per cent). Variability was significantly less in the two older groups, with 49 and 47 different profiles of action demonstrated by those in their forties and fifties, respectively. This represents about 19–20 per cent of the possible combinations.

As a result of these three studies of older children and teens, younger and middle-aged adults, it is possible to examine age differences in movement patterns across a broad period of the life span. As evident in Table 4.8, the far upper limb pattern Double Push pattern predominated in the teens and middle-aged adults, with the Push pattern found to be most common among young adults. In the near upper limb, the Grasp and Push pattern and the Push pattern alternated dominance across the ages studied. Grasp and Push was predominant in the early teen years, during the twenties and thirties, and again among those in their fifties. The push pattern predominated among 17-year-old subjects and those in their forties. It is important to note that, because these two patterns were quite common at all ages, it is not clear if there is a developmental change in patterns that can be expected for this component of the rising action.

In the axial region, a clearer sequence of age differences can be seen. The lateral roll pattern is

Table 4.8 Incidence of movement patterns for the task of rising from bed

	Mean age (years) (n = ~30 each age group)						
	11	14	17	24	34	44	54
Far Upper Limb							
Lateral Lift and Push	1.5	0	0	18.3	0	1	0
Double Push	72	83	63	13.1	44	47	60
Push	16.5	16.5	20	63.4	36	40	29
Lift and Push	8	0.5	15	4	10	9	8
Lift and Reach	2	0	3.5	1.2	10	2	3
Near Upper Limb							
Lateral Lift and Push	25	9.5	10.5	22.5	10	9	8
Grasp and Push	36.5	48.5	42	59	61	44	53
Push	38	42	47	18.5	29	47	39
Lift and Reach	0.5	0	0.5	0	0	0	0
Axial Region							
Pelvis Leads	5	0	4.5	3	1	4	10
Lateral Roll	34.5	10	1.5	5	4	1	1
Come to Sit	43	75.5	70	41	66	65	75
Roll Off	17.5	14.5	24	51	29	30	15
Lower Limbs							
Asynchronous with Leg Extension	44.5	28	47.5	25	22	22	16
Step Off	10.5	32.5	17	30.8	10	5	2
Asynchronous	32.5	26	28.5	33.8	41	36	35
Synchronous	12.5	13.5	7	10.4	27	37	47

most common in the later childhood, the come to sit pattern predominated among teens, and the roll off pattern was most common among the young adults. The come to sit pattern predominates with increasing incidence across the middle adult years. In the lower limbs, the Asynchronous and Step Off patterns are common during later childhood, the teen and young adult years. The Asynchronous pattern of later childhood and the teen years involves extension of one limb when the legs are being lowered from the bed to the floor. In adulthood the Asynchronous pattern involves an asynchronous lift, but legs then become aligned and are moved synchronously as they are lowered to the floor. The Synchronous lifting pattern becomes predominant with increasing age across middle adulthood.

Since these studies have been reported, Sherwin (1993) has completed a study of individuals with low back pain rising from bed. She observed the movement patterns of 29 individuals with chronic low back pain when rising from bed, and also documented their level of pain. She identified additional movement patterns for each body region that had not been observed in studies of healthy adults. The new movement patterns involve repetitive pushes of the upper limbs, and a pattern she termed the Crossover Push, in which the far upper limb reached across the body and pushed off the surface on the contralateral side of the body. The multiple push patterns were most common among subjects reporting the highest levels of pain.

In the axial region, two patterns not seen in healthy individuals were identified. The first involved a shoulder leading pattern, that appears to be the complement of the pelvis leading pattern identified by Sarnacki (1985). A new pattern titled Lateral Roll–Sit–Slide was identified, which is characterized by a fragmentation of the elements of trunk action. The new pattern was similar to the

Lateral Roll pattern seen in healthy subjects. The subjects demonstrating Lateral Roll–Sit–Slide rolled to side facing with minimal flexion of the trunk. They then elevated the trunk with minimal rotation, and after achieving sitting they slid forward on the buttocks to the edge of the bed. Sherwin suggested that her findings of a higher incidence of the Lateral Roll pattern than that reported for healthy adults and the use of the Lateral Roll–Sit–Slide were likely evidence of strategies used by those with pain to reduce the amount of stress placed on the trunk during rising. She noted the similarity to the 'log roll' pattern often taught by physical therapists to individuals with low back pain.

New lower limb patterns were also reported, including a Walk-Off pattern and a Slide pattern. In the Walk-Off strategy, the lower limbs slide to the side from which the subject will exit the bed, and first one and then the other limb is lowered over the edge. In the Slide pattern, the near LL slides toward the buttocks, and the far LL slides to a position parallel to the thigh of the near LL. The lower limbs are then moved together over the edge of the bed and lowered to the floor. Again, as in the other body regions, subjects who reported higher pain levels were more likely to use these strategies. Sherwin suggested that they may be used in conjunction with limited trunk flexion, and thus might possibly require less force to be generated by the abdominal muscles and thus produce less stress on the lower back.

At the current time, an additional study is under way of movement patterns used by pregnant women when rising from bed (Allard, work in progress). The rising movement is being examined during each of the three trimesters of pregnancy. The strategies used by women as they approach the term of pregnancy will probably lead to the identification of additional movement patterns used to perform this task of daily life.

In summary, for the tasks of rising from the floor and rising from bed, sets of movement patterns have been identified. Studies of healthy individuals of various ages have permitted development of a life-span model of movement for the task of rising from the floor. A life-span model of movements used to rise from bed is being constructed.

More recent studies are providing information regarding the change in movement patterns expected when external constraints are added to healthy young adults rising from the floor. We are also extending our work to include various populations with disabling conditions performing the rising tasks. Increasingly, we are using dynamic pattern theory to inform our studies of these tasks. We are particularly interested in studying the physical parameters of our subjects that influence their performance.

Table 4.9 Rolling from supine to prone: Upper Limb movement pattern categories*

Movement pattern	Description
Lift and Reach at or Below Shoulder Level	The right upper extremity is lifted off the supporting surface and reaches across the body with the right hand at or below shoulder level. The left arm stays at the side of the body, or abducts, or may be lifted off the mat. The left shoulder or upper limb contacts the supporting surface as the subject rolls over the left shoulder or upper limb.
Lift and Reach Above Shoulder Level	The right upper limb is lifted off the suporting surface. The right hand is brought above shoulder level. The left arm may stay at the side of the body. The subject rolls over the left upper limb or shoulder.
Push and Reach	At the start of the movement, part of the right upper limb appears to push while in contact with the supporting surface, as the right shoulder flexes, reaching toward a position parallel to or in front of the body at the time the subject reaches the side-lying position. The left arm may stay at the side of the body and the left shoulder or upper limb remains in contact with the surface as the subject rolls.
Push	The right upper limb maintains contact with the supporting surface as the right shoulder extends. The right arm remains behind the body until the subject reaches the side-lying position. The left arm may stay at the side of the body, abduct or flex. The left shoulder or upper limb remains in contact with the supporting surface as the subject rolls past the side-lying position.

* Adapted from Richter (1985). These categories are written to allow classification of movement patterns when the subject rolls from supine to prone over the left side of the body.

Rolling from supine to prone

Richter *et al.* (1989) provided the first study of movement patterns used to move from the supine to the prone position. He videotaped 36 young healthy adults performing the rolling task, and developed categorical descriptions of movement patterns for three components of body action: the upper limbs, lower limbs and axial region. He described common forms of rolling in young adults, and proposed a developmental sequence for each component of body action. Four patterns of action were identified for each component. Those pattern descriptions can be found in Tables 4.9, 4.10 and 4.11.

Richter and colleagues (1989) found 32 different combinations of action demonstrated by the 36 subjects, representing 50 per cent of the possible movement pattern combinations. It is indicative of a greater degree of variability in the performance of this task than has been observed in the rising

Table 4.10 Rolling from supine to prone: Axial Region movement pattern categories*

Movement pattern	Description
Aligned Pelvis and Shoulder Girdle	The head and trunk turn to the left. The head may be raised from the supporting surface and the trunk may flex as the subject rolls. The right pelvis and shoulder girdle remain aligned with each other beyond the side-lying position.
Pelvis Leads	The head may be raised off the supporting surface and may turn to the left. The trunk turns to the left. The right pelvis leads the right shoulder girdle, and this relationship stays the same beyond the side-lying position. The trunk becomes extended prior to reaching the side-lying position.
Relationship between Pelvis and Shoulder Girdle Changes	The head may be raised off the supporting surface and may turn as the trunk rotates to the left. The right shoulder may initially lead the movement or the right shoulder girdle and right pelvis may be aligned. Before or when the side-lying position is reached, the relative position of the right pelvis and right shoulder girdle changes.
Right Shoulder Girdle Leads	The head may be raised from the supporting surface and may turn to the left. The trunk rotates to the left and may flex prior to reaching the side-lying position. The right shoulder girdle leads the right pelvis, and this relationship stays the same beyond the side-lying position.

* Adapted from Richter (1985). These categories are written to allow classification of movement patterns when the subject rolls from supine to prone over the left side of the body.

Table 4.11 Rolling from supine to prone: Lower Limb movement pattern categories*

Movement pattern	Description
Bilateral Lift	Both lower limbs are simultaneously lifted off the support surface, with the knees either flexed or extended, and then carried to the left.
Unilateral Lift without a Push	One lower limb is lifted off the support surface. The other lower limb may flex and assume a position as if to push, or may remain extended. The extremity contacting the surface slides or moves and does not maintain a fixed point of contact with the support surface.
Unilateral Push	One or both lower limbs are flexed, and assume a position as if to push. One foot may be lifted off or moves across the support surface, while the other maintains a fixed point of contact, pushing against the surface.
Bilateral Push	Both lower limbs are flexed and assume a position to push against the support surface. Both feet maintain a fixed point of contact simultaneously as the hips extend. The uppermost thigh may remain behind the lower thigh when approaching the side-lying position.

* Adapted from Richter (1985). These lower limb categories were revised from Richter's original work by the author, to promote reliable classification when using a side and foot view camera to record performance. These categories are written to allow classification of movement patterns when the subject rolls from supine to prone over the left side of the body.

tasks, where typically 20–30 per cent of the possible combinations of action have been observed in samples of comparable size. Five forms of movement were found to occur on approximately 10 per cent of the subjects' trials. These represented various combinations of two trunk patterns: Pelvis Leads, or the Relationship between Pelvis and Shoulder Girdle changes,

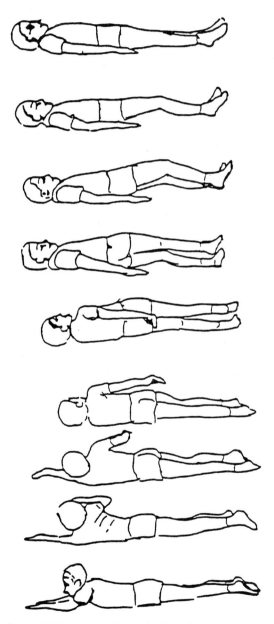

Figure 4.5 A common form of rolling from supine to prone exhibited by young adults (from Richter *et al.,* 1989)

coupled with the UL Lift and Reach above Shoulder Level pattern in four instances, and the Push pattern in one instance. Three different LL limb patterns contributed to these five common profiles, and one of these is illustrated in Figure 4.5.

Lewis (1987) continued the study of rolling movements in a sample of children aged 6, 8, and 10 years. Because the original study reported by Richter (1985) was completed using a single video camera, the movement pattern categories of the lower limbs were revised to reflect the perspective obtained when a foot-view camera was used. The categorical descriptions in Table 4.11 represent this altered perspective, and are the descriptions that have been used in all studies since Richter's original work. Lewis found the most common form of rolling in young children to be comprised of a Push pattern in the ULs, a Pelvis Leads pattern of the trunk and a Unilateral Lift pattern of the LLs. This pattern was seen on about 35 per cent of the trials of the 6-year-old subjects, 40 per cent of the 8-year-old children's trials and 20 per cent of the 10-year-old children's rolling trials. It is interesting to note, however, that when component action was examined the 6-year-old children were found to more commonly use a LL Unilateral Push pattern across their trials. It is not uncommon for a pattern that is most common across trials not to be part of the most common combination of actions for that group. Often the most common pattern is seen in combination with a variety of patterns of other components.

Inspection of the incidence of each component pattern with respect to age led Lewis to conclude that movement patterns used to roll from supine to prone vary with age across childhood. Her findings led to a new developmental sequence for each of the three components of rolling.

Boucher (1987) completed a study of adolescents (13-, 15- and 17-year-olds) performing the rolling task. Her study revealed that the younger teens rolled using different patterns to those of the older teens. Thirteen-year-old subjects most commonly rolled using either an Upper Limb Push and Reach or a Push pattern; they demonstrated a Relationship between Pelvis and Shoulder Girdle Changes or a Pelvis Leads AR pattern, and a Unilateral Push or Bilateral Push pattern in the LLs. The two older groups commonly demonstrated two different forms of rolling. One pattern was similar to that of the younger subjects, and one was distinctly different. The latter involved

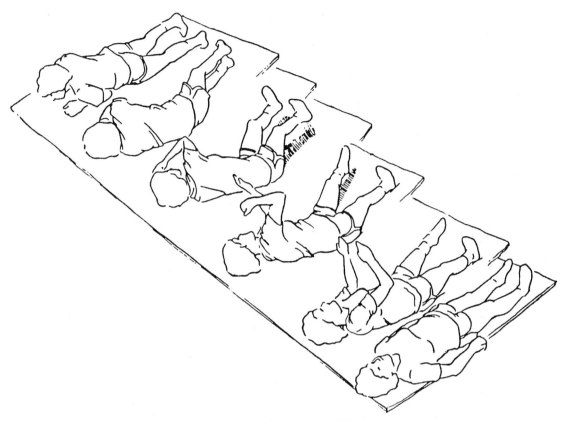

Figure 4.6 Most common form of rolling in children (from Lewis, 1987)

Lifting and Reaching Below Shoulder Level as the leading UL moved across the body, the Shoulder Girdle Leads pattern in the AR, and a Bilateral Lift pattern of the LLs. The combination of actions that was similar to the younger teens involved an UL Push and Reach pattern, a changing relationship between the pelvis and shoulder girdle in the AR, and a Unilateral Push pattern in the LLs.

MacDonald (1991) completed a longitudinal study of the rolling movements of infants who were aged 6–9 months. In that study, as in studies of rising in toddlers, new patterns were identified. These new pattern descriptions describe a common practice in these young subjects – fractionating the movement into parts. Infants often pause in the intermediate side-lying position during the process of rolling, and also appear to try out various combinations of movement patterns in search of an efficient form of rolling.

At the present time, a study of movement patterns of older adults completing the rolling task is being undertaken. In addition to our descriptive work, we explored therapists' thoughts regarding the use of the prone position for older adults. We await the outcome of this study to add to our understanding of life-span development in the rolling task. As with the rising tasks, we predict that external constraints and the internal constraints provided by body shape and size may be contributing to performance in the rolling task. We look forward to studies of individuals with disabling conditions performing this task.

Summary

The component approach to movement pattern analysis has proved to be a very useful method for the study of righting movements. It is a relatively inexpensive approach that leads to greater understanding of these movements, and allows testing of various theories of motor development and control. The body of knowledge regarding performance in these tasks is growing as additional studies of individuals with and without disabilities are carried out. We are also beginning to understand the factors that influence performance in righting. As we understand these factors better, we will improve the application of knowledge of motor performance in the fundamental tasks of daily life to the clinical practice of physical therapy.

References

Bobath, B. (1965). *Abnormal Postural Reflex Activity Caused by Brain Lesions*. Heinemann.

Bobath, K. and Bobath, B. (1972). Cerebral palsy. In *Physical Therapy Services in the Developmental Disabilities* (P. H. Pearson and C. E. Williams, eds.), pp. 31–185. Charles C. Thomas.

Boucher, J. (1987). *Age-related Differences in Adolescent Movement Patterns during Rolling from Supine to Prone*. Master's thesis, Medical College of Virginia.

Dhawan, L. D. and VanSant, A. F. (1995). The effect of two levels of added weight on the movement patterns used to rise from supine to standing. Poster Presentation, 12th Congress of the World Confederation of Physical Therapy, Washington DC.

Ford-Smith, C. and VanSant, A. F. (1993). Age differences in movement patterns used to rise from a bed: a study of middle adulthood. *Phys. Ther.*, **73**, 300–9.

Green, L. and Williams, K. (1992). Differences in developmental movement patterns used by active versus sedentary middle-aged adults coming from a supine position to erect stance. *Phys. Ther.*, **72**, 560–67.

King, L. A. and VanSant, A. F. (1995). The effect of solid ankle foot orthotics on movement patterns used in a supine to stand rising task. *Phys. Ther.*,**75**, 952–64.

Lawrence, D. G. and Kuypers, H. G. (1968a). The functional organization of the motor system in the monkey. I. The effects of bilateral pyramidal lesions. *Brain*, **91**, 1–14.

Lawrence, D. G. and Kuypers, H. G. (1968b). The functional organization of the motor system in the monkey. II. The effects of lesions of the descending brainstem pathways. *Brain*, **91**, 15–36.

Lewis, A. M. (1987). *Age-related Differences in Component Action during Rolling in children*. Master's thesis, Medical College of Virginia.

Luehring, S. (1989). *Component Movement Patterns of Two Groups of Older Adults in the Task of Rising to Standing from the Floor*. Master's thesis, Medical College of Virginia.

Marsala, G. and VanSant, A. F. (1998). Age-related differences in movement patterns used by infants and toddlers to rise from supine to erect standing. *Phys. Ther.*, **78**, 149–59.

MacDonald, J. (1991*). Developmental Ordering of the Movement Patterns in Infants rolling Supine to Prone*. Master's thesis, Medical College of Virginia.

McCoy, J. O. and VanSant, A. F. (1993). Movement patterns of adolescents rising from a bed. *Phys. Ther.*, **73**, 182–93.

McGraw, M. B. (1945). *Neuromuscular Maturation of the Human Infant*. New York: Haefner.

Richter, R. R. (1985). *Developmental Sequences for Rolling from Supine to Prone: A Prelongitudinal Study*. Master's thesis, Medical College of Virginia.

Richter, R. R., VanSant, A. F. and Newton, R. A. (1989). Description of adult rolling movements and hypothesis of developmental sequences. *Phys. Ther.* **69**, 63–71.

Roberton, M. A. (1977). Stability of stage categorizations across trials: implications for the 'stage theory' of overarm throw development. *J. Hum. Mov. Stud.*, **3**, 49–59.

Roberton, M. A. (1978). Longitudinal evidence for developmental stages in the forceful overarm throw. *J. Hum. Mov. Stud.*, **4**, 167–75.

Sarnacki, S. J. (1985). *Rising from Supine on a Bed: A Description of Adult Movement and Hypothesis of Developmental Sequences*. Master's thesis, Medical College of Virginia.

Schaltenbrand, G. (1928). The development of human motility and motor disturbances. *Arch. Neur. Psychiatry*, **20**, 720–30.

Scholtz, J. P. (1990). Dynamic pattern theory – some implications for therapeutics. *Phys. Ther.*, **70**, 827–43.

Sherwin, V. M. (1993). *The Task of Rising out of Bed in Individuals with Chronic Low Back Pain*. Master's project report, College of Allied Health Professions, Temple University, PA.

VanSant, A. F. (1976). *The Relationship between Standing Posture and Equilibrium Abilities in Children with Spastic Cerebral Palsy*. Master's thesis, Medical College of Virginia.

VanSant, A. F. (1988a). Children's body action in righting from supine to erect stance: pre-longitudinal screening of developmental sequences. *Phys. Ther.*, **68**, 1330–8.

VanSant, A. F. (1988b). Adults' body action in rising from supine to erect stance: a developmental hypothesis. *Phys. Ther.*, **68**, 185–92.

VanSant, A. F. (1989a). Rising from the floor: age differences in movement patterns, a life-span perspective. In *Proceedings of the Forum on Neurological Physical Therapy Assessment, Combined Sections Meeting. Alexandria VA*. Neurology Section, American Physical Therapy Association.

VanSant, A. F. (1989b). A life-span concept of motor development. *Quest: The Journal of the National Association for Physical Education in Higher Education*, **41**, 224–34.

VanSant, A. F. (1990). Life-span development in functional tasks. *Phys. Ther.*, **70**, 788–98.

VanSant, A. F. (1991a). Life-span motor development. In *II STEP Proceedings: Contemporary Concepts in the Management of Motor Control Problems* (M. Lister, ed.). Foundation for Physical Therapy, Alexandria VA.

VanSant, A. F. (1991b). Use of developmental sequences with adults. In *II STEP Proceedings: Contemporary Concepts in the Management of Motor Control Problems* (M. Lister, ed.). Foundation for Physical Therapy, Alexandria VA.

VanSant, A. F. (1991c). Life-span development of movement patterns in a righting task. In *Proceedings of the World Confederation for Physical Therapy 11th International Congress Book III*, pp. 1286–88. World Confederation for Physical Therapy, London.

VanSant, A. F. (1991d). Recovery of movement patterns following traumatic head injury. In *Proceedings of the World Confederation for Physical Therapy 11th International Congress Book II*, pp. 992–4. World Confederation of Physical Therapy, London.

VanSant, A. F. (1993). Analysis of movement dysfunction: usefulness of a component approach. *Proceedings of the 13th Annual Eugene Michels Researchers' Forum* (Section on Research), pp. 15–22. American Physical Therapy Association, Alexandria VA.

VanSant, A. F. (1997). A life-span perspective of age differences in righting movements. In *Motor Development: Research & Reviews, Volume 1* (J. E. Clark and J. H. Humphrey, eds.), pp. 46–63. National Association for Sport and Physical Education, Reston VA.

Wild, M. (1938). The behaviour pattern of throwing and some observations concerning its course of development in children. *Res. Q.*, **9**, 20–24.

5 Rising to stand and sitting down

G. D. Baer and B. R. Durward

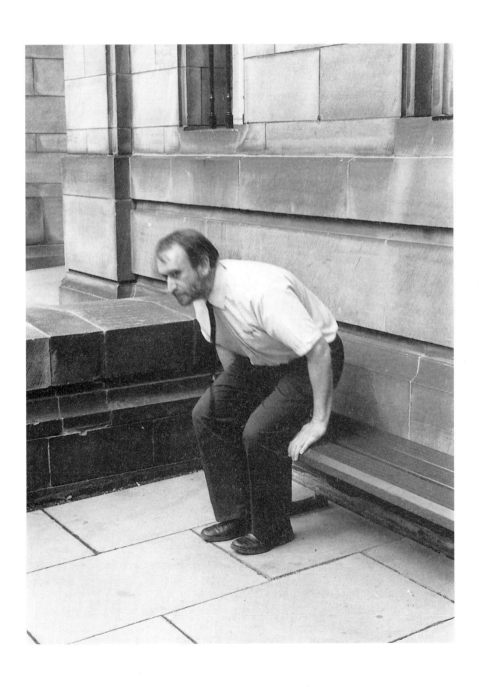

Introduction

The importance of rising to stand (RTS) and sitting down (SitD) may be associated with upright bipedal walking. It may also be argued that both functions represent essential movements in their own right.

The movements of RTS and SitD are performed routinely many times in the course of a day, and represent essential prerequisites for the successful completion of other functional tasks such as walking, climbing stairs and getting in and out of bed. Despite this basic functional requirement, many individuals report difficulties in completing these movements (Munton *et al.*, 1981; Kerr *et al.*, 1991).

While functional tasks such as gait have received extensive attention, there remains a paucity of objective scientific evidence related to the characteristic features of RTS and SitD. Recent studies investigating the movements indicate that, under controlled conditions, motion is highly reproducible and therefore conducive to scientific examination (Berger *et al.*, 1989a, 1989b; Schenkman *et al.*, 1990).

General description of rising to stand and sitting down

The RTS and SitD movements are characterized by gross changes in the shape of body mass and body segment alignment, which occur within a brief time period of approximately 1.6–1.8 s (Nuzik *et al.*, 1986; Baer and Ashburn, 1995). The successful completion of these movements is dependent upon muscle activity, joint angle displacements, joint moments of force and movement of the position of the centre of body mass (COM).

The gross angular changes in body segment motion during RTS have been described as initially flexion, followed by extension (Kelley *et al.*, 1976; Nuzik *et al.*, 1986). These gross patterns of movement are sequential, and terminate once the body has adopted an upright position. In comparison, SitD starts from a position of generalized extension, but is followed by a pattern of controlled descent into a flexed alignment of body segments. Although these gross descriptions generally represent lower limb joint angle changes, they do not reflect the complex associated interactions of flexor and extensor movement that occurs throughout the body.

Essential features of both RTS and SitD movements are alterations in the supporting area of base that occur during each movement. The changes in the supporting area of base comprise magnitude, location and the anatomical structures providing support. For example, when standing the supporting area of base is relatively small and encompasses the boundary surrounding the feet. During SitD, the size and location of this supporting area of base is maintained until the thighs contact the supporting surface of the seat. At this point the original supporting area of base is extended to include the feet, thighs and buttocks.

Scientific studies of rising to stand and sitting down

The remaining sections will provide an overview of scientific research related to RTS and SitD, and include details of the measurement techniques adopted.

Qualitative studies

There are limited qualitative data to describe normal activity or the problems experienced by patient groups. A study of the nature and extent of seating difficulties experienced by the elderly and patients with rheumatic diseases was undertaken by Munton *et al.* (1981). Analysis of 379 completed questionnaires revealed that 42 per cent of people had 'some degree of difficulty in rising from an easy chair at home and of these 18 per cent either expressed great difficulty or could not rise unaided'; 34 per cent of this sample declared that their easy chair caused either pain or discomfort. Roorda *et al.* (1996) argued that there was a need to develop a comprehensive self-administered questionnaire capable of identifying functional limitations in RTS and SitD. Their questionnaire included five tasks related to rising from and sitting down on a high chair, low chair, toilet, bed and car seat. Initial studies revealed that the questionnaire was both valid and reliable, and appeared to be capable of assessing degrees of limitation in RTS and SitD.

The suitability of chairs appropriate for the elderly was investigated by Finlay *et al.* (1983). Ninety-two elderly subjects were assessed using a pass or fail scoring system and an 11 point rating scale to determine their ability to stand up from a dining chair, armchair and a chair designed to assist the elderly (Haypark chair). Chairs appropriately configured for the elderly were found to enable independent RTS when previously it had not been possible.

The major RTS manoeuvres used by patients with various forms of neuromuscular dystrophy were observed by Butler *et al.* (1991). The group was found to exhibit different movement patterns compared to normal subjects and, in each case, compensatory strategies were adopted that maximized remaining useful muscle activity. It was proposed that the prevention of joint contractures was of prime importance in order for weakened muscles to continue effectively to provide a balance of joint moments and thereby enable RTS.

Age-related differences in the RTS movement pattern have been identified from analysis of videotapes of children and adults performing the movement (VanSant, 1990). The analysis entailed categorizing and plotting body segment movement patterns to describe developmental sequences. This process revealed that age factors may influence variability of performance.

There is little evidence from qualitative research to describe normal or abnormal activity. Knowledge of the nature and extent of difficulties associated with RTS is limited and, in the case of SitD, non-existent.

Temporal characteristics of rising to stand and sitting down

Rising to stand time

The time taken by normal subjects to stand up in an unpaced manner is approximately 1.8 s. Times reported from a number of studies are summarized in Table 5.1. These time values were established using different measurement techniques and test protocols. Where times were measured using interrupted light photography, cinefilm and video, the start and end of motion were visually estimated from the filmed records. Alexander *et al.* (1989) also used video, but added a light source and event markers triggered by switches attached to the backrest and seat of a chair. This technique provided an objective means of identifying the temporal components of movement. The start and end of RTS and SitD motion have been successfully identified by observation and the use of a hand-held switch by Engardt and Olsson (1992). The reliability of this technique was established by comparing time values acquired using the hand-held switch with data from a motion analysis system (ELITE).

The results from some studies of healthy older subjects suggest that the elderly require approximately 10 per cent more time to stand up (Wheeler *et al.*, 1985; Millington *et al.*, 1992; Engardt and Olsson, 1992). The reason why the elderly take longer to RTS is uncertain, but it may be due to a need to stabilize anteroposterior sway. In contrast, Alexander *et al.* (1989) report similar RTS time values for young and old subjects. It remains inconclusive whether there are age-related differences associated with the time to rise to stand in normal subjects.

There are instances when RTS time may be reduced. Coghlin and McFadyen (1994) identified that people with back pain took less time to RTS than normal subjects. It was speculated that the reduction in time was due, in part, to a modified movement strategy that distributed the moments required to stand up more evenly throughout the lower back.

It is more typical for patients to demonstrate increased RTS times. The time to RTS in hemiplegic subjects reveal great discrepancies when compared to normal values (Table 5.2). Forty-two hemiplegic subjects, tested between 1 week and 3 months following stroke, took a mean time of 3.7 s to rise to stand (Engardt and Olsson, 1992).

During rehabilitation, the RTS time has been found to decrease. Ada and Westwood (1992) used video to record the performance of eight hemiplegic patients at the point when they were first able to RTS independently, and at a later stage in their rehabilitation programme. The patients' mean initial time was 2.28 s, and by the later stage the times had reduced to 1.57 s. This reduction in time was confirmed by Baer (1991). RTS times were measured in a group of six recovering hemiplegic patients, when they could perform the movement independently and then 4 and 8 weeks later. Median rise to stand times of 3.0, 2.14 and 1.67 s were reported at each stage. Although small samples were tested, the results highlight the possibility that hemiplegics may have the potential to move more effectively and achieve time values approaching those of normal subjects.

Sitting down time

Compared to RTS, there are few reports of normal times for sitting down. The mean SitD time for normal subjects has been reported to be between 2.5 s (Engardt and Olsson, 1992) and 4.62 s (Kralj *et al.*, 1990). The reported differences in these time values could be due to a number of reasons such as differences in test protocols, variability within

Table 5.1 Rising time values (unpaced) from studies of normal subjects

Author	Type of subjects	N	Age (years)	Measurement technique	Test position	Mean (seconds)	Range (seconds)	SD (seconds)
Jones et al., 1959	Normal males	6	20–26	Interrupted light photography	Unspecified	~1.8		
Wheeler et al., 1985	Normal females females	10 10	22–28 67–81	Video	Self selected	1.5 1.9		0.16 0.68
Nuzik et al., 1986	Normal	55	20–48	Cinefilm	Armless chair	1.8	1.3–2.5	0.3
Fleckenstein et al., 1988	Normal	10	25.4 mean	Cinefilm	Knees flexed at 105° Knees flexed at 75°	1.37 1.57		0.32 0.16
Alexander et al., 1989	Normal	15 21	20–24 ~63–75	Video and event markers	With hands No hands With hands No hands	1.5 1.6 1.5 1.6		0.2 0.3 0.3 0.3
Kralj et al., 1990	Normal	20	32.6 mean	Force platform and electrogoniometry	Normalized backrest	3.33		0.56
Pai et al., 1991	Normal	8	26–38	WATSMART motion analysis	Standard chair	1.6		0.2
Engardt and Olsson, 1992	Normal	16	59 mean	Force plates and hand-held switch	Normalized height	2.3		~0.3
Millington et al., 1992	Normal	10	65–76	Video, EMG and force platform	Standard chair	2.03	1.62–2.54	0.34
Coghlin and McFadyen, 1994	Normal	5	32 mean	Video, EMG and force platform	Normalized height	1.95	1.68–2.28	0.05
Hanke et al., 1995	Normal	18	31.7	WATSMART motion analysis, 2 force platforms	Chair with fixed height	1.85		0.28
Baer and Ashburn, 1995	Normal	30	61.6	CODA and event marker	Fixed height stool	1.67	1.26–2.13	0.27
Weighted mean						1.8		0.45

Table 5.2 Time to stand values from clinical studies

Author	Type of subjects	N	Mean age (years)	Measurement technique		Test position	Mean (seconds)		Range (seconds)	SD (seconds)
Baer, 1991	Hemiplegic	6	64.5	CODA and event marker		Fixed height stool				
					Initial		median 3		2.13–5.36	
					4 weeks		median 2.14		1.57–2.83	
					8 weeks		median 1.67		1.50–2.82	
Ada and Westwood, 1992	Hemiplegic	8	65	Videotape		Dining chair				
					MAS2		2.28			0.68
					MAS6		1.57			0.24
Engardt and Olsson, 1992	Hemiplegic	42	64	Forceplates and hand-held switch		Normalized height	3.7			0.9
Coghlin and McFadyen, 1994	Low back pain	5	36.7	Video EMG, force platform		Normalized height	1.7		1.4–2.23	0.06

subject groups, and the different measurement methods used to time the motion. These values indicate that the movement of SitD requires more time than RTS.

Effects of paced and unpaced activity

A number of studies have imposed a fixed time period during which the movement of RTS must be completed (Jeng *et al.*, 1990; Schenkman *et al.*, 1990; Ikeda *et al.*, 1991; Riley *et al.*, 1991). The purpose of pacing the movement was to investigate joint moments and changes in momentum during RTS under controlled conditions. The time allocated to complete the RTS movement varied from 1.15–1.3 s, which is approximately 0.5 s faster than the reported normal subject times.

Phases of movement

One of the problems in comparing studies of RTS and SitD is the variety of conventions used to describe separate phases of the movement cycles. At one extreme, the entire movement has been considered to be a continuous cycle (Jones *et al.*, 1959; Ellis *et al.*, 1984; Fleckenstein *et al.*, 1988; Pai and Rogers, 1991a, 1991b), but many investigators have devised divisions that allow the motion to be described relative to discrete phases in a manner similar to gait.

Initially Kelley *et al.* (1976) divided the RTS movement cycle into two phases. A light bulb was mounted on the side of a chair and connected to a switch sensitive to body contact. With this technique, the light bulb remains unlit during the initial phase when the thighs are in contact with the chair. The second phase is identified when the mass of the subject is no longer in contact with the chair, causing the switch to open and activate the light bulb.

Components of movement have also been used to identify phases associated with RTS. Two distinct phases have been detected by visual examination of video data (Nuzik *et al.*, 1986). The first division, termed the 'flexion phase', includes the forward motion of the trunk prior to lifting the thighs off the seat. The second phase, the 'extension phase', begins as the head starts to extend on the cervical spine and describes the remainder of the rising movement. Rodosky *et al.* (1989) adopted a similar division, but the phases were termed the forward-thrust phase and the extension phase. In this case, the division between phases was detected when the external moments tending to flex the hip and knee reached maximum values simultaneously.

Three phases that can be identified from video data have been proposed by Millington *et al.* (1992). Phase one, 'weight shift', occurs when trunk movement is initiated and continues until knee extension starts. Phase two, 'transition', is detected from the initiation of knee extension and ends with the reversal of trunk flexion to trunk extension. Phase three, 'lift', begins from the reversal of trunk motion and ends when trunk motion can no longer be detected.

The behaviour of forces measured beneath the subject has also been used to define phases for RTS and SitD. Kralj *et al.* (1990), using a force platform, defined six identifiable events for RTS and six for SitD by measuring changes in the horizontal (Fy) and vertical forces (Fz) during motion. Although it is possible to detect these phases of movement in normal subjects, this procedure has not been used in the clinical setting, where the behaviour of horizontal and vertical forces may be altered and the technology is usually unavailable.

Full biomechanical analysis using a force platform, three-dimensional motion analysis system and control software has also been used to define phases for RTS. Schenkman *et al.* (1990) was instrumental in developing a four-phase description. Phase one is designated the 'flexion momentum phase', and begins with initiation of movement and ends before the buttocks leave the seat ('lift off'). The second phase, 'momentum transfer', begins at 'lift off' and ends when maximum ankle dorsiflexion is detected. Phase three, the 'extension phase', follows maximum ankle dorsiflexion and ends when the hips cease to extend. The final 'stabilization phase' begins just after the hip extension velocity reaches zero degrees per second. These divisions have been adopted in a number of subsequent studies that have attempted to describe the rising motion using combined kinetic and kinematic data (Riley *et al.*, 1991; Ikeda *et al.*, 1991; Hughes *et al.*, 1994).

The differences in phase definitions and test protocols make comparing results between studies difficult. Despite these differences, there are some identifiable trends in the RTS cycle; notably, the movement prior to thighs off represents approximately 35 per cent of the RTS cycle. The remaining 65 per cent comprises phases associated with extension and body stabilization. The identification of completion of the RTS cycle, which may include the process of stabilizing the body, remains problematic.

RTS under constrained conditions

Many investigators have adopted test protocols designed to standardize components of the RTS activity. These components include elimination of upper limb activity, normalizing seat height with reference to limb segment lengths or joint angles and standardizing the position of the feet. Studies that have attempted to constrain upper limb activity by requiring test subjects to fold their arms across the chest as they performed the RTS movement include those by Rodosky *et al.* (1989), Schenkman *et al.* (1990), Riley *et al.* (1991), Ikeda *et al.* (1991), Kerr *et al.* (1994a), Hughes *et al.* (1994) and Hanke *et al.* (1995). This technique was employed to prevent direct assistance from the arms during movement or indirect activity, such as arm swing, which could affect the body momentum characteristics.

The orientation of the feet, in both the sagittal and frontal planes, has also been standardized. The most common position entails placing the feet parallel, 10 cm apart and with 18° of ankle dorsiflexion (Schenkman *et al.*, 1990; Riley *et al.*, 1991; Ikeda *et al.*, 1991; Kerr *et al.*, 1994a, 1994b).

In many instances the seat height has been adjusted to 80 per cent of the distance measured between the floor and the knee joint (Schenkman *et al.*, 1990; Riley *et al.*, 1991 and Ikeda *et al.*, 1991). Other investigators have attempted to set the seat height with reference to knee joint flexion; 90° (Millington *et al.*, 1992) and 95–100° (Kerr *et al.*, 1994a).

These techniques have been adopted to eliminate all possible sources of variance that might effect movement performance. However, constraining upper limb movement and adjusting the seat height and alignment for individual subjects may lead to movement that is unnatural and not a true reflection of normal human activity.

Kinematics of rising to stand and sitting down

A description of RTS and SitD motion, without regard to the forces generated to complete each movement, provides a wealth of information. RTS and SitD have generally been investigated in the sagittal plane, with an underlying assumption that the body is maintained in a symmetrical alignment (Rodosky *et al.*, 1989).

General body motion

Generalized descriptions of body motion during RTS and, in particular, the trajectory of specific body segments have been the subject of a number of studies (Jones *et al.*, 1959; Jones, 1963; Kelley *et al.*, 1976; Nuzik *et al.*, 1986; Stevens *et al.*, 1989; Pai and Rogers, 1990, 1991a).

In an early study by Jones *et al.* (1959), interrupted light photography was used to observe differences in head, trunk and thigh trajectory during rising when the head was maintained in three different orientations: 'relaxed habitual', 'best sitting' and an 'experimental' posture controlled by the investigator. Sagittal plane analysis was undertaken by measuring the linked locations of three anatomical landmarks. The study is important for having provided the first description of curvilinear head motion linked with thigh translation during rising.

A similar measurement technique was employed in a further study of eight male patients with a range of neurological diseases and an undisclosed number of normal subjects (Jones, 1963). Trajectories were established for head, neck, chest, arm and leg, using six sit to stand movements from each subject. Initial velocity and acceleration values for vertical and horizontal components of head motion for normal subjects were reported in graphical form as $\sim 1.18 \, ms^{-1}$ for maximum horizontal head velocity and $\sim 0.35 \, ms^{-2}$ for vertical head acceleration.

Variations in the execution of rising to stand, as performed by six normal subjects of different sizes, has been investigated (Kelley *et al.*, 1976). The thigh–knee angle was standardized at 75° and the subjects performed a paced movement (2 s) when rising. The path of the centre of mass in relation to the ankle was plotted for the entire movement and related to muscle activity. An example of the trajectory for one subject is shown (Figure 5.1).

The vertical line crossing the x-axis at 0 cm indicates the point of thighs off. Pai and Rogers (1990) confirmed this description of the trajectory of the centre of mass and identified two distinct portions; the horizontal body mass transfer associated with the flat section of the curve, followed by a vertical ascent represented by the steep section of the curve.

Kinematic and kinetic data have been used to model the trajectory of the body centre of mass (COM) while RTS. The location of the COM while sitting is above that associated with the standing anatomical position, and lies approximately at the thoracolumbar junction (Roebroeck, 1994). During RTS the movement of the COM, although at some instances considered to be displaced anteriorly outwith the body mass, remains within the supporting area of base (Kelley *et al.*, 1976; Roebroeck

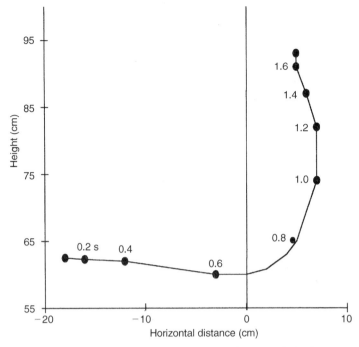

Figure 5.1 The height and horizontal position of the whole body centre of mass in relation to the ankle joint in a normal subject during standing up (from Kelley *et al.*, 1976)

et al., 1994). The trajectory of the centre of mass in specific patient groups has not been described.

A comprehensive kinematic analysis of rising to stand has been reported by Nuzik *et al.* (1986). The relative motion of eight body segments was analysed from cinefilm records of 55 healthy young subjects. Mean angular positions for each segment were computed at 5 per cent intervals of the RTS movement cycle. Figure 5.2 shows the trajectory paths of selected anatomical structures in the sagittal plane throughout the movement. Some of the key features identified were that:

the horizontal excursion of the head was greater than that of the acromion
the horizontal displacement of the knee was greater than vertical displacement
the curvilinear displacement for the pelvis and hip region was 'S' shaped, while that of the head and shoulder region was 'C' shaped.

There are few descriptions of changes in body motion in the frontal plane. Baer and Ashburn (1995) described the lateral displacement of the shoulders and pelvis in a group of 30 normal subjects, and a mean displacement of 36.1 mm at

the shoulder and 29.6 mm at the pelvis was reported. These values indicate the extent to which normal subjects deviate laterally during the RTS movement and provide data against which patient performance may be compared.

Joint motion
Normal joint motion during rising to stand has been the subject of a number of investigations (Kelley *et al.*, 1976; Nuzik *et al.*, 1986; Wheeler *et al.*, 1985; Burdett *et al.*, 1985; Fleckenstein *et al.*, 1988; Rodosky *et al.*, 1989; Alexander *et al.*, 1989; Ikeda *et al.*, 1991; Millington *et al.*, 1992; Ada and Westwood, 1992).

The characteristics of hip and knee joint motion during RTS in normal subjects were investigated using cinematography by Kelley *et al.* (1976). In general, a constant relationship was found to exist between hip and knee joint motion from the point of thighs off until completion of the movement. The mean angle of the knee joint was reported as 115.8° extension when the hip joint angle was at 120° extension, indicating that knee extension lagged behind hip extension.

A similar angular measurement technique was used by Nuzik *et al.* (1986) to investigate the

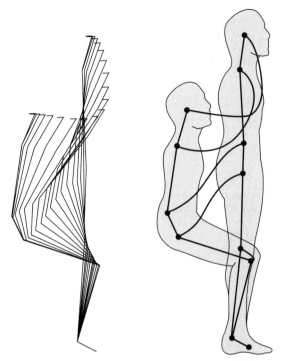

Figure 5.2 Left diagram depicts a representative movement pattern. Data points are joined by lines to form 21 stick figures (sampling rate). The enhanced line on the left indicates the initial position; the enhanced line on the right indicates the final position. Right diagram depicts trajectories of data points at the tragus, acromion, midiliac crest, hip and knee. (Reprinted from Nuzik *et al., Phys. Ther. 1986* with permission from the American Physical Therapy Association)

relationship between hip and knee joint motion. From a sample of 55 normal subjects, video analysis of movement indicated that the hip flexed during the first 40 per cent of the sit to stand movement cycle and extended during the last 60 per cent. The knee was found to extend throughout the cycle, and ankle dorsiflexion was complete by 45 per cent of the movement cycle. The knee alignment adopted by the normal group (mean knee extension angle) at the beginning of the movement cycle was 95°.

Differences in body motion in young and old healthy subjects have been reported. Comparison of peak joint angles, moments and velocities of 11 body segments revealed few differences. The timing and order of kinematic events were generally similar apart from head position, where the elderly group showed decreased (−15°) head to trunk extension angles during the RTS movement

(Ikeda *et al.*, 1991). It was identified that older subjects preferred to place their feet further back at the point of initiating the rising movement, and that total hip (elderly 106°; young 104°) and knee joint (elderly 100°; young 106°) ranges of motion were less when compared to those of young subjects. It remains unclear whether problems of rising to stand in the elderly may be partly associated with reduced range of motion in the hip and knee joint, thereby restricting trunk motion at the onset of the movement.

Maximum angular velocity changes occur during initial trunk flexion and onset of trunk and lower limb extension. Maximum trunk flexion, hip flexion and head extension angular velocities have been measured during the 'flexion momentum' phase, and maximum trunk extension, hip extension, knee extension and head flexion angular velocities in the 'extension phase' (Schenkman *et al.*, 1990). Ikeda *et al.* (1991) reported similar angular velocity values for young and elderly normal subjects while completing RTS as a paced movement (1.15 s).

Kinematic data were reported in only one clinical study of rising to stand. The performances of eight stroke patients were recorded with video at the start and end of a training programme for RTS (Ada and Westwood, 1992). Digitized x and y co-ordinates were measured and angular displacement patterns plotted for the hip and knee joint, and angular velocity values were then derived from this data. The results showed that, as performance of RTS improved, peak angular velocities increased at the knee (1.33 rad s^{-1} to 2.07 rad s^{-1}) and the hip (1.47 rad s^{-1} to 2.01 rad s^{-1}). The velocity profiles also changed, and were comparable to normal values with distinct acceleration and deceleration phases. These findings indicate that training strategies that target the temporal characteristics of RTS may be beneficial.

Kinetics of rising to stand and sitting down

The movements of RTS and SitD require co-ordinated muscle activity to generate forces against the chair and ground. The forces, acting around joints and then transmitted to either the chair or floor, serve to propel the body mass and provide stability, or control the body mass during descent. Measurement of the ground reaction forces and joint forces can provide an understanding of how each movement is performed and highlight differences between normal and abnormal activity.

Joint forces

The forces in the knee during rising were studied initially by Seedhom and Terayama (1976), using a combination of force platform and cine data to calculate knee forces in normal subjects. The forces acting through the heels and forefeet were determined separately, and this allowed the investigators to estimate approximately the line of action of the total force acting on the foot. Results from two subjects indicated that, during movement, the maximum forces along the tibial axis were 2.45 times the body weight, and, in an anteroposterior perpendicular direction to that axis, 1.07 times the body weight. The patellofemoral joint force was 2.36 times the body weight. While these forces were found to be similar to those occurring during activities such as level walking, the use of arms when RTS caused a considerable reduction in all knee forces.

The same technique was employed to compare the knee forces while rising from a normal chair without the use of arms with those with assistance from a motorized chair (Ellis *et al.*, 1979). It was found that, when rising from a normal chair without the aid of arms, the tibiofemoral force could rise to seven times body weight at the point of thighs off and the patellofemoral force increased to between two and six times body weight. The use of a motorized chair was found to reduce the tibiofemoral force to about twice body weight.

A chair capable of measuring the forces between a subject and the seat was added to the test procedure to compare rising with and without the use of arms, and rising from high and low chairs (Ellis *et al.*, 1984). The results confirmed that the knee joint and muscle forces were considerably reduced when rising with the aid of arms. It was also found that the calculated knee joint forces and muscle tensions were between 8 per cent and 56 per cent less when rising from a high chair compared with a low chair, irrespective of arm activity. Similar findings when using high and low arm rests were reported by Wretenberg *et al.* (1993).

Ground reaction forces

A force platform has been used by a number of investigators to determine ground reaction forces (GRF) during RTS (Bajd and Kralj, 1982; Stevens *et al.*, 1989; Kralj *et al.*, 1990; Pai and Rogers, 1990; Pai and Rogers, 1991b; Millington *et al.*, 1992; Wretenberg *et al.*, 1993; Vander Linden *et al.*, 1994; Hanke *et al.*, 1995; Yoshida *et al.*, 1983).

Vertical ground reaction forces have received specific attention in a number of studies, and are reported to reach over 100 per cent of body weight during RTS (Figure 5.3).

Peak vertical ground reaction forces tend to occur immediately following the point of thighs off (Millington *et al.*, 1992; Kralj *et al.*, 1990), and reach around 111 per cent of body weight. These maximum forces immediately decrease after thighs off (Yoshida *et al.*, 1983; Pai and Rogers, 1990; Kralj *et al.*, 1990). Following these changes, and near completion of the RTS activity, the ground reaction forces stabilize at body weight. This distinctive pattern is due to the initial requirement to create a force greater than body weight that will

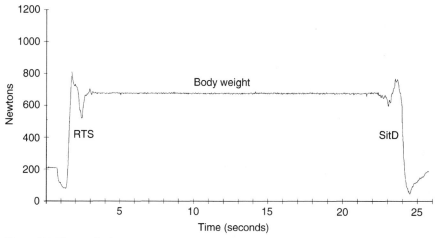

Figure 5.3 The vertical ground reaction force during rising to stand and sitting down (from Durward, 1994)

cause upward acceleration of the body. Once the body is moving at the required velocity, the force can be reduced to body weight.

The behaviour of vertical ground reaction forces during SitD has received less attention, but appears to follow a similar pattern (Figure 5.3). Initially the vertical ground reaction forces decrease below body weight by approximately 5 per cent of the body weight, and are followed by an increase to a level of 110 per cent body weight prior to seat contact (Durward, 1994). This increase may be related to the braking activity required to control the descent.

The anteroposterior forces during RTS and SitD are considerably smaller than the vertical forces. During RTS, prior to thighs off, propulsive forces (approximately 10 per cent body weight) are generated in a posterior direction and are followed by anterior forces of a similar magnitude that serve to counter the momentum of the body. During SitD the pattern is reversed, but the forces in this case are around 5 per cent body weight (Kralj *et al.*, 1990).

The changes in lateral forces are even smaller than the vertical or anteroposterior forces, and are reported to fluctuate from side to side (Stevens *et al.*, 1989).

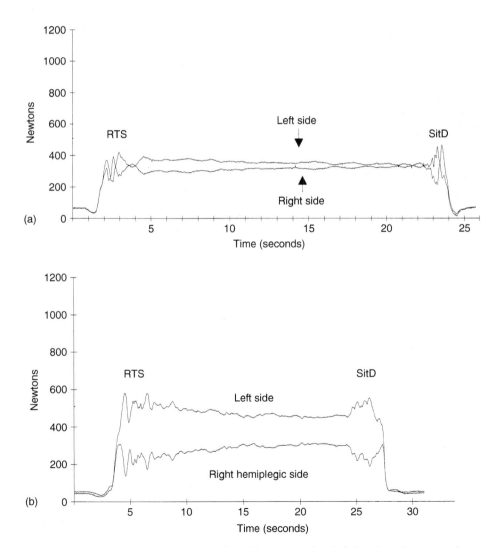

Figure 5.4 Lateral weight distribution during rising to stand and sitting down in a normal subject and hemiplegic patient (from Durward, 1994)

Distribution of forces

Direct measurement of forces related to specific body parts during RTS and SitD can indicate force differentials and the interactions of body segments during each movement. Direct techniques have been used to measure forces beneath the left and right sides, the hands and the feet.

The lateral distribution of body weight beneath the feet while rising and sitting down is relatively even, and values of 49.7 per cent and 50.3 per cent body weight have been reported by Engardt and Olsson (1992). This force differential compares closely to the values of normal subjects when standing (Sackley and Lincoln, 1991). In comparison with normal subjects, hemiplegic subjects demonstrate a characteristic lateral force asymmetry (Figure 5.4). The body weight distribution during rising for the stroke group indicated that 37.5 per cent of body weight was borne on the hemiplegic leg (Engardt and Olsson, 1992).

Although the normal lateral distribution of forces is almost equal, there are differences in the separate forefoot and hindfoot forces. Durward (1994), in a study of 120 subjects, reported that following thighs off, maximum forces beneath each heel reached 40 per cent body weight. Throughout RTS the mean force value beneath each heel was 26%. In contrast, data from 36 recovering hemiplegic patients showed that the maximum forces beneath the affected side heel were 37 per cent body weight and that the mean affected side heel value was 21%. In the unaffected side, maximum forces beneath the heel were 63 per cent body weight and that the mean heel value was 42%. These values indicate that, in hemiplegic patients, there is a disproportionate amount of force directed beneath the unaffected side heel during RTS. Although not so pronounced, a similar trend was identified during SitD (Figure 5.5).

The use of armrests has been found to affect the distribution of forces during RTS and SitD. Durward (1994) reported maximum vertical force values of 15 per cent body weight beneath each hand during RTS and 11 per cent body weight during SitD. Alexander *et al.* (1989) has proposed that the use of hands causes a reduction in the amount of trunk flexion during RTS. While there is some evidence that use of armrests can reduce the hip and knee joint moments, it remains uncertain whether the height of the armrests or the position of the hands have any influence, (Wretenberg *et al.*, 1993).

Joint moments

During RTS and SitD the lower limb joint moments are influenced by foot position, seat height, movement speed, the use of armrests, age and body mass.

The alteration of different knee joint angles and therefore foot position has been found to cause changes in joint moments and body movement (Fleckenstein *et al.*, 1988). Ten normal subjects stood up under two conditions; knees flexed at 75° and 105°. The results revealed that the peak hip extension moments increased significantly when the initial knee flexion was limited to 75°. In this alignment, subjects were found to accentuate the forward movement of the arms and trunk to help them stand up. The peak hip extension moments were calculated to be much greater when knee flexion was limited to 75°, and the differences were most marked at initiation of movement. Similar changes in joint moments and trunk motion due to alterations in foot position have been reported by Shepherd and Koh (1996).

The influence of chair height on lower limb mechanics during rising has been investigated by Burdett *et al.* (1985) and Rodosky *et al.* (1989). Burdett *et al.* (1985) compared joint moments and ranges of motion during rising from two types of chair of differing heights (0.43 metres and 0.64 metres) with and without the use of arms. In 10 healthy subjects, the higher seat and the use of arms decreased joint moments at the hip and knee. Results from four disabled subjects confirmed the general findings for the healthy subjects. Rodosky *et al.* (1989) also studied the effects of four different seat heights (65 per cent, 80 per cent, 100 per cent and 115 per cent of sitting knee height). As chair height was increased, maximum range of motion in the hip, knee and ankle decreased. The maximum hip flexor moment decreased by less than 12 per cent, while the maximum knee flexor moment decreased by 50 per cent.

The effect of variation in movement speed on resultant joint moments during rising to stand has been investigated. Bajd *et al.* (1982) measured approximately 50 per cent reduction in the resultant peak joint moments in the knee joint when a normal subject stood up at a slow pace compared to a rapid pace, even though no difference was found in the peak hip joint moments. Pai and Rogers (1991b) compared fast and slow rising and confirmed that, when speed of ascent increased progressively, the resultant joint moments for peak hip flexion, knee extension, and ankle dorsiflexion increased disproportionately.

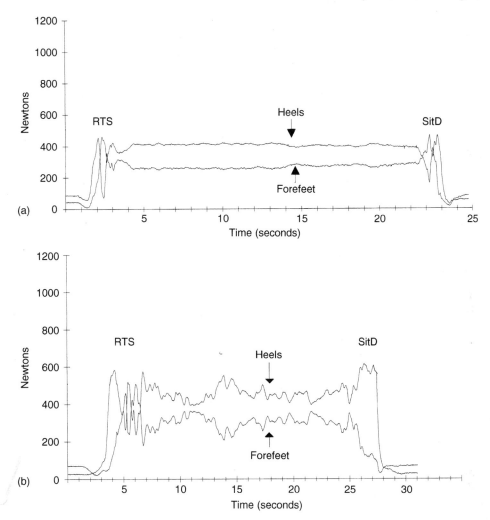

Figure 5.5 Heel and forefoot hand forces during rising to stand and sitting down in a normal subject and a hemiplegic patient (from Durward, 1994)

Propulsive use of the arms has been found to have an influence on ground reaction forces. Alexander *et al.* (1989) found that, when using hands, elderly females exerted peak horizontal forces later (0.78 s) than elderly males (0.046 s) and young females (0.46 s). When the arms were used, elderly males exerted forces (231 N) that were double those exerted by elderly females (115 N), and were also larger than those generated by young males (134 N). The ˙ young females produced forces that were more vertical (63°) than those of either the elderly females (50°) or the young males (46°).

Schultz *et al.* (1992) also identified that hand use, exerting approximately 150 N at an angle of

50° with respect to the horizontal, decreased the required hip and knee moments by up to 35 Nm. It remains uncertain whether the use of arms to rise to stand serves to reduce joint moments or, rather, to provide increased postural stability.

While the effects of body mass, morphology, anthropometric factors and gender may also influence RTS and SitD performance, there have been few studies examining these issues.

EMG activity during rising to stand and sitting down

Detailed knowledge of the muscle activity involved in initiating and completing RTS is incomplete; however, there are emerging trends from EMG studies.

Although the initial movement involves generalized flexion, Coghlin and McFadyen (1994) and Vander Linden *et al.* (1994) have reported that rectus abdominus activity is minimal and inconsistent. By comparison, tibialis anterior is active throughout RTS and peaks prior to the body losing contact with the seat of the chair (Roebroeck *et al.*, 1994). This activity is associated with the flexion of the tibia with regard to a fixed, weight-bearing foot.

Many of the lower limb antagonist muscles, such as gastrocnemius and semitendinosus, demonstrate continuous low level activity throughout the movement, and this may be related to the need to provide stability or eccentric activity to enable joint motion (Roebroeck *et al.*, 1994).

The most consistent feature during RTS is that knee extensor muscle activity peaks when body weight is transferred from the chair to the feet (Kelley *et al.*, 1976; Wheeler *et al.*, 1985; Millington *et al.*, 1992; Roebroeck *et al.*, 1994). Initially, Kelley *et al.* (1976) observed cocontraction in vastus medialis, rectus femoris, biceps femoris and gluteus maximus during RTS, and this feature has since been confirmed by Millington *et al.* (1992) and Roebroeck *et al.* (1994).

Erector spinae activity has been reported to commence at around 20 per cent of the motion (Millington *et al.*, 1992; Vander Linden *et al.*, 1994), and to peak prior to the thighs leaving the seat of the chair (Coghlin and McFadyen, 1994). Upper limb muscle activity has received little attention. Triceps activity has been studied by Wheeler *et al.* (1985) and found to peak prior to the thighs leaving contact with the chair.

A description of muscle activity during SitD has been provided by Munton *et al.* (1984). When standing, the biceps femoris, gastrocnemius and soleus muscles were found to be active. As subjects sat down, rectus femoris and biceps femoris were active throughout the motion and, once descent had commenced, gluteus maximus and tibialis anterior became active.

Effects of age and seat height

Most biomechanical studies have described RTS in a young population, and there is a need to establish age-related baseline data. In a study of healthy men and women aged 65 to 76, Millington *et al.* (1992) used video combined with force platform and EMG data to describe the rising motion in the elderly. Mean joint angles and moments were calculated for the different stages of motion and related to muscle activity. The peak vertical forces, normalized to body mass, were then related to the stage of motion (per cent). The mean peak vertical force occurred at 39.9 ± 3.2 per cent of the movement cycle. This value related to a point following the lifting of thighs from the seat (27 per cent) when hips and knees were extending simultaneously.

Age-related differences in head alignment and trunk to pelvis flexion during RTS have been found by Ikeda *et al.* (1991). An older group (mean age 66.9 years) demonstrated less trunk to pelvis flexion and greater head to ground flexion than a group of young healthy women (mean age 28.9 years). These differences may be related to balance and control factors and, therefore, could have clinical implications. Wheeler *et al.* (1985) have suggested that rising from a standard chair is more difficult for the elderly than the young and that, to complete the task, the elderly prefer to place their feet further back.

Differences in joint range of motion due to chair height have been identified (Rodosky *et al.*, 1989; Schenkman and Riley, 1991).

The relationship between chair height and lower limb joint motion was investigated by Rodosky *et al.* (1989) and Schenkman and Riley (1991), who experimentally manipulated the height of the test chair. A Selspot motion analysis system was used by Rodosky to record joint movement in healthy subjects while rising from four seat heights corresponding to 65, 80, 100, 115 per cent of knee joint height. Under these test conditions, the maximum range of flexion at the hip, knee and ankle significantly decreased $(p < 0.05)$ with increasing chair height.

In the Schenkman and Riley study the same test protocol was adopted, but subjects were paced using a metronome (set at 52 beats per minute) as they rose from a chair with their arms folded. The results of this study showed no significant differences in any of the kinematic parameters measured at each seat height. These conflicting results may be due to differences in testing procedures and, in particular, the adoption of a standardized paced test.

Little is known of the effects of inclined seating, where the supporting surface is angled in either an anterior or posterior alignment. There is some evidence that a high seat with an anterior inclination may reduce lower limb joint moments and therefore make the RTS motion less physically demanding for the elderly (Naqvi and Stobbe, 1992).

Future needs and development issues

It is evident throughout this chapter that, while rising to stand has received some attention, the movement of sitting down has had little systematic examination. While intuitively the RTS movement would seem directly linked to gait and therefore important in functional terms, an ability to complete the SitD movement in a safe and controlled manner is also a basic requirement for normal daily living. There is a need for research that addresses the temporal, kinematic and kinetic features of SitD. Such studies should also consider age, gender and environmental factors affecting performance.

A major difficulty in undertaking comparisons of investigations of either RTS or SitD has been the lack of agreed protocols for defining the phases of movement. Unlike gait, which is characterized by an identifiable pattern of contact between the feet and ground, RTS and SitD are complicated by difficulties in establishing the beginning and end of each movement. The consistent feature of each function is when the body either leaves (*thighs off*) or regains contact (*thighs on*) with a supporting surface. These spatial variables should be a central feature of phase definition for each movement. The problem remains that there is a need to develop simple techniques capable of establishing the beginning and end of each movement.

It is unlikely that protocols such as those proposed by Kralj *et al.* (1990), which are dependent upon expensive instrumentation, technical support and complex data analysis techniques, will be appropriate for a clinical setting. The development of a simple timed test, similar to the 10 m walking test for gait (Wade, 1992) but based on identifiable features of movement, would have considerable value for clinical evaluation purposes.

While many investigations have described components of movement, little work has been done to establish the control mechanisms related to RTS and SitD. Furthermore, there remains a need to identify RTS and SitD profiles for specific groups of patients. An understanding of control factors and the main features of patient groups would influence the development of rehabilitation strategies for individuals with difficulties in completing RTS or SitD.

References

Ada, L. and Westwood, P. (1992). A kinematic analysis of recovery of the ability to stand up following stroke. *Aust. J. Physiother.*, **38(N2)**, 135–42.

Alexander, N., Schultz, A., Warwick, D. and Ashton-Miller, J. (1989). Rising from a chair: performance biomechanics of healthy elderly and young adult subjects. *Symp. Biomech.* (ASME Annual Meeting). ADM – 89, 333–6.

Baer, G. (1991) *A Study of Sitting to Standing in Normal Subjects and Hemiplegic Subjects.* MSc thesis, University of Southampton.

Baer, G. D. and Ashburn, A. M. (1995). Trunk movements in older subjects during sit to stand. *Arch. Phys. Med. Rehabil.*, **76**, 844–9.

Bajd, T., Kralj, A. and Turk, R. (1982). Standing up of a healthy subject and a paraplegic patient. *J. Biomech.*, **15(1)**, 1–10.

Berger, R. A., Schenkman, M. L., Riley, P. O. and Hodge, W. A. (1989a). Advantages of rising from a chair to quantitate human performance. In *Proceedings of 35th Annual Meeting, Orthopaedic Research Society*, February 6–9, Las Vegas, Nevada.

Berger, R. A., Schenkman, M. L., Riley, P. O. and Hodge, W. A. (1989b). The chair model and its advantages for quantifying human functional performance. *Orthop. Trans.*, **13**, 275.

Burdett, R. G., Habasevich, R., Pisciotta, J. and Simon, S. R. (1985). Biomechanical comparison of rising from two types of chairs. *Phys. Ther.*, **65**, 1177–83.

Butler, P. B., Nene, A. V. and Major, R. E. (1991). Biomechanics of transfer from sitting to the standing position in some neuromuscular diseases, *Physiotherapy*, 77, 521–25.

Coghlin, S. S. and McFadyen, B. J. (1994). Transfer strategies used to rise from a chair in normal and low back pain subjects. *Clin. Biomech.*, **9**, 85–92.

Durward, B. R. (1994). *The Biomechanical Assessment of Stroke Patients in Rising to Stand and Sitting Down.* PhD dissertation, University of Strathclyde, Glasgow.

Ellis, M. I., Seedhom, B. B. and Wright, V. (1984). Forces in the knee joint whilst rising from a seated position. *J. Biomed. Eng.*, **6**, 113–20.

Ellis, M. I., Seedhom, B. B., Amis, A. A. *et al.* (1979). Forces in the knee joint whilst rising from normal and motorized chairs. *Eng. Med.*, **8**, 33–40.

Engardt, M. and Olsson, E. (1992). Body weight-bearing while rising and sitting down in patients with stroke. *Scand. J. Rehabil.*, **24**, 67–74.

Finlay, O. E., Bayles, T. E., Rosen, C. and Milling, J. (1983). Effects of chair design, age and cognitive status on mobility. *Age and Ageing*, **12**, 329–35.

Fleckenstein, S. J., Kirby, R. L. and MacLeod, D. A. (1988). Effect of limited knee-flexion range on peak hip moments while transferring from sitting to standing. *J. Biomech.*, **21**, 915–18.

Hanke, T. A., Pai, Y.-C. and Rogers, M.W. (1995). Reliability of measurements of body centre of mass momentum during sit to stand in healthy adults. *Phys. Ther.*, **75(N2)**, 105–18.]

Hughes, M. A., Winer, D. K., Schenkman, M. L. *et al.* (1994). Chair rise strategies in the elderly. *Clin. Biomech.*, **9**, 187–92.

Ikeda, E. R., Shenkman, M. L., Riley, P. O. and Hodge, W. A. (1991). Influence of age on dynamics of rising from a chair. *Phys. Ther.*, **71**, 473–81.

Jeng, S.-F., Schenkman, M., Riley, P. O. and Lin, S.-J. (1990). Reliability of a clinical kinematic assessment of the sit-to-stand movement. *Phys. Ther.*, **70**, 511–20.

Jones, F. P., Gray, F. E., Hanson, J. A. and O'Connell, D. N. (1959). An experimental study of the effect of head balance on patterns of posture and movement in man. *J. Psychol.,* **47,** 247–58.

Jones, F. P., Hanson, J. A., Miller, J. F. and Bossom, J. (1963). Quantitative analysis of abnormal movement: the sit-to-stand pattern. *Am. J. Phys. Med.,* **42,** 208–18.

Kelley, D. L., Dainis, A. and Wood, G. K. (1976). Mechanics and muscular dynamic of rising from a seated position. In *International Series on Biomechanics: Biomechanics V-B* (P. V. Komi, ed.) pp. 127–34. University Park Press.

Kerr, K. M., White, J. A., Mollan, R. A. B. and Baird, H. E. (1991). Rising from a chair: a review of the literature. *Physiotherapy,* **77,** 15–19.

Kerr, K. M., White, J. A., Barr, D. A. and Mollan, R. A. B. (1994a). Analysis of the sit-to-stand movement cycle: development of a measurement system. *Gait and Posture,* **2(3),** 173–181.

Kerr, K. M., White, J. A., Barr, D. A. and Mollan, R. A. B. (1994b). Standardization and definitions of the sit-to-stand movement cycle. *Gait and Posture,* **2(3),** 182–90.

Kralj, A., Jaeger, R. J. and Munih, M. (1990). Analysis of standing up and sitting down in humans: definitions and normative data presentation. *J. Biomech.,* **23,** 1123–38.

Millington, P. J., Myklebust, B. M. and Shambes, G. M. (1992). Biomechanical analysis of the sit-to-stand motion in elderly persons. *Arch. Phys. Med. Rehabil.,* **73,** 609–17.

Munton, J. S., Ellis, M. I. and Wright, V. (1984). Use of electromyography to study leg muscle activity in patients with arthritis and in normal subjects during rising from a chair. *Ann. Rheum. Dis.,* **43,** 63–5.

Munton, J. S., Ellis, M. I., Chamberlain, M. A. and Wright, V. (1981). An investigation into the problems of easy chairs used by the arthritic and the elderly. *Rheum. Rehabil.,* **20,** 164–73.

Naqvi, S. A. and Stobbe, T. J. (1992). Influence of chair features on ease of egress. *J. Hum. Move. Stud.,* **23,** 151–64.

Nuzik, S., Lamb, R., VanSant, A and Hirt, S. (1986). Sit-to-stand movement patterns, a kinematic study. *Phys. Ther.,* **66,** 1708–13.

Pai, Y.-C. and Rogers, M. W. (1990). Control of body mass transfer as a function of speed of ascent in sit-to-stand. *Med. Sci. Sports Exer.,* **22,** 378–84.

Pai, Y.-C. and Rogers, M. W. (1991a). Segmental contributions to total body momentum in sit-to-stand. *Med. Sci. Sports Exer.,* **23,** 225–30.

Pai, Y.-C. and Rogers, M. W. (1991b). Speed variation and resultant joint torques during sit-to-stand. *Arch. Phys. Med. Rehabil.,* **72,** 881–5.

Riley, P. O., Schenkman, M. L., Mann, R. W. and Hodge, W. A. (1991). Mechanisms of a constrained chair rise. *J. Biomech.,* **24,** 77–85.

Rodosky, M. W., Andriacchi, T. P. and Andersson, G. B. J. (1989). The influence of chair height on lower limb mechanics during rising. *J. Orthop. Res.,* **7,** 266–71.

Roebroeck, M. E., Doorenbosch, C. A. M., Harlaar, J. *et al.* (1994). Biomechanics and muscular activity during sit to stand transfer. *Clin. Biomech.,* **9,** 235–44.

Roorda, L. D., Roebroeck, M. E., Lankhorst, G. J. *et al.* (1996). Measuring functional limitations in rising and sitting down: development of a questionnaire. *Arch. Phys. Med. Rehabil.,* **77(7),** 663–9.

Sackley, C. M. and Lincoln, N. B. (1991). Weight distribution and postural sway in healthy adults. *Clin. Rehabil.,* **5,** 181–6.

Schenkman, M. L. and Riley, P. O. (1991). Influence of chair height on the dynamics of rising from sit to stand. *Phys. Ther.,* **71(S55)** (suppl.).

Schenkman, M. L., Berger, R. A., Riley, P. O. *et al.* (1990). Whole-body movements during rising to standing from sitting. *Phys. Ther.,* **70,** 638–51.

Schultz, A. B., Alexander, N. B. and Ashton-Miller, J. A. (1992). Biomechanical analysis of rising from a chair. *J. Biomech.,* **25,** 1383–91.

Seedhom, B. B. and Terayama, K. (1976). Knee forces during the activity of getting out of a chair with and without the aid of arms. *Biomed. Eng.,* August, 278–82.

Shepherd, R. B. and Koh, H. P. (1996). Some biomechanical consequences of varying foot placement in sit to stand in young women. *Scand. J. Rehabil. Med.,* **28,** 79–88.

Stevens, C., Bojsen-Moller, F. and Soames, R. W. (1989). The influence of initial posture on the sit-to-stand movement. *Eur. J. Appl. Physiol.,* **58,** 687–92.

Vander Linden, D. W., Brunt, D. and McCulloch, M. U. (1994). Variant and invariant characteristics of the sit to stand task in healthy elderly adults. *Arch. Phys. Med. Rehabil.,* **75,** 653–60.

VanSant, A. F. (1990). Life-span development in functional tasks. *Phys. Ther.,* **70(12),** 788–98.

Wade, D. T. (1992). *Measurement in Neurological Rehabilitation.* Oxford University Press.

Wheeler, J., Woodward, C., Ucovich, R. L. *et al.* (1985). Rising from a chair, influence of age and chair design. *Phys. Ther.,* **65,** 22–6.

Wretenberg, P., Lindberg, F. and Arborelius, U. P. (1993). Effect of arm rests and different ways of using them on hip and knee load during rising. *Clin. Biomech.,* **8,** 95–101.

Yoshida, K., Iwakura, H. and Inoue, F. (1983). Motion analysis in the movements of standing up from and sitting down on a chair. *Scand. J. Rehabil. Med.,* **15,** 133–40.

6 Walking

J. C. Wall

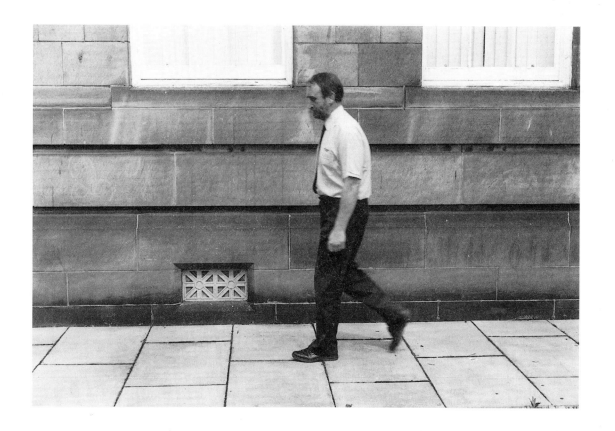

Introduction

Definition and basic description

Walking is defined as a form of bipedal progression in which the repetitive movements of the lower limbs include periods of double support, when both feet are in contact with the ground, followed by periods when only one foot is supporting the body (single support) while the other is being moved above the ground (swing). A diagram representing the periods of time that the feet are in contact with the ground during walking is shown in Figure 6.1.

The right foot makes contact with the ground at right heel contact (RHC) while the left foot is still on the ground, and, as indicated in the diagram, this is a period of double support. When the left foot leaves the ground at left toe off (LTO), the right foot alone maintains contact during a period of single support. This sequence of double support followed by single support repeats when the left foot again makes contact with the ground at left heel contact (LHC). During each of the single support phases, the opposite limb is in its swing phase; however, unlike running, there is no time when both feet are off the ground at the same time (see Chapter 8).

Importance

Walking is of major importance when one considers activities of daily living. Obviously it is central to human locomotion, but the ability to stand and move on two feet is also a prerequisite for many other tasks. If one considers the limitations imposed by a wheelchair, it is easier to understand just how important the ability to ambulate independently is for everyday tasks, whether for independent living, occupation or recreation. Thus it is hardly surprising that physiotherapists and other health care professionals involved in the rehabilitation of patients with locomotor disabilities focus so much of their attention on attaining independent ambulation.

The search for objectivity – brief history

From a clinical standpoint, it is essential that the therapist be able to assess a patient's ability to walk in order to determine which treatments would be appropriate and also to measure if those treatments are working. Traditionally this assessment has been subjective in nature, and perhaps

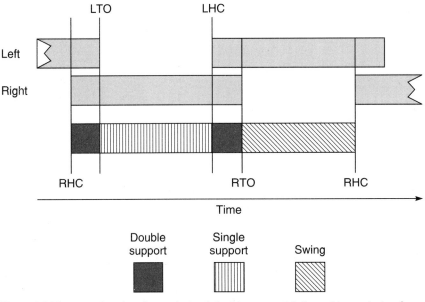

Figure 6.1 Diagram showing the periods of double support followed by periods of single support when the opposite limb is in swing. The diagram shows that, unlike running, there is no period when both feet are not in contact with the ground at the same time

the following quote sums up the most commonly cited reasons for this:

The method of recording gait used by the author is essentially a subjective one, inasmuch as it does not use instrumentation. Its lack of true objectivity is by far outweighed by its practical aspects; no time-consuming preparations are needed, very little space is required, and it is easy to administer. The experienced gait observer can evaluate and record the gait without the patient's knowing that he is being 'tested', which has definite advantages.

(Brunnstrom, 1970)

These points are well taken and it may well be more pragmatic to assess gait by eye, but the information so obtained has some major drawbacks. First and foremost is that the quality of the assessment will vary widely and will be dependent upon the experience of the clinician (Goodkin and Diller, 1973). Once the clinician has observed the gait, observations must then be recorded, usually in the form of a summary statement placed in the patient's notes. Here again there are difficulties for the clinician, because there is no standard terminology (Wall *et al.*, 1987). Thus, what may be a clear description to therapists making the notes may be less clear to others – or even to themselves at some later date. However, the greatest problem with visual assessment of gait is that it is of questionable validity and reliability (Saleh and Murdoch, 1985; Krebs *et al.*, 1985; Eastlack *et al.*, 1991; Patla *et al.*, 1987). To overcome these problems, there have been a number of checklists and rating scales developed which focus the attention of the therapist on deviations. These can range from the one developed at Roncho Los Amigos Hospital in Downey, California (Norkin, 1994), which can be used for any condition, to those developed for specific diagnoses. Perhaps the best use of these rating scales is for screening patients. Good examples are the *Duke Mobility Skills Profile* and the *Dynamic Gait Index*, which are used to screen elderly patients at risk of falling (Shumway-Cook and Woollacott, 1995). However, because the grading of these and other similar instruments is so coarse (often on a three-, four- or five-point scale), small but significant changes in gait may be missed. This is particularly troublesome when dealing with conditions in which change occurs slowly, most notably in patients with neurological conditions such as stroke. In an era of managed care where many insurance companies will only reimburse for treatment while the patient is improving, it is critical that therapists have at their disposal objective measurements which are sensitive to small changes.

Objective analysis of human locomotion is a rapidly developing field of endeavour, which has seen dramatic advances since it became possible to record and replay moving images. Initially this was achieved by the capture of rapidly sequenced still photographic images using multiple cameras, a technique developed by Eadweard Muybridge. He used this successfully to show that there were times in the gait cycle that all four limbs of a trotting horse were off the ground simultaneously (Muybridge, 1979). Cinephotography lead to techniques for determining the movements of body segments from frame to frame, and, knowing the frame rate, determining the velocities and accelerations of these movements. The electronic age brought us videography and the subsequent ability to digitize these analogue images and analyse them by means of computers (Winter *et al.*, 1972; Jarret *et al.*, 1976). With the use of multiple cameras it is possible to determine movements in three dimensions. Along with the kinematic information produced by this process, computers are also used to obtain kinetic data from force platforms and electromyographic information from electrodes.

A child will normally start to walk at around 12 months of age and, through musculoskeletal and neural development and much practice, will develop a mature walking pattern (Sutherland *et al.*, 1988). At the other end of the age spectrum one sees declines in performance (O'Brien *et al.*, 1983; Wall *et al.*, 1991; Oberg *et al.*, 1993, 1994). From a clinical standpoint it is important to understand these changes in walking across the life span, particularly the declines with increasing age, since it may be possible to intervene and prevent or slow these through appropriate exercise and lifestyle changes.

Gait assessment

Walking speed

Measurements of how the position of the body or body segments change with time are referred to as the temporal and spatial parameters. Perhaps the most fundamental of these measures is how much time it takes for a person to walk a set distance, i.e. walking speed. From a clinical standpoint this is perhaps the single most important objective measure of functional mobility. It is clearly a global indicator of ability, or, more importantly, disability, since it is the one measure that is affected in virtually all patients with gait abnormalities. In general, the more severe the impairment the slower the patient will walk. The other reason that this measurement is so important is that almost all other gait measurements are speed dependent (Andriacchi *et al.*, 1977) – for example, as speed increases the hip range of motion increases. Therefore, when dealing with patients that are walking very slowly because of some impairment, it is important to be able to separate what has changed in the gait pattern simply as a result of the reduced speed from changes caused by the impairment. For healthy young adults walking at their self-selected medium speed, walking speed is typically about $1.4 \, \text{ms}^{-1}$. This equates to a little more than 3 mph or 5 kph.

Fortunately, the measurement of this parameter is extremely simple. All that is required is for a known distance to be marked off and a stopwatch to time how long it takes a subject to walk that distance. The other clinically important feature of this measurement is that it can easily be used to determine how patients function under different environmental conditions, such as walking over a variety of surfaces or under different lighting conditions.

During the gait cycle there are changes in the instantaneous velocity of the body; it speeds up and slows down. The peak velocities and accelerations occur when the foot is pushing off against the ground in order to swing the leg through. Ganguli and Mukherjee (1973) used a method that involved string, attached to the subject at the level of the centre of mass, passing around a pulley on a DC generator. As the subject walked the generator rotated, producing a voltage proportional to the rate of rotation and reflecting the instantaneous velocity. Knowing how velocity changes with time allows for the calculation of instantaneous accelerations. Another way of determining this

parameter is with the use of accelerometers, some of which are triaxial, allowing for measurement in three planes (Duncan *et al.*, 1992).

Spatial gait parameters

The spatial parameters refer most often to the relative positions of the feet when walking, although they could also include other body segments. The basic measurements that are made to indicate the relative positions of the feet when walking are shown in Figure 6.2.

The distance from the point of heel contact to the next heel contact by the same foot is termed stride length. Each stride is made up of two steps. By definition, left step length is the distance that the left foot is placed in front of the right, as shown in Figure 6.2. Similarly, the distance that the right foot is placed in front of the left is called right step length. Note that measures of step and stride lengths are made along the line of progression, i.e. in the direction that the subject is walking. The separation of the feet at right angles to the line of progression is a measure of step width. In all of these spatial parameters it is important to ensure that the same anatomical landmarks are used on both feet; most commonly this is the centre of the heel. The alignment of the foot with reference to the line of progression defines the step angle, as shown in Figure 6.2 for the second right footfall. Here, the right foot is shown as toeing out; the left foot, however, is parallel with the line of progression and therefore has a step angle of zero.

For healthy young adults walking at their self-selected medium speed, stride length is about 1.4 m with a step length of 0.7 m.

These measurements can be determined from a record of where the feet were placed when walking. This record could be from painted feet walking across blank newsprint, or the attachment of markers to the heels (Cerny, 1983). Notice that

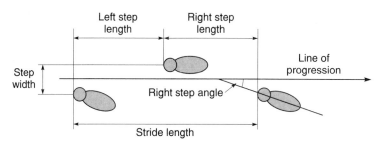

Figure 6.2 Diagram showing the spatial parameters of gait that define the relative positions of the feet during a stride

in order to measure step angle there must be two marks for each foot, one on the heel and the other on the forefoot.

Temporal gait parameters

Stride and steps can also be timed. The interval between right heel contact (RHC) and the next RHC is stride time. From the instant of right heel contact to that of left heel contact (LHC) is left step time. Right step time is the interval between LHC and the next RHC, as shown in Figure 6.3. A measure commonly used to reflect step time is cadence, which is a measure of frequency and is most often expressed in terms of the number of steps taken per minute (Wall and Ashburn, 1979). For healthy young adults walking at their self-selected walking speed a stride lasts approximately 1 s and the steps are of equal duration. Each step therefore lasts 0.5 s, giving a cadence of 120 steps per minute.

A stride includes two major phases; stance and swing, as shown in Figure 6.3. The stance phase for a given foot is when that foot is in contact with the ground; thus right stance starts at RHC and terminates when the foot breaks contact with the ground at right toe off (RTO). When the foot leaves the ground the swing phase commences. Right swing phase starts at RTO and ends when the foot again makes contact with the ground at the next RHC. For healthy young adults walking at their self-selected medium walking speed, stance lasts for 60 per cent of the gait cycle with swing accounting for the other 40 per cent.

The stance phase can be further subdivided into three phases; (a), (b) and (c). During phases (a) and (c) both feet are in contact at the same time, and during phase (b) only one foot is in contact. As indicated in Figure 6.3, when the right foot makes contact at RHC the left foot is still on the ground. This then is a double support phase, which terminates when the left foot breaks contact at left toe off (LTO). The name given to this phase is right braking double support (RBDS). As we shall see later, during this time the right foot is plantar flexing and the right knee is flexing to help cushion the impact of the limb with the ground when contact is made. This has been referred to as the braking mechanism, hence explaining the terminology used to name this phase of the gait cycle (Wall *et al.*, 1987). When the left foot leaves the ground at LTO, the right foot alone is in contact with the ground in what is called appropriately right single support (RSS). This phase ends at LHC, an event that also starts a second double support phase, right thrusting double support (RTDS). This is the phase during which the right foot is pushing off and accelerating the limb into swing. RTDS terminates when the swing phase starts at RTO. Consider now what is happening to the left foot during these phases. In RBDS, as indicated by (a) in Figure 6.3, the left foot is about to push off into the swing phase and this is therefore left thrusting double support (LTDS). When the left foot is in swing, the right is in single support, as indicated by (b). When the right foot is about to push off in RTDS, shown as (c), the braking mechanism is occurring on the left in LBDS. When the right foot is in swing, the left foot is in single support (LSS). Notice that all of the temporal phases are defined with reference to make and break of foot floor contact. In normal walking these are heel contacts and toe offs and, because they define the phases, they have been referred to as the 'key events' of the gait cycle

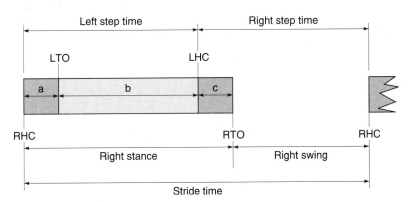

Figure 6.3 Diagram showing the temporal phases of gait cycle and the key events of heel contact and toe off that define them

(Wall and Brunt, 1996). Each of the double support phases accounts for 10 per cent of the gait cycle for healthy young adults walking at their self-selected medium walking speed. Since single support and contralateral swing are defined by the same key events, each of these phases lasts for 40 per cent of stride time. However, it is critical to remember that the duration of these phases changes with walking speed, and that the figures quoted are approximately those associated with a medium speed walk.

Step and stride times can readily be measured with a stopwatch. However, the phases of the gait cycle are too short to be measured in this way in real time. To overcome this difficulty a number of techniques have been developed based on the use of stop action and slow motion video. Wall (1991) used a time code generator to mark each field of video. The fields are a known interval apart so, by determining from the code how many fields separated the key events shown in Figure 6.3, the duration of the phases could be determined. The validity and reliability of this technique were determined in a later study (Wall and Crosbie, 1996). Using slow motion video and a multi-memory stopwatch, Wall and Scarbrough (1997) obtained the duration of the phases as percentages of stride time. Using the same principles, Wall and Crosbie (1997) showed how a computer could be used in exactly the same way as the multimemory stopwatch to determine the duration of the temporal phases. The obvious advantage of this approach is that the computer can then do all the calculations and plot the graphs of the results, saving a great deal of time and reducing potential errors. It is also possible to use footswitches or force plates to determine the times that the feet are in contact with the ground (Wall and Crosbie, 1996). Again, if these are interfaced with a computer, the results can be obtained automatically.

A number of systems have been developed to provide simultaneous measurement of the temporal and spatial parameters, such as resistive grid walkways (Wall *et al.*, 1976; Gifford and Hughes, 1983; Crouse *et al.*, 1987). Law and Minns (1989) describe a novel low-cost method in which two punched tapes pass through a reading head assembly and are attached to the subjects' heels. As the subjects walk, the heads determine the rate and distance that the tapes move and hence the temporal and spatial parameters can be determined. A relatively recent introduction into the gait analysis field has been the Gait Trak system developed by CIR Systems Inc. (CIR Systems Inc.,

Clinton NJ 07012). This is a mat that can be rolled out on a flat surface, and embedded in the mat are small pressure-sensitive switches that determine the position of the feet and the time that they are in contact with the ground. Again a computer is used to collect, analyse, print and store the data. However, to date no studies have been published based on the use of this system.

Angular displacements

Linear motion of the body from point A to point B is achieved primarily through angular displacements of the joints of the lower limbs. These joints can and do move in all planes during walking, but the major excursions are in the sagittal plane. Graphs showing angular movements of the joints are commonly referred to as goniograms. The sagittal plane motions of the hip, knee and ankle are shown in Figure 6.4.

The hip is flexed when contact is made with the ground, and it extends through neutral at mid stance to reach maximum extension at about 50 per cent of the gait cycle when contralateral heel contact occurs. From this point, through swing phase, the hip flexes. Using vertical as the reference, the hip moves from 25° of flexion to 20° of extension. Again, caution must be emphasized when quoting these figures since the excursion of the hip will change with walking speed.

The knee is close to neutral (the anatomical position) when heel contact is made, at which time it flexes about 20° through the braking double support phase, as shown in Figure 6.4. During single support the knee extends, coming close to neutral at approximately 40 per cent of the gait cycle, after which it again flexes rapidly reaching a maximum of approximately 65° of flexion at mid swing. This action, along with hip flexion and ankle dorsiflexion, effectively shortens the limb to allow for foot clearance during swing phase. Once past mid swing, the knee rapidly extends in preparation for heel contact.

As can be seen from the ankle goniogram shown in Figure 6.4, when the heel makes contact with the ground, the ankle is close to neutral. Once contact is made, the ankle plantarflexes as the foot is lowered to the ground to support body weight. This rotation is about the heel and has been referred to as first or heel rocker (Perry, 1992). This motion, of about 7°, occurs in the braking double support phase. As the tibia rotates about the ankle joint during the second or ankle rocker the ankle is dorsiflexing, and continues to do so till about the time of contralateral heel contact at 50 per cent of

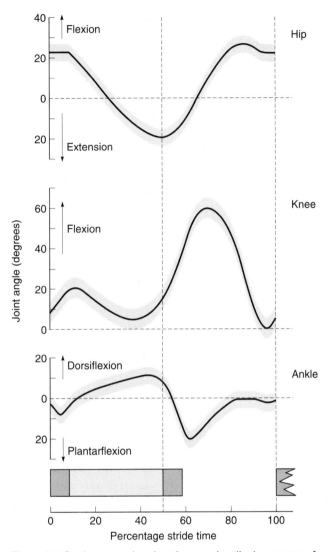

Figure 6.4 Goniograms showing the angular displacements of the hip, knee and ankle in the sagittal plane

the gait cycle, when it reaches about 10°. During this time the heel leaves the ground and rotation is about the metatarsal heads. This rotation is called third or forefoot rocker. During thrusting double support, the ankle rapidly plantarflexes, reaching a maximum of 20° as the toe breaks contact with the ground. The ankle then dorsiflexes in order to clear the ground at mid swing.

If these angular displacements are recorded with respect to time then it is possible to determine angular velocities and accelerations. These measurements are important considerations when assessing or treating a patient with a joint problem using an isokinetic dynamometer. Not only should

the therapist be aware of the range that a joint must move through for normal walking, but the speed at which it moves must also be considered.

In terms of measurement of joint angles there are really only two alternatives: electrogoniometers and optoelectronic systems. Originally, electrogoniometers were constructed using a potentiometer at the centre of two arms that were attached to the body segments on either side of the joint being measured (Karpovich *et al.*, 1960). These simple devices had one fixed centre of rotation, which somewhat limited their use for measurement of joints with centres that changed through the range of motion. Later electrogoniometers were made that incorporated linkage systems designed to overcome this limitation (Lamoreux, 1971). Further developments had electrogoniometers with three potentiometers arranged in orthogonal planes to record movements in those planes (Hannah and Cooper, 1980; Pratt, 1991). Flexible electrogoniometers, which are far less bulky and restrictive to the subject, have also been used to measure joint angular displacements (Rowe and Nicol, 1991). However, all electrogoniometers still have a major drawback in that they must be mounted on the subject, often with wires from the potentiometers attached to the recording device.

The most widely accepted means of measuring joint displacements are optoelectronic systems, which track markers placed on joints or body segments (Winter *et al.*, 1972; Jarret *et al.*, 1976). There are several of these systems commercially available that will measure movements in two or three dimensions, depending on the number of cameras used. From a clinical standpoint, their major drawbacks are cost and complexity. They also require that markers be attached to the subject, which may interfere with the subject's walking pattern.

Kinetics

Kinetics is the study of the forces causing movement, which may be internal or external. The internal forces can be generated by the contractile elements (muscle) or in non-contractile tissue (such as ligaments and joint capsules). These forces can be positive when they produce movement, or negative when movement is resisted. The external forces that must be considered are gravity and the ground reaction forces that are generated when the foot is in contact with the walking surface. In terms of measurement of kinetic parameters, gait analysts focus on ground reaction forces. It is also possible, through electromyography (EMG), to determine when in the gait cycle a given muscle or muscle group is active, and the intensity of that activity. However, EMG measurements do not allow determination of the force being generated as a result of the muscle activity. Since muscles are generating forces, they are here considered under kinetics.

Muscle activity during gait

Perry (1992) provides a very detailed description of muscle activity through the gait cycle. Only a very brief description of this activity is herein provided. Electromyography (EMG) patterns for the major muscle groups that move the joints of the lower limbs in the sagittal plane are shown in Figure 6.5.

The hip extensors, primarily gluteus maximus, are most active just after heel contact. Although, as can be seen from Figure 6.4, the hip is extending during this time, the role of this muscle group is to control the forward momentum of the trunk at this time. The activity just prior to heel contact is probably slowing the swinging limb. Activity of the hip flexors, particularly iliopsoas, commences during the thrusting double support phase and coincides with the initial flexion of the hip. The hamstrings, which flex the knee, are active towards the end of the swing phase and, like gluteus maximus, are working to slow the swing limb. The quadriceps are most active just after heel contact when the knee is flexing. This activity is therefore to control rather than cause this movement. This controlled knee flexion is part of the braking mechanism referred to earlier. The plantarflexors, soleus and gastrocnemius, work during the initial part of the single support phase to control the dorsiflexion that is occurring as a result of momentum causing the tibia to rotate about the ankle joint during second rocker. Peak activity of this group is seen towards the end of the single support phase when the ankle is plantarflexing. The second part of the braking mechanism that was mentioned earlier was the controlled lowering of the foot to the ground following heel contact. It was seen in Figure 6.4 that plantarflexion does occur in this phase. Figure 6.5 also indicates that this coincides with the maximum activity of the dorsiflexor group, primarily tibialis anterior. Again this muscle is actively controlling this movement in much the same way as gluteus maximus is controlling trunk flexion and the quadriceps control knee flexion.

For a detailed treatise on electromyography, consider the texts *Muscles Alive: Their Functions Revealed by Electromyography* (Basmajian, 1978) or *Gait Analysis: Normal and Pathological Function* by Perry (1992). The electrical activity of the muscle is detected by means of electrodes, either surface mounted or indwelling. These signals are amplified and input to a computer for processing and analysis. Muscles are rarely completely inactive, and therefore one has to decide upon a threshold signal that indicates when the muscle is 'active'. Since it is not possible to determine with any accuracy what force the muscle is generating during this activity, the signal is usually expressed

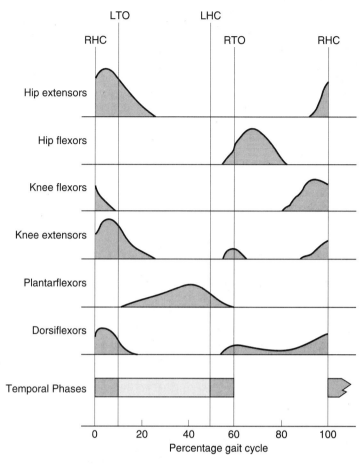

Figure 6.5 Graphs showing the activity of the major muscle groups of the lower extremity during the gait cycle

as a percentage of that generated when the subject performs a maximal isometric contraction of that muscle.

Ground reaction forces

When quietly standing, the body's mass, accelerated by gravity, exerts a force on the floor and, because the body is not moving, it must be in a state of equilibrium. The force due to bodyweight must therefore be opposed by an equal and opposite force from the floor, and this is termed the ground reaction force. Components of this force act in the horizontal plane, both anterior/posterior and medial/lateral, as well as in the vertical direction. All three components are essential for walking, and these are shown in Figure 6.6.

In terms of magnitude, the vertical component is by far the greatest. As can be seen from Figure 6.6, once contact has been made with the floor

the vertical component rapidly rises to approximately 125 per cent bodyweight. Through mid stance the vertical component drops to around 75 per cent bodyweight before again exceeding bodyweight during the thrusting double support phase just prior to swing. The horizontal component in the anterior/posterior direction acts for a very brief period anteriorly on the foot at heel contact. This is a result of the foot moving backwards at this instant. However, this force very rapidly becomes directed posteriorly on the foot as the foot starts to accept weight, and reaches a maximum value of approximately 25 per cent bodyweight. The magnitude of the force decreases till it is zero at about mid stance, at which point the force starts to act anteriorly on the foot and reaches a maximum of about 25 per cent of bodyweight during thrusting double support. Apart from a very brief period following

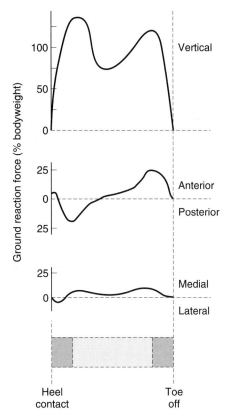

Figure 6.6 Graphs showing the ground reaction forces in the vertical, anterior/posterior and medial/lateral directions during the stance phase of the gait cycle

heel contact, the horizontal force acts medially and has peaks of less than 10 per cent bodyweight during the two double support phases of the gait cycle. Again, the values given for the magnitudes of these forces are only approximate and will change with speed of walking.

The primary method of collecting data on ground reaction forces is with the use of force platforms. Notice that these platforms provide information on the single force vector between the foot and the ground during stance, but do not provide information relative to where under the foot the force is acting. This may be of interest, for example, to the clinician treating a patient with ulceration resulting from peripheral vascular disease. Determination of the distribution of forces under the foot requires that there be multiple force transducers beneath the plantar surface. This can be done with special insoles (Wu and Chiang, 1996) or a multisensor platform (Kernozek and

LaMott (1995). Several of these are commercially available, with software available for data collection and analysis. As with the optoelectronic systems for measuring kinematics, the main drawbacks of these systems for clinical use are cost and complexity.

Examples of clinical gait measurements

It has been stated earlier that perhaps the most important single measure of gait is walking speed. This measurement was used by Martin and Cameron (1996) to evaluate patients in a geriatric day hospital. A significant reduction in walking speed and the range of walking speeds could be a clinically important method of determining patients with balance problems who may be at potential risk of falling (Wall et al., 1991). Not all clinical studies use the term walking speed but, rather, look at the measurement that was actually made. Thus results are quoted as either the time taken to walk a given distance or the distance covered in a given time. For example, Collin et al. (1992) measured the time taken to walk 10 m as a functional outcome in amputees. The two-minute timed walking test was used by Stewart et al. (1990) as an index of mobility in the rehabilitation of elderly patients. To make comparisons simpler, both across studies and within the clinical setting, it would be preferable also to quote the results of these tests as walking speeds. Measurements of the instantaneous velocity have been used to demonstrate asymmetries in amputees (Ganguli and Mukherjee, 1973).

The use of subjective rating scales can be useful clinically, although they do suffer from lack of sensitivity. For this reason, a growing number of studies are using these in conjunction with a measure of walking speed in an attempt to show more subtle changes. Functional ambulation categories, which rate a subject's ability to walk on a five-point scale, were used with walking speed to assess patients in a geriatric day hospital (Martin and Cameron, 1996). The study demonstrated how both measures could be used to show whether or not patients improved or deteriorated. Since these measurements were found to be simple to obtain, it was suggested that they were suitable for routine clinical use. Shumway-Cook et al. (1997) included the Dynamic Gait Index and the Three-Minute Walk Test along with other measures of balance to show how a multidimensional exercise programme can improve balance and mobility and reduce the risk of falls in the elderly.

The temporal and distance parameters, which have been labelled the 'vital signs' of walking (Wall and Brunt, 1996), have been used in many clinical studies. Murray and co-workers (1975) included these measures in a study designed to show how patients recover from total hip arthroplasty over a two-year period. The techniques used were precursors of those used today, and are probably no longer relevant since the data can now be collected in more clinically acceptable ways. However, this study is an excellent example of the use of objective gait measurement to assess outcome. In the neurological field these same measures, collected from a resistive grid walkway, were used to show how they could be used as outcome measures for clinicians treating stroke patients (Wall and Ashburn, 1979).

The temporal phases have been shown to be useful measures of asymmetry in amputees and in stroke (Cheung *et al*., 1983; Wall and Turnbull, 1986). This is important clinically since, in many cases, the therapy is directed at reducing these asymmetries. For example, the relatively static exercises designed to improve weight-bearing ability on the hemiplegic lower limb are aimed at more symmetrical weight bearing in functional activities such as walking. The other clinical use of measurements of the temporal phases is to help identify where in the gait cycle an abnormality exists. Such information can assist the clinician in selecting treatment protocols that target the specific problem. It has been found, for example, that elderly subjects who have either fallen or have a fear of falling spend longer in the double support phases and less in single support, and that they also take shorter steps than elderly people without these criteria (Wall *et al*., 1991). With this information the clinician can direct exercises that improve single support and encourage increased step lengths, which will also lead to an increased walking speed. Equally important is that these objective measurements can then be used to monitor outcomes of such treatment protocols.

For physiotherapists, joint range of motion is an important measurement that is most often done in a static position. When it comes to looking at these movements during functional tasks such as walking, the therapist has had to rely on subjective assessment. Systems that remove this subjectivity and provide objective data on joint movements are finding more widespread clinical application, and these angular measures are extremely useful for assessment and for directing treatment. An example might be a patient who has sufficient active range of knee movement when assessed while standing but through measurements of angular kinematics is revealed to be unable to use that range in a dynamic function such as walking. If these measurements indicate that this is due to an inability to move the joint at sufficient speed, then this information will assist the clinician with treatment decision-making. These measurements may be used to assess outcome. For example, angular kinematics were measured with a flexible goniometer by Rowe and Nicol (1991) in a study of patients following total hip replacement. Assistive devices are often prescribed by therapists who should be aware that they dramatically alter joint kinematics (Crosbie, 1993a). Knowing the joint ranges of movement required to use such devices can help the therapist prepare patients for the new mode of locomotion that will be expected of them.

Commonly, therapists are charged with the task of strengthening muscles to allow a patient to be able to complete a functional task more independently. Therefore, clinically it is important to know the phasic muscle activities through the task and how these may change in gait abnormalities. For example, it has been shown in static tests that muscle activity, as determined by surface EMG, may show changes in multiple sclerosis patients before there is significant evidence of neural motor dysfunction (Jones *et al*., 1994). This type of information could be particularly useful to the clinician in deciding what anticipated effect this might have on gait, knowing the role and the phase in the gait cycle that the particular muscle group is active. When considering strength for walking, one tends to think primarily of the musculature of the lower extremities; however, when using an assistive device, the activity of the musculature around the shoulder must also be considered since these muscles are fundamental to gait (Crosbie, 1993b). Since the kinematics and EMG activities when using an assistive device are not the same as in walking without devices, it is not surprising to hear that the kinetics also change (Winter *et al*., 1993).

Another clinically important use of objective gait measurement is to improve our understanding of the course of a pathology. An excellent example of this can be seen in a pair of review articles that looked at what the literature has to say about hemiparetic gait following stroke (Olney and Richards, 1996; Richards and Olney, 1996). These articles cover the whole gamut of objective gait measurements, including such kinetic measures as joint moments and powers and mechanical energy. Such comprehensive gait analyses are now being routinely done in clinical settings, thanks in large part to the commercially available systems that allow for the integrated collection of data from multiple sources including videocameras, EMG electrodes and force platforms. Software packages are also readily available to handle all these data and produce a report for the clinician. Perhaps the area that is receiving the greatest attention in terms of the growth of clinical gait laboratories is that of paediatrics, particularly cerebral palsy. The basic reason for this is the growing need to understand exactly what muscle patterns the patient is using before making decisions about which surgeries should be performed. It is not surprising, therefore, that there are many comprehensive clinical studies and publications dealing with gait in this condition (Sutherland, 1984; Gage, 1991; Ounpuu *et al.*, 1996).

As the power of technology increases, there will be better and faster methods of collecting objective measurements of gait. Eventually such measurements will become part of the routine clinical assessment process in much the same way as dynamometry is now used to measure muscle strength.

References

Andriacchi, T. P., Ogle, J. A. and Galante, J. O. (1977). Walking speed as a basis for normal and abnormal gait measurements. *J. Biomech.*, **10**, 261–8.

Basmajian, J. V. (1978). *Muscles Alive: Their Functions Revealed by Electromyography.* Williams & Wilkins.

Brunnstrom, S. (1970). *Movement Therapy in Hemiplegia: A Neurophysiological Approach.* Harper Row.

Cerny, K. (1983). A clinical method of quantitative gait analysis. *Phys. Ther.*, 1125–6.

Cheung, C., Wall, J. C. and Zelin, S. (1983). A microcomputer based system for measuring the temporal phases of amputee gait. *Prosth. Orthot. Int.*, **7**, 131–40.

Collin, C., Wade, D. T. and Cochrane, G. M. (1992). Functional outcome of lower limb amputees with peripheral vascular disease. *Clin. Rehabil.*, **6**, 13–21.

Crosbie, J. (1993a). Kinematics of walking frame ambulation. *Clin. Biomech.*, **8**, 31–6.

Crosbie, J. (1993b). Muscle activation patterns in aided gait. *Clin. Rehabil.*, **7**, 229–38.

Crouse, J. G., Wall, J. C. and Marble, A. E. (1987). Measurement of the temporal and spatial parameters of gait using a microcomputer based system. *J. Biomed. Eng.*, **9**, 64–8.

Duncan, G., Currie, G. D., Evans, A. L. and Gilchrist, W. (1992). Gait analysis: a step in the right direction. *Clin. Rehabil.*, **6**, 111–16.

Eastlack, M. E., Arvidson, J., Snyder-Mackler, L. *et al.* (1991). Inter-rater reliability of videotaped observational gait-analysis assessments. *Phys. Ther.*, **71**, 465–71.

Gage, J. R. (1991). *Gait Analysis in Cerebral Palsy.* MacKeith Press.

Ganguli, S. and Mukherjee, P. (1973). A gait recording technique suitable for clinical use. *Biomed. Eng.*, **8**, 60–63.

Gifford, G. and Hughes, J. (1983). A gait analysis system in clinical practice. *J. Biomed. Eng.* **5**, 297–301.

Goodkin, R. and Diller, L. (1973). Reliability among physical therapists in diagnosis and treatment of gait deviations in hemiplegics. *Perceptual and Motor Skills*, **37**, 727–34.

Hannah, R. E. and Cooper, D. (1980). Electrogoniometry and symmetry: an approach to clinical gait analysis. *Proc. Int. Conf. Rehabil. Eng., Toronto*, 271–73.

Jarret, M. O., Andrews, B. J. and Paul, J. P. (1976). A television/computer system for the analysis of human locomotion. In *Applications of Electronics in Medicine*, pp. 357–70. The Institute of Electronic and Radio Engineers.

Jones, R., Rees, D. P. and Campbell, M. J. (1994). Tibialis anterior surface EMG parameters change before force output in multiple sclerosis patients. *Clin. Rehabil.*, **8**, 100–106.

Karpovich, P. V., Harden, E. L. and Asa, M. M. (1960). Electrogoniometric study of joints. *U.S. Armed Forces Med. J.*, **11**, 424–50.

Kernozek, T. W. and LaMott, E. E. (1995). Comparisons of plantar pressures between the elderly and young adults. *Gait and Posture*, **3**, 143–8.

Krebs, D. E., Edelstein, J. E. and Fishman, S. (1985). Reliability of observational gait analysis. *Phys. Ther.*, **65**, 1027–33.

Lamoreux, L. W. (1971). Kinematic measurements in the study of human walking. *Bull. Prosth. Res.*, **10–15**, 3–84.

Law, H. T. and Minns, R. A. (1989). Measurement of the spatial and temporal parameters of gait. *Physiotherapy*, **75**, 81–84.

Martin, B. J. and Cameron, M. (1996). Evaluation of walking speed and functional ambulation categories in geriatric day hospital patients. *Clin. Rehabil.*, **10**, 44–6.

Murray, M. P., Brewer, B. J., Gore, D. R. and Zuega, R. C. (1975). Kinesiology after McKee-Farrar total hip replacement: A two year follow-up of one hundred cases. *J. Bone Jt. Surg.*, **57A**, 337–42.

Muybridge, E. (1979). *Muybridge's Complete Human and Animal Locomotion. All 781 Plates from the 1887 Animal Locomotion.* Dover Publications.

Norkin, C. C. (1994). Gait analysis. In *Physical Rehabilitation Assessment and Treatment* (S. B. O'Sullivan and T. J. Schmitz, eds.). F. A. Davis.

Oberg, T., Karsznia, A. and Oberg, K. (1993). Basic gait parameters: reference data for normal subjects, 10–79 years of age. *J. Rehabil. Res. Dev.*, **30**, 210–23.

Oberg, T., Karsznia, A. and Oberg, K. (1994). Joint angle parameters in gait: reference data for normal subjects, 10–79 years of age. *J. Rehabil. Res. Dev.*, **301** 199–213

O'Brien, M., Power, K., Sanford, S. *et al.* (1983). Temporal gait patterns in healthy young and elderly females. *Physio. Can.*, **35**, 323–6.

Olney, S. J. and Richards, C. (1996). Hemiparetic gait following stroke. Part I: Characteristics. *Gait and Posture*, **4**, 136–48.

Ounpuu, S., Davis, R. B. and DeLuca, P. A. (1996). Joint kinetics: methods, interpretation and treatment decision-making in children with cerebral palsy and myelomeningocele. *Gait and Posture*, **4**, 62–78.

Patla, A. E., Proctor, J. and Morson, B. (1987). Observations on aspects of visual gait assessment: a questionnaire study. *Physio. Can.*, **39**, 311–16.

Perry, J. (1992). *Gait Analysis: Normal and Pathological Function*. Thorofare, SLACK.

Pratt, D. J. (1991). Three-dimensional electrogoniometric study of selected knee orthoses. *Clin. Biomech.*, **6**, 67–72.

Richards, C. and Olney, S. J. (1996). Hemiparetic gait following stroke. Part II: Recovery and physical therapy. *Gait and Posture*, **4**, 149–162.

Rowe, P. J. and Nicol, A. C. (1991). A new computerized system of electrogoniometry for movement analysis. *Proc. World Confed. Phys. Ther.*, 11th International Congress, London, pp. 1398–1400.

Saleh, M. and Murdoch, G. (1985). In defence of gait analysis: observation and measurement in gait assessment. *J. Bone Jt. Surg.*, **67B**, 237–41.

Shumway-Cook, A. and Woollacott, M. (1995). *Motor Control: Theory and Practical Applications*. Williams & Wilkins.

Shumway-Cook, A., Gruber, W., Baldwin, M. and Liao, S. (1997). The effect of multidimensional exercises on balance, mobility and fall risk in community-dwelling older adults. *Physical Therapy*, **77**, 46–57.

Stewart, D. A., Burns, J. M. A., Dunn, S. G. and Roberts, M. A. (1990). The two-minute walking test: a sensitive index of mobility in the rehabilitation of elderly patients. *Clin. Rehabil.*, **4**, 273–6.

Sutherland, D. H. (1984). *Gait Disorders in Childhood and Adolescence*. Williams & Wilkins.

Sutherland, D. H., Olshen, R. A., Biden, E. N. and Wyatt, M. P. (1988). *The Development of Mature Walking*. Blackwell Scientific Publications.

Wall, J. C. (1991). Measurement of temporal gait parameters from videotape using a field counting technique. *Int. J. Rehabil. Res.*, **14(4)**, 344–7.

Wall, J. C. and Ashburn, A. (1979). Assessment of gait disability in hemiplegics. *Scand. J. Rehabil. Med.*, **11**, 95–103.

Wall, J. C. and Brunt, D. (1996). Clinical gait analysis: temporal and distance parameters. In *Assessment in Occupational Therapy and Physical Therapy* (J. V. Van Deusen and D. Brunt eds.), pp. 435–47. Philadelphia.

Wall, J. C. and Crosbie, J. (1996). Accuracy and reliability of temporal gait measurement. *Gait and Posture*, **4**, 293–6.

Wall, J. C. and Crosbie, J. (1997). Temporal gait analysis using slow motion video and a personal computer. *Physiotherapy*, **83**, 109–15.

Wall, J. C. and Scarbrough, J. (1997). Use of a multimemory stopwatch to measure the temporal gait parameters. *J. Orthop. Sports Phys. Ther.*, **25**, 277–81.

Wall, J. C. and Turnbull, G. I. (1986). Gait asymmetries in residual hemiplegia. *Arch. Phys. Med. Rehabil.*, **67**, 550–53.

Wall, J. C., Dhenedran, M. and Klenerman, L. (1976). A method of measuring the temporal/distance factors of gait. *Biomed. Eng.*, **11**, 409–12.

Wall, J. C., Charteris, J. and Turnbull, G. I. (1987). Two steps equals one stride equals what? The applicability of normal gait nomenclature to abnormal walking patterns. *Clin. Biomech.*, **2**, 119–25.

Wall, J. C., Hogan, D. B., Turnbull, G. I. and Fox, R. A. (1991). The kinematics of idiopathic gait disorder of the elderly: a comparison with healthy young and elderly females. *Scand. J. Rehabil. Med.*, **23**, 159–64.

Winter, D. A., Greenlaw, R. K. and Honson, D. A. (1972). Television–computer analysis of kinematics of human gait. *Comp. Biomed. Res.*, **5**, 498–504.

Winter, D. A., Deathe, A. B., Halliday, S. *et al.* (1993). A technique to analyse the kinetics and energetics of cane assisted gait. *Clin. Biomech.*, **8**, 37–43.

Wu, G. and Chiang, J. (1996). The effects of surface compliance on foot pressure in stance. *Gait and Posture*, **4**, 122–129.

7 Stairs

C. M. Myles

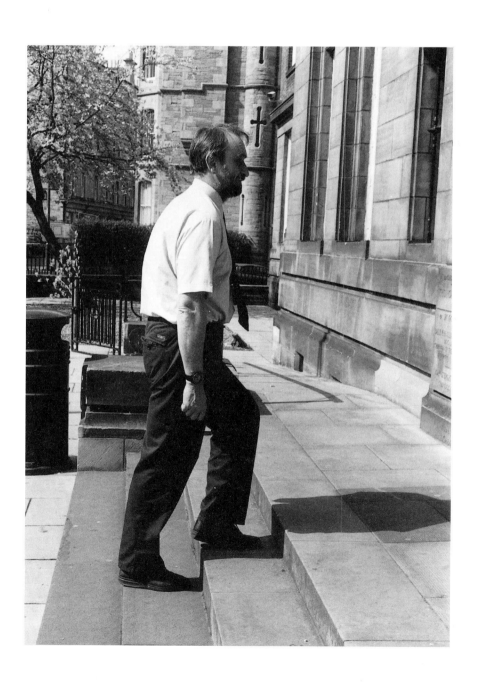

Introduction

Ascending and descending stairs are functional activities common to normal daily life. Confidence and competence in negotiating stairs allow an individual to go shopping, use public transport, access public buildings and visit relatives and friends (Gill *et al.*, 1994). While modern public buildings are required to locate disabled access in the main entrance, many older buildings are out of bounds to the individual who is unable to negotiate stairs.

It would appear that the elderly are particularly affected by disability on stairs (Lundgren-Lindquist *et al.*, 1983). In 1991, Goldstein found 12.1 per cent of the elderly population in the USA was unable to negotiate stairs without help. Many elderly people avoid using stairs altogether, which can result in social isolation and a reduction in their quality of life (Williams, 1996).

Current evaluations of disability on stairs made in the clinical field are largely qualitative. Therapists are commonly required to categorize elderly people on their stair-climbing ability, often as part of one of many functional mobility assessment scales. Many of these scales are simple to use, but offer little information on the quality of movement and possible causes of disability.

To date there has been a poverty of published literature on the biomechanics of stair ascent (SA) and stair descent (SD). Only a small number of authors have attempted to study stair-climbing ability in an objective manner. These have ranged from surveys and questionnaires that include a section on ability to negotiate stairs to detailed kinematic and kinetic movement studies. These will be discussed later in the chapter.

General description of stair ascent and stair descent

There are many ways to ascend and descend stairs, the most common method being foot over foot where the lower limbs move in a cyclic pattern similar to that of level walking. McFadyen and Winter (1988) found that, although strategies may vary, a basic biomechanical pattern is adopted in normal stair ascent and descent. They found the knee in particular demonstrates stereotypical kinetic and kinematic characteristics.

Both level walking and ascending and descending stairs involve periods of support (stance) and non-support (swing). In stair ascent (SA), the leading leg moves from the ground to the first step, then to the third step, then the fifth, and so on, and the following leg moves from the ground to the second step, then to the fourth step, then to the sixth step, etc. Stair descent (SD) follows a similar pattern of foot over foot from the top down.

Physically disabled individuals often employ other methods of moving up or down stairs. The method which will be referred to as 'step to' involves ascending or descending one step at a time, with periods where both feet are placed on the same step. This method is commonly used by individuals who have asymmetrical functional ability of their lower limbs. It is not uncommon, however, to see individuals ascending and descending stairs sideways, on their bottom or, in the case of descent, backwards. Most of the published literature has focused on the conventional method of foot over foot, and this chapter will therefore concentrate on this method.

Sagittal plane motions are dominant in SA and SD, and thus most studies have concentrated on movements in this plane (Andriacchi *et al.*, 1980). Movements such as hip abduction, hip rotation, tibial and ankle rotation and movements of the trunk and arms should not be forgotten, despite a poverty of published data on these parameters.

The activity of ascending and descending stairs is often compared to level walking. Jevsevar *et al.* (1993) compared mean values for maximum knee range of movement in the sagittal plane in five normal young subjects ascending stairs, descending stairs and level walking. They found 98.6 degrees of knee flexion was required to ascend stairs, 90.3 degrees of knee flexion was required to descend stairs and 64.6 degrees of knee flexion was required to walk on level ground. Andriacchi *et al.* (1982) measured maximum moments in the knee during stair negotiation and level walking in 14 normal subjects. They found maximum flexion moments in the knee while ascending stairs to be 1.5 times greater than during level walking. During stair descent, the maximum knee flexion moment found was 4.1 times greater than level walking.

The method of foot contact employed in SA and SD is markedly different to that of level walking. In a description of the biomechanics of normal SA, Loy and Voloshin (1991) found only the metatarsal part of the foot made contact with the step. Joseph and Watson (1967) described the foot contact in SD as toe–heel, with the weight being transferred along the outer border of the foot.

The marked differences between SA, SD and level walking warrant separate investigation of these functional activities. Detailed analysis of SA and SD is necessary in order for therapists to clearly define the level of functioning of a subject and to analyse the effect of treatment through precise outcome measures. An overview of the available literature will be presented in the rest of the chapter.

Functional outcome scales and assessments

Assessment and restoration of function has long been seen as the goal in rehabilitation medicine. Over the years a number of functional assessment scales have been developed in the effort to standardize the collection of data. Most of these scales include a section relating to stairs.

In 1965, Mahoney and Barthel published a simple index of independence, the Barthel Index. The scale includes stair ascending and descending activity, with three identified levels. A maximum score is attributed for independence, a reduced score for the requirement for help or supervision, and zero for inability. The total score comprises the sum of the points attributed to 10 functional activities, including feeding, transfers, toileting, bathing, grooming, walking, dressing and bowel and bladder control. Stair climbing contributes to 10 per cent of the total points score. The Barthel Index is commonly used in rehabilitation settings today, but serves poorly as an indicator of quality of movement as it fails to detect subtle changes in function over a period of time.

Similarly, the Functional Independence Measure scale (FIM) addresses ascending and descending stairs as one function (Rankin, 1993). FIM looks at the movement in slightly more detail, using a seven-point ordinal scale to record the amount of help required and the use of handrails. Once again, ascending and descending stairs is the topic of only one question in a functional assessment scale, in this case contributing to 5.5 per cent of the total score, and indicates little about the quality of the subject's movement.

The Physical Performance Test (Reuben and Siu, 1990) scores the patient on the time taken to climb one flight of stairs, giving a score of zero to four. The highest score is given to subjects who are able to climb one flight of stairs in 5 s or less. The number of flights a subject is able to climb is also recorded and scored from zero to four, with four corresponding to a maximum of four flights climbed. In this scale, stair climbing contributes to 22 per cent of the total functional assessment score. An attempt is made in this study to attribute a temporal measure to stair climbing ability, but it gives the user little indication as to the cause of disability on stairs or possible therapeutic intervention.

Other mobility scales, such as the Elderly Mobility Scale (Smith, 1994), do not assess stairs at all, despite the need for many frail elderly people to negotiate stairs on discharge from hospital.

These are only a few of the functional assessment scales available to the therapist. They do, however, indicate the poverty of clinical data available regarding the quality of movement of subjects on stairs.

As an alternative to the global functional assessment scales, Lundgren-Lindquist *et al.* (1983) looked at the step climbing capacity of a group of normal 79-year-old people in Scandanavia. Subjects were asked to climb up and down a number of steps of differing heights, and the maximum height climbed with and without a rail was recorded along with their heart rate and the subjects' own related perception of exertion for each step. One hundred and twelve women and 93 men were investigated, and all were found to be able to climb up and down a 20 cm step using a handrail. However, 20 per cent of the women and 6 per cent of the men were unable to climb up and down a 40 cm high step, even when using the handrail. Swedish public transport step heights range from 30 to 40 cm, and this would therefore, account for the fact that many of the subjects reported difficulty negotiating public transport.

Subjects' perception of their ability to negotiate stairs may play an important part in stair-climbing ability. Konczak *et al.* (1992) asked a group of 24 young and 24 older adults to identify what height of step they thought was the highest they could climb from a choice of eight step heights, and then to attempt to climb that step. They found the group of older adults made fewer mistakes in their initial perceptual assessment than the younger adults. A possible explanation of this behaviour is that older adults operate within a smaller range of functional capabilities and therefore learn to be sensitive to changes in the environment around them.

Temporal characteristics

A number of authors have attempted to define the temporal characteristics of SA and SD. The most detailed studies in this area on normal subjects have been by McFadyen and Winter (1988) and Zachazewski *et al.* (1993). McFadyen and Winter (1988) identified the subphases of stance and swing for SA and SD according to different objectives for progression using a force plate inserted into the second step of a five-step staircase. These subphases were then further defined by Zachazewski *et al.* (1993) using two force plates located under steps two and three of a four-step staircase.

Zachazewski *et al.* (1993) divided SA and SD into phases, defining one cycle as first contact of a foot with the step to subsequent contact of the same foot. During SA the stance phase was found to represent 65 per cent of the cycle, with the remaining 35 per cent representing the swing phase. Zachazewski *et al.* (1993) then divided stance into a number of subphases. These included weight acceptance (0–17 per cent SA cycle); vertical thrust (2–37 per cent SA cycle)

and forward continuance (37–51 per cent SA cycle); double limb support, which occurs at the start of the stance phase (0–17 per cent SA cycle), followed by single limb support (17–48 per cent SA cycle) and then double support to the end of the stance phase (48–65 per cent SA cycle). The swing phase consists of foot clearance (65–82 per cent SA cycle) and foot placement (82–100 per cent SA cycle). The phases of SA can be seen in Figure 7.1.

Stair descent (Figure 7.2) is described by Zachazewski *et al.* (1993) as being divided into a stance and swing phase, comprising of 68 per cent and 32 per cent of the total SD cycle respectively. The stance phase is divided into weight acceptance (0–14 per cent SD cycle), forward continuance (14–34 per cent SD cycle) and controlled lowering (34–68 per cent SD cycle). Single limb support is defined as contributing to 39 per cent of the stance phase (14–53 per cent of each cycle). Double

STANCE PHASE 65%				SWING PHASE 35%	
WEIGHT ACCEPTANCE (0–17%)	VERTICAL THRUST (2–37%)	FORWARD CONTINUANCE (37–51%)		FOOT CLEARANCE (65–82%)	FOOT PLACEMENT (82–100%)

DOUBLE SUPPORT (0–17%)	SINGLE LIMB SUPPORT (17–48%)	DOUBLE SUPPORT (48–65%)	SINGLE OPPOSITE LIMB SUPPORT (65–100%

Figure 7.1 Phases of stair ascent (based on data from Zachazewski *et al.*, 1993)

STANCE PHASE 68%			SWING PHASE 32%	
WEIGHT ACCEPTANCE (0–14%)	FORWARD CONTINUANCE (14–34%)	CONTROLLED LOWERING (34–68%)	LEG PULL THROUGH (68–84%)	FOOT PLACEMENT (84–100%)

DOUBLE SUPPORT (0–14%)	SINGLE LIMB SUPPORT (14–53%)	DOUBLE SUPPORT (53–68%)	SINGLE OPPOSITE LIMB SUPPORT (68–100%)

Figure 7.2 Phases of stair descent (based on data from Zachazewski *et al.*, 1993)

support is said to occur at the start and end of the stance phase (0–14 per cent and 53–68 per cent). The swing phase accounts for the remaining 32 per cent of SD, and is divided into leg pull through (68–84 per cent SD cycle) and foot placement (84–100 per cent SD cycle).

Cheaper and portable alternatives to force plates that can be used to record temporal characteristics of SA and SD are footswitches, which can be attached directly to the sole of the foot (Torburn *et al.*, 1994). These identify when contact is made with the ground by a pressure-sensitive resistor located in the footswitch which, when pressed, results in a flow of current and a positive reading. Livingston *et al.* (1991) used a similar device, called a switchmat, which was mounted on the treads of the steps and triggered the on and off record of three digital clocks. From this they were able to identify total stride time, stance phase duration and the period of double-limb support in a group of 15 normal women.

The values for stance to swing ratios in normal subjects identified by Zachazewski *et al.* (1993) are similar to those found by other authors. McFadyen and Winter (1988) identified stance to swing ratios for SA and SD as 64 : 36 per cent; Powers *et al.* (1997), using insoles containing compression-closing footswitches, found SA to be 63 : 37 per cent and SD to be 61.7 : 38.3 per cent.

SA and SD speeds in normal populations have been quoted by some authors. Andriacchi *et al.* (1982) identified speeds of $0.32 \pm 0.09 \, \mathrm{ms^{-1}}$ for both SA and SD; Powers *et al.* (1997) found SA speeds of $33.4 \, \mathrm{mmin^{-1}}$ ($0.557 \, \mathrm{ms^{-1}}$) and SD speeds of $35.2 \, \mathrm{mmin^{-1}}$ ($0.587 \, \mathrm{ms^{-1}}$). Zachazewski *et al.* (1993) used cycle time as a measure of speed. They identified cycle times of $1.662 \pm 0.371 \, \mathrm{s}$ for SA and $1.621 \pm 0.269 \, \mathrm{s}$ for SD.

Comparisons between studies are difficult as the parameters measured vary and are undoubtedly affected by factors such as step height, pitch of the stairs and subject height and leg length. These factors are not always identified in the published literature. The parameters published in a number of stair-climbing studies can be seen in Table 7.1.

Temporal characteristics in patient groups

Only a small number of studies of patient groups negotiating stairs have been conducted. Powers *et al.* (1997) used temporal characteristics to determine the symmetry between prosthetic and normal legs in a group of 10 transtibial amputees, along with a group of 14 non-disabled subjects. They found the amputees demonstrated stance asymmetry between the sound and residual limbs in SA and SD, in addition to significantly slower SA and SD velocities, when compared with the control group. SA velocity in the control group was $33.4 \, \mathrm{mmin^{-1}}$ (sd 3.6) and $29.6 \, \mathrm{mmin^{-1}}$ (sd 3.6) in the amputee group. The SD velocity was $35.2 \, \mathrm{mmin^{-1}}$ (sd 3.6) in the control group and $29.6 \, \mathrm{mmin^{-1}}$ (sd 5.4) in the amputee group.

Marks (1994) studied six women with osteoarthritis in their knees, and recorded stair-walking time with a stopwatch on a four-step staircase. He

Table 7.1 Parameters of stair-climbing studies

Author	Subject type	Number	Age (years)	Step height (cm)	Number of steps	Measurement method
McFadyen and Winter, 1988	normal	3		22	5	kinetic, kinematic, EMG
Livingston *et al.*, 1991	normal	15	19–26	20.3	5	kinematic
Andriacchi *et al.*, 1980	normal	10	20–34	21	3	kinetic, kinematic, EMG
Jevsevar *et al.*, 1993	normal knee-replacements	11 15	26–88 61–78	18	4	kinetic, kinematic
Laubenthal *et al.*, 1972	normal	30	x = 25		2	kinematic
Powers *et al.*, 1997	normal amputees	14 10	x = 34 x = 51	15	4	kinematics, EMG
Moffet *et al.*, 1993	normal load carrying	15	21–35	16	3	kinematic, EMG

found walking time on stairs significantly corre-lated with pain (r = 0.84; *p* = 0.033). The stair dimensions used in this study are not given, making it difficult to compare these data with other studies.

Paced versus unpaced activity

The majority of studies have permitted the subjects to ascend and descend stairs at their own pace, allowing as natural a movement as possible. This, however, results in variability in the length of SA and SD cycles, and makes direct comparison of the raw data difficult. Therefore, most authors inter-polate SA and SD cycles, plotting the parameter of interest against a percentage of the total cycle, and this allows for direct comparison of data between cycles of varying length. Figure 7.3 shows electro-goniometry data from the right hip, knee and ankle of a normal subject ascending stairs. One cycle from foot contact with the step to successive foot contact has been interpolated with the x axis representing the percentage of the cycle. Other examples of interpolated data are provided by Andriacchi *et al.* (1980), Andriacchi *et al.* (1982), McFadyen and Winter (1988) and Zachazewski *et al.* (1993).

In an unusual attempt to pace activity in a kinematic study of SA and SD, Krebs *et al.* (1992) investigated trunk kinematics in 11 normal sub-jects by using an optoelectric camera system. The subjects ascended and descended the four-step staircase to the beat of a metronome set at 80 beats per minute. The SA speed was found to be $0.39 \pm 0.05\,\text{ms}^{-1}$ with a cycle time of $1.60 \pm 0.29\,\text{s}$, and the SD speed was $0.36 \pm 0.07\,\text{ms}^{-1}$ with a cycle time of $1.58 \pm 0.25\,\text{s}$. The SA and SD cycles were interpolated for analysis in this paper. The reasons for pacing the activities in this paper are unclear, although it is assumed the purpose was to attempt to standardize time between tests. This factor may, however, be outweighed by the falsity of the movement created by removing the subjects' natural speed of motion.

Kinematics

A small number of studies have been carried out to investigate the kinematics involved in normal subjects during SA and SD. These have involved a variety of measurement systems, including:

Advanced optoelectronic systems (Zachazewski *et al.*, 1993; Andriacchi *et al.*, 1980; Krebs *et al.*, 1992)
Cinematography (Livingston *et al.*, 1991; McFad-yen and Winter, 1988; Cooper *et al.*, 1989)
35 mm cameras (Mital *et al.*, 1987)
Polarized light goniometry (Grieve *et al.*, 1978);

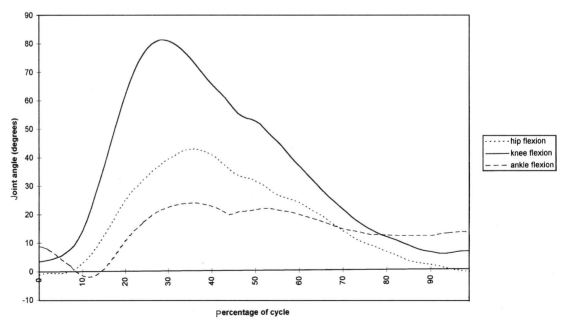

Figure 7.3 Normal subject ascending stairs (Myles *et al.*, 1995)

Electrogoniometry (Laubenthal *et al.*, 1972; Moffet *et al.*, 1993 and Myles *et al.*, 1995) and Mathematical modelling (Shinno, 1971 and Townsend and Tsai, 1976).

Only a small number of studies have investigated kinematics in pathological groups. Examples include Powers *et al.* (1997), who used a three-dimensional optoelectronic camera system to investigate SA and SD in subjects with a transtibial amputation, and Andriacchi *et al.* (1982), Kelman *et al.* (1989) and Jevsevar *et al.* (1993), who used optoelectronic systems to investigate knee motion during SA and SD in patients who had received knee replacements.

Stair ambulation involves movement of the lower limbs, trunk, neck and upper limbs in the sagittal, frontal and horizontal planes of motion. Sagittal plane motions are dominant in normal (and abnormal or aided) SA and SD (Townsend and Tsai, 1976), and hence the focus of almost all studies is on movement in the sagittal plane.

Andriacchi *et al.* (1980) described the movements of the hip, knee and ankle joints of one leg in 10 normal subjects when moving from step 1 to step 3 (Figure 7.4). When the foot strikes step 1, the hip and knee joints are flexed and the ankle joint is plantar flexed. As the limb moves from foot-strike to mid stance, the hip and knee joints extend and the ankle joint dorsiflexes slightly. From mid stance towards toe-off, the hip and knee

continue to extend and the ankle plantar flexes during toe-off. The hip and knee then flex to a maximum during mid-swing, while the ankle reaches maximum dorsiflexion. The hip and knee then move towards extension and the ankle towards plantar flexion to foot-strike.

Descending from step 3 to step 1 is also described clearly by Andriacchi *et al.* (1980), and is represented in Figure 7.5. At toe-off from step 3, the hip and knee are flexed and the ankle is dorsiflexed close to maximum. During the swing phase, hip and knee flexion decreases and the ankle moves into plantar flexion. When the foot strikes step 1, the hip joint is only slightly flexed and the knee is almost fully extended and the ankle plantar flexed. As the limb moves towards mid stance on step 1, the hip extends and the knee flexes slightly. The ankle moves towards dorsiflexion after mid stance, and the hip remains near full extension. Prior to toe-off, the knee begins to flex and maximum dorsiflexion at the ankle occurs.

The kinematic parameters quoted by Andriacchi *et al.* (1980) are the mean values for the maximum sagittal plane motions of the hip, knee and ankle joints. For SA, these were 41.9° (sd = 9.9), 83.3° (sd = 5.2) and 13.6° (sd = 8.6) respectively. The ankle value represents dorsiflexion. Livingston *et al.* (1991) found (mean) maximum hip flexion was 58° (sd = 13.5), knee flexion 101° (sd = 1) and ankle dorsiflexion 17° (sd = 7.5) for SA in normal subjects of medium height.

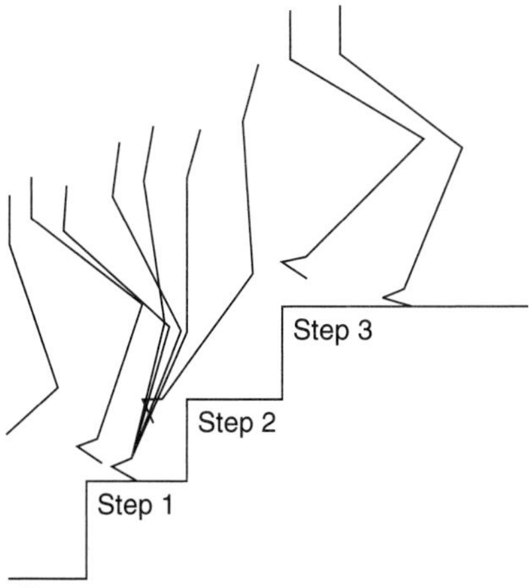

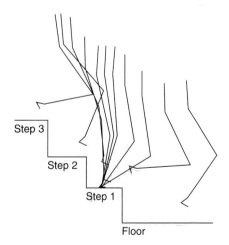

Figure 7.4 Sagittal plane flexion–extension movements of the hip and knee and plantar flexion–dorsiflexion movements of the ankle in one limb of a subject ascending from Step 1 to Step 3. (Reproduced from Andriacchi *et al.*, 1980, *J. Bone Jt. Surg.* **62A**, 749–57, by kind permission of the authors and publishers)

Figure 7.5 Sagittal plane flexion–extension movements of the hip and knee and plantar flexion–dorsiflexion movements of the ankle in one limb of a subject descending from Step 3 to Step 1. (Reproduced from Andriacchi *et al.*, 1980, *J. Bone Jt. Surg.* **62A**, 749–57, by kind permission of the authors and publishers)

For SD, Andriacchi *et al.* (1980) found values of 28.2° (sd = 12.9) for hip flexion, 87.9° (sd = 4.4) for knee flexion and 27.0° (sd = 11.4) for ankle flexion. Livingston *et al.* (1991) quoted 37° (sd = 0.5) flexion at the hip, 93° (sd = 0.5) at the knee and 21° (sd = 7) at the ankle.

When we examine the step heights used in these two studies, we find they are similar. Andriacchi *et al.* (1980) used a step height of 21 cm, and Livingston *et al.* (1991) one of 20.3 cm. However, on closer examination the slope of the 20.3 cm step was 45° and the 21 cm step only 38°, and it is therefore not advisable to make direct comparisons between these two sets of data. Some other studies give less comprehensive information on the stair dimensions used, or other factors such as subject age and height, which may prevent external comparison.

Another common method of presenting kinematic data is in graphical form, showing the mean values for repeated tests on an individual or a group along with the standard deviation bands (McFadyen and Winter, 1988; Powers *et al.*, 1997; Moffet *et al.*, 1993). This allows the reader to view the pattern of the motion in addition to the peak values. It is useful, however, to give the maximum, minimum and range values as well, as it is often difficult to read precise values from small graphs in published literature.

Kinetics

Ascending and descending stairs are complex functional activities, requiring control and co-ordination of a number of muscle groups, and an awareness of the forces and moments involved is necessary to broaden our understanding of the underlying mechanisms involved in SA and SD.

Ground reaction forces

Ground reaction forces (GRF) have been measured using force plates located directly under one or more step treads (Andriacchi *et al.*, 1980; Jevsevar *et al.*, 1993; McFadyen and Winter, 1988; Zachazewski *et al.*, 1993). These forces are clearly described by Zachazewski *et al.* (1993), who used a four-step staircase with two force plates located directly under steps two and three and studied 11

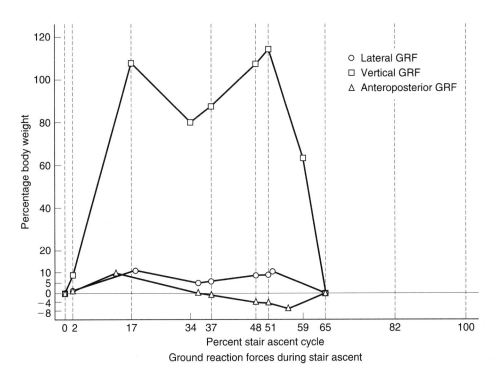

Ground reaction forces during stair ascent

Figure 7.6 Ground reaction forces during stair ascent. GRFs during stair ascent as a percentage of body weight are graphed. Points indicated on the graph are data. (Reproduced from Zachazewski *et al.*, 1993, *J. Rehabil. Res. Dev.* **30**, 412–22, by kind permission of the authors and publishers)

normal subjects. During SA (Figure 7.6) it is suggested there is a rapid increase in the vertical GRF on foot contact, reaching a maximum at the start of single limb support. The vertical GRF then gradually decreases until mid stance, after which it increases again to reach a second maximum at the start of double support. The lateral GRF is said to increase from foot contact until single limb support, where it reaches a maximum. It then gradually reduces until mid stance, before increasing again to reach a second maximum at the initiation of double support. The anterior–posterior GRF is initially directed posteriorly, but by the end of this foot contact phase it reverses direction to become anterior. Similar findings were discussed by McFadyen and Winter (1988). Zachazewski *et al.* (1993) suggest maximum anterior shear is reached during weight acceptance, and immediately before single limb support the A/P GRF is directed posteriorly again with the greatest posterior shear force reached 56 per cent into SA.

Zachazewski *et al.* (1993) also describe in detail the GRF found during descent (Figure 7.7). They suggest foot contact results in a rapid increase in vertical GRF to a maximum at the start of single limb support. There is then a gradual decrease in vertical GRF until mid stance. After mid stance the vertical GRF increases, reaching a maximum value at approximately the time of initiation of the second double support phase. Lateral GRF increases from foot contact until the start of single limb support, when it gradually reduces until mid stance. After mid stance the lateral GRF increases, reaching a maximum at the start of the second double support phase. Anterior–posterior GRF demonstrates maximum anterior shear during weight acceptance immediately prior to the start of single limb support. Posterior shear forces are apparent just prior to single limb support, with maximum posterior shear being reached just prior to double limb support.

Jevsevar *et al.* (1993) compared mean and standard deviations of right and left leg vertical GRF during SA and SD in 11 normal subjects. He found the right leg values for ascent to be 116.7 per cent body weight (sd = 12.5) and left leg 108.3 per cent body weight (sd = 10.6). For SD, he found the right leg vertical GRF was 133.7 per cent body weight (sd = 31.3) and the left leg 145.2 per cent body weight (sd = 24.2). Zachazewski *et al.* (1993)

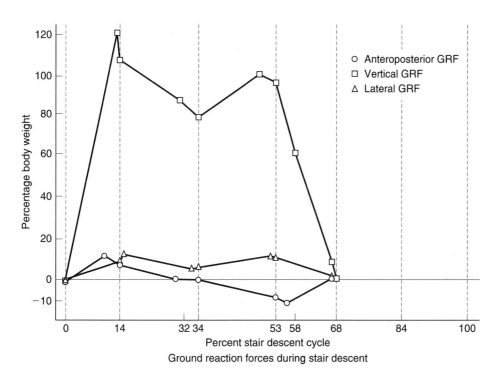

Figure 7.7 Ground reaction forces during stair descent. GRFs during stair descent as a percentage of body weight are graphed. Points indicated on the graph are data. (Reproduced from Zachazewski *et al.*, 1993, *J. Rehabil. Res. Dev.* **30**, 412–22, by kind permission of the authors and publishers)

found the maximum vertical GRF represent approximately 110 per cent body weight for SA and 120 per cent body weight for SD. Once again caution must be employed when comparing different studies, as variability in a large number of parameters can influence the results.

Moments

McFadyen and Winter (1988) found similarities in the patterns of the support moments of both SA and SD with level walking, which were all predominantly positive in stance and of a similar two-peaked pattern. However, SA and SD resulted in higher magnitude moments than level walking, and the need for higher antigravity activity is offered as the explanation for this result. Andriacchi *et al.* (1980) demonstrated the highest moments occurring in normal subjects while descending stairs, and found that the flexion–extension moments correlate with the activity of the major flexor–extensor muscle groups. The flexion moments found at the knee were largest during SD when the knee was in about 50° of flexion, resulting in a large force in the knee extensor muscles to offset this. The knee joint contact forces are equated to more than six times body weight in this study. This offers an explanation as to why therapists commonly observe patients with arthritis in the knee struggling with stair descent and often resorting to a 'step to' gait. Andriacchi *et al.* (1980) also found that, as with level walking, the ankle joint was subject to relatively large dorsiflexion moments during both SA and SD. The inversion moments at the ankle during both functions were of greater magnitude than those observed during level walking. As with the knee joint, they found the flexion–extension moments at the hip were larger during SD by the 'foot over foot' method than by the 'step to' method. During the normal method of SD (foot over foot), the largest moments were found when the hip was in 30–40° of flexion. These moments were identified as 1.5 times greater than those found in the hip during level walking. McFadyen and Winter (1988) suggest some caution should be employed when examining the values given for joint moments in the study by Andriacchi *et al.* (1980). It is suggested that the method used to calculate the moments, which involves performing the cross product of the ground reaction force vector and the joint centre's positional vector, is problematic in that it neglects the contribution made by segment weight and inertial forces, thus increasing the size of errors for

the hip and knee joint. The poverty of other published literature in this area means there is little other evidence with which to compare these values, and highlights the need for further work.

Centre of mass

Centre of mass (COM) was first addressed in detail by Zachazewski *et al.* (1993). In SA, the whole body COM was found to be displaced vertically during vertical thrust in the stance phase. During forward continuance, no further vertical CM displacement occurred. The COM lateral displacement is described as following a sinusoidal curve in the frontal plane. Maximum COM displacement is said to occur at mid stance during the vertical thrust subphase, representing 4.4 ± 1.2 cm. A rapid direction reversal follows, with weight being transferred to the opposite extremity following opposite foot strike. Throughout SA and SD, Zachazewski *et al.* (1993) describe the COM as being displaced anteriorly. Similarly, McFadyen and Winter (1988) describe periods of concurrent movement of the trunk in both the vertical and horizontal directions as well as periods of horizontal translation in both SA and SD.

For SD, Zachazewski *et al.* (1993) found the COM vertical position descends during the weight acceptance phase of stance then remains level until controlled lowering, where it descends again. As with SA, the COM follows a sinusoidal curve in the frontal plane with maximum medio-lateral displacement occurring at mid stance (4.2 ± 1.4 cm).

EMG characteristics

The majority of work to date on stair negotiation has been in the field of electromyography (EMG) to investigate muscle activity (Joseph and Watson, 1967; Shinno, 1971; Townsend *et al.*, 1978; Andriacchi *et al.*, 1980; Freedman and Craik, 1981; McFadyen and Winter, 1988; Cooper *et al.*, 1989; Moffet *et al.*, 1993; Powers *et al.*, 1997).

Joseph and Watson (1967) were the first authors to shed light on the pattern of activity of muscles of the lower limbs and back in six normal male subjects. They found that, in order to raise the body onto the step above in SA (Figure 7.8), contraction of soleus, quadriceps femoris, hamstrings and gluteus maximus occurs. The gluteus medius was active at the same time, preventing the body falling onto the unsupported side. The swing phase was found to involve tibialis anterior to dorsiflex the

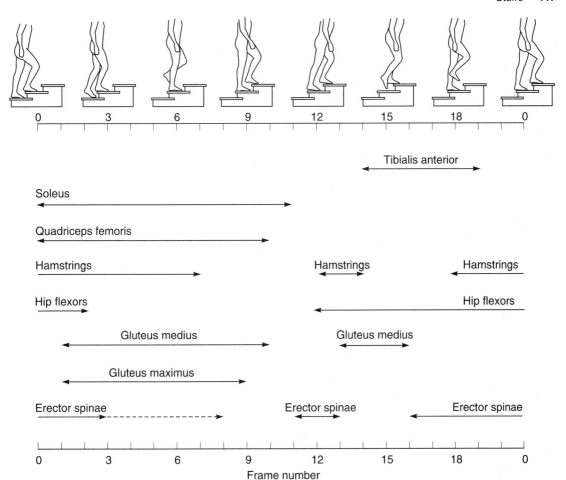

Figure 7.8 A summary of the results obtained from the muscles investigated during walking up stairs. The arrows indicate the beginning and end of the phase of activity. The dotted line indicates a marked decrease in activity found in only half the subjects. (Reproduced from Joseph and Watson 1967, *J. Bone Jt. Surg.* **49B**, 774–80, by kind permission of the authors and publishers)

foot and clear the step. During the early part of the swing phase the hamstring was observed to flex the knee and, at the end of the swing phase, to control the terminal part of extension. The erector spinae muscles were active twice in each step, controlling the forward bending of the body.

Joseph and Watson (1967) observed the following features of EMG activity during SD (Figure 7.9). The body was found to be lowered down onto the step below by controlled lengthening of soleus and quadriceps femoris, with the gluteus medius at the same time showing electrical activity in order to prevent the body from falling onto the unsupported side. The tibialis anterior was thought to dorsiflex the foot in the middle of the swing phase, and invert the foot at the beginning of the support

phase as the toe is placed on the step below. The hamstring was shown to be active during the middle of the swing phase, controlling extension of the knee. As with SA, both erector spinae were found to contract twice in each step, preventing forward flexion of the trunk.

The difference in muscular activity levels between SA and SD was investigated by McFadyen and Winter (1988). The mean EMG activity for vastus lateralis, semitendinosus, gluteus maximus, medial gastrocnemius, soleus and tibialis anterior was determined to be greater for SA than SD. Only rectus femoris and gluteus medius were found to be higher for SD. This is explained by the body centre of mass being closer to the point of support during SD, thus optimizing the

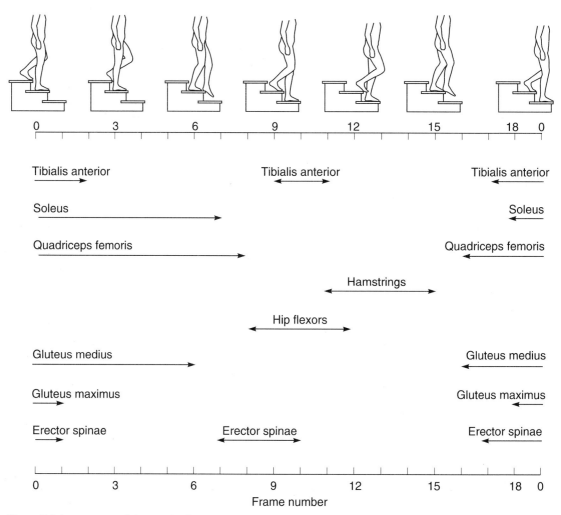

Figure 7.9 A summary of the results from muscles investigated during walking down stairs. (Reproduced from Joseph and Watson 1967, *J. Bone Jt. Surg.* **49B**, 774–80, by kind permission of the authors and publishers)

position. Similarly, Shinno (1971) found the activity of the extensors of the knee was smaller during SD than SA. He found the amplitude of the biceps femoris to be slightly greater in SD than SA.

Investigating the trunk muscle EMG activity during SA and SD, Cooper *et al.* (1989) found a significantly greater ($p < 0.01$) amount of EMG activity occurred in erector spinae during SA when compared with SD and level walking. SD was found to have the least amount of EMG activity in erector spinae. Rectus abdominus electrical activity was observed to be low during all activities.

Environmental factors affecting the ability to ascend and descend stairs

A number of environmental factors may influence the ability of an individual to ascend and descend stairs safely and efficiently.

The elderly are particularly susceptible to falls on stairs that are poorly lit, uneven under foot, and unfamiliar to them. Despite the health hazards associated with negotiating stairs, research on stair activities has predominantly been limited to healthy young subjects (Simoneau *et al.*, 1991).

Table 7.2 Scottish Office Technical Standards for Building (1990): newly built stairs

Description of stairs	Maximum rise (mm)	Maximum going (mm)	Minimum width (mm)	Maximum pitch (degrees)
Private stair	220	225	800	42
Access stairs and public buildings	190	250	800	38

In one of the few studies of elderly people on stairs, Simoneau *et al.* (1991) suggested that the small amount of foot clearance exhibited by elderly women during stair descent indicates that the use of properly fitting footwear is essential to prevent accidents. Other environmental factors highlighted in this study as being in need of more investigation were illumination, step and wall covering characteristics, and the use of bifocal lenses (which may blur vision during SD).

Stair dimensions

Stair dimensions have altered little in the past three centuries. The formula used for calculating stair riser and tread dimensions was derived by Francis Blondel in 1672. The formula specifies the total of the tread and two times the height of the step should be equivalent to 24 inches (Livingston *et al.*, 1991). Despite an increase in the average height and shoe size, little has been done to alter the architectural guidelines, which are still used today. The Scottish Office Technical Standards for Building (1990) dimensions for rise, going and width of stair can be seen in Table 7.2.

Future needs and development issues

It is clear from the work presented in this chapter that stair ascent and descent are complex functional activities, and are sufficiently different from level walking to warrant separate investigation. The number of studies carried out in this area to date has been limited, but they serve as a good basis for the understanding of this function and indicate the need for further investigation.

Many of the studies to date have been carried out on a small number of subjects (Table 7.1). Further investigation of kinetics, kinematics and electromyography in larger groups of normal subjects is required. As it is often the elderly population who experience difficulty on stairs,

studies on normal elderly populations are needed.

Few studies have reported stair ascent and descent in pathological groups. Therapists commonly rehabilitate elderly, orthopaedic and neurological patients on stairs, and detailed investigation into the difficulties patients have on stairs is required in order to identify problems and to develop and evaluate rehabilitation programmes.

References

Andriacchi, T. P., Galante, J. O. and Fermier, R. W. (1982). The influence of total knee-replacement design on walking and stair climbing. *J. Bone Jt. Surg.*, **64A(9)**, 1328–35.

Andriacchi, T. P., Andersson, G. B. J., Fermier, R. W. *et al.* (1980). A study of lower-limb mechanics during stair-climbing. *J. Bone Jt. Surg.*, **62A(5)**, 749–57.

Cooper, J., Quanbury, A., Grahame, R. and Dubo, H. (1989). Trunk kinematics and trunk muscle EMG activity during five functional locomotor types. *Can. J. Occup. Ther.*, **56(3)**, 120–27.

Freedman, W. and Craik, R. (1981). Effects of altered sensory input on stair descent. *Bull. Prosth. Res.*, **18(1)**, 239–40.

Gill, D. L., Kelley, B. C., Williams, K. and Martin, J. J. (1994). The relationship of self-efficacy and perceived well-being to physical activity and stair climbing in older adults. *Res. Q. Exer. Sport*, **65(4)**, 367–71.

Goldstein, T. (1991). *Geriatric Orthopaedics, Rehabilitative Management of Common Problems*. Aspen Publications.

Grieve, D. W., Leggett, D. and Wetherstone, B. (1978). The analysis of normal stepping movements as a possible basis for locomotor assessment of the lower limbs. *J. Anat.*, **127(3)**, 515–32.

Jevsevar, D. S., O Riley, P., Hodge, W. A. and Krebs, D. E. (1993). Knee kinematics and kinetics during locomotor activities of daily living in subjects with knee arthroplasty and in healthy control subjects. *Phys. Ther.*, **73(4)**, 229–42.

Joseph, J. and Watson, R. (1967). Telemetering electromyography of muscles used in walking up and down stairs. *J. Bone Jt. Surg.*, **49B(4)**, 774–80.

Kelman, G. J., Biden, E. N., Wyatt, M. P. *et al.* (1989). Gait laboratory analysis of a posterior cruciate-sparing total knee arthroplasty in stair ascent and descent. *Clin. Orthop. Rel. Res.*, **248**, 21–6.

Konczak, J., Meeuwsen, H. J. and Cress, M. E. (1992). Changing affordances in stair climbing: the perception of maximum climbability in young and older adults. *J. Exp. Psychol: Hum. Percep. Perf.*, **18(3)**, 691–7.

Krebs, D. E., Wong, D., Jevsevar, D. *et al.* (1992). Trunk kinematics during locomotor activities. *Phys. Ther.*, **72**, 505–14.

Laubenthal, K. N., Smidt, G. L. and Kettlekamp, D. B. (1972). A quantitative analysis of knee motion during activities of daily living. *Phys. Ther.*, **52(1)**, 34–42.

Livingston, L. A., Stevenson, J. M. and Olney, S. J. (1991). Stair-climbing kinematics on stairs of differing dimensions. *Arch. Phys. Med. Rehabil.*, **72**, 398–402.

Loy, D. J. and Voloshin, A. S. (1991). Biomechanics of stair walking and jumping. *J. Sports Sci.*, **9**, 137–49.

Lundgren-Lindquist, B., Aniansson, A. and Rundgren, A. (1983). Functional studies in 79-year-olds. III. Walking performance and climbing capacity. *Scand. J. Rehabil. Med.*, **15**, 125–31.

McFadyen, B. J. and Winter, D. A. (1988). An integrated biomechanical analysis of normal stair ascent and descent. *J. Biomech.*, **21(9)**, 733–44.

Mahoney, F. I. and Barthel, D. W. (1965). Functional evaluation: the Barthel Index. *MD State Med. J.*, **Feb.**, 61–5.

Marks, R. (1994). An investigation of the influence of age, clinical status, pain and position sense on stair walking in women with osteoarthrosis. *Int. J. Rehabil. Res.*, **17**, 151–8.

Mital, A., Fard, H. F. and Khaledi, H. (1987). A biomechanical evaluation of staircase riser heights and tread depths during stair-climbing. *Clin. Biomech.*, **2**, 162–4.

Moffet, H., Richards, C. L., Malouin, F. and Bravo, G. (1993). Load-carrying during stair ascent: a demanding functional test. *Gait and Posture*, **1**, 35–44.

Myles, C., Rowe, P. J., Salter, P. and Nicol, A. C. (1995). An electrogoniometry system used to investigate the ability of the elderly to ascend and descend stairs. *Physiotherapy*, **81(10)**, 639–40.

Powers, C. M, Boyd, L. A., Torburn, L. and Perry, J. (1997). Stair ambulation in persons with transtibial amputation: an analysis of the Seattle Lightfoot. *J. Rehabil. Res. Dev.*, **34(1)**, 9–18.

Rankin, A. (1993). Functional independence measure. *Physiotherapy*, **79**, 842–3.

Reuben, D. B. and Siu, A. L. (1990). An objective measure of physical function of elderly outpatients, the physical performance test. *J. Am. Geriatr. Soc.*, **38**, 1105–12.

Scottish Office (1990). *Technical Standards*. HMSO.

Simoneau, G. G., Cavanagh, P. R., Ulbrecht, J. S. *et al.* (1991). The influence of visual factors on fall-related kinematic variables during stair descent by older women. *J. Geront.*, **46(6)**, M188–195.

Shinno, N. (1971). Analysis of knee function in ascending and descending stairs. *Med. Sport*, **6**, 202–7.

Smith, R. (1994). Validation and reliability of the elderly mobility scale. *Physiotherapy*, **80(11)**, 744–7.

Torburn, L., Schweiger, G. P., Perry, J. and Powers, C. M. (1994). Below-knee amputee gait in stair ambulation. *Clin. Orthop. Rel. Res.*, **303**, 185–92.

Townsend, M. A. and Tsai, T. C. (1976). Biomechanics and modelling of bipedal climbing and descending. *J. Biomech.*, **9**, 227–39.

Townsend, M. A., Lainhart, S. P. and Shiavi, R. (1978). Variability and biomechanics of synergy patterns of some lower-limb muscles during ascending and descending stairs and level walking. *Med. Biol. Eng. Comput.*, **16**, 681–8.

Williams, K. (1996). Intralimb co-ordination of older adults during locomotion: stair climbing. *J. Hum. Move. Stud.*, **30**, 269–84.

Zachazewski, J. E., O Riley, P and Krebs D. E. (1993). Biomechanical analysis of body mass transfer during stair ascent and descent of healthy subjects. *J. Rehabil. Res. Dev.*, **30(4)**, 412–22.

8 Running

A. Lees

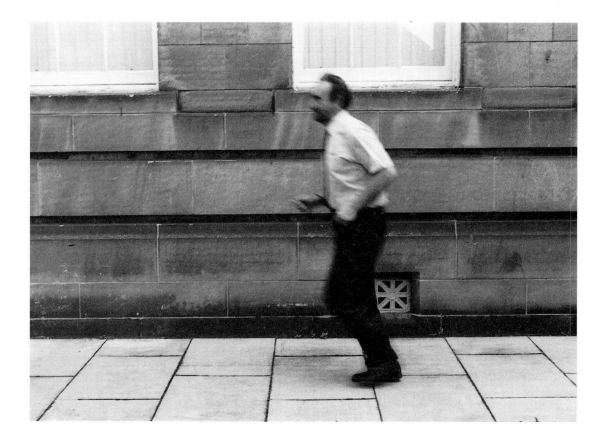

Introduction

Running is a form of locomotion which enables humans to progress from one place to another more quickly than they would if they chose to walk. The running action is distinct from walking in that it has a period of non-contact (or flight phase) and a support phase where only one leg is in contact with the ground. Running can be performed at speeds up to $11\,ms^{-1}$, but a typical running speed is $4\,ms^{-1}$ and most research has been conducted at this speed.

Slow running (up to about $3\,ms^{-1}$) is termed jogging while very fast running (over $7\,ms^{-1}$) is termed sprinting, although in all of these the action has essentially the same form. Those who run regularly develop a fluency of movement, and athletes involved in running events demonstrate both speed and economy in their movements. These movements can be scientifically described in a variety of ways. Principally they are to do with the temporal, kinematic and kinetic characteristics of the movement. This chapter will seek to provide an understanding of the running action from these points of view.

Descriptive and temporal characteristics of running

The running cycle is depicted in Figure 8.1, and can be divided into the flight and support phases. The flight phase begins at take-off (defined as the moment one leg leaves the ground) and ends at touch-down (defined as the moment that the opposite leg touches the ground). The support phase is the period between touch-down and take-off. The first third (approximately) of the support phase is termed impact, where the force of touch-down is absorbed. The latter third of the support phase is termed drive-off, where effort is expended to propel the body into the next stride. The arms move in opposition to the legs, such that when the right leg is brought forward, the right arm is taken backwards. The difference in the position of the take-off foot at take-off and the landing foot at touch-down is known as the step length, and the sum of two successive step lengths is known as the stride length. The time it takes for one step is the step time, but often its reciprocal (the step frequency) is the preferred term.

The running step can be characterized by the flight and support periods during which the body rises and falls in an oscillatory motion. It is also characterized by the step length and step frequency. These all vary as a function of speed, and are illustrated in Figure 8.2 and Table 8.1. It can be seen that a runner increases speed by increasing both the step length, through increasing the joint range of motion, and the step frequency, by more rapid movements.

There is a physical limit to the range of motion and hence the step length, which is illustrated by a tendency for the step length to reach a plateau at higher running speeds (Dillman, 1975; Luhtanen and Komi, 1978). As running speed is determined by the product of step length and step frequency, in order to run faster still the runner must increase the

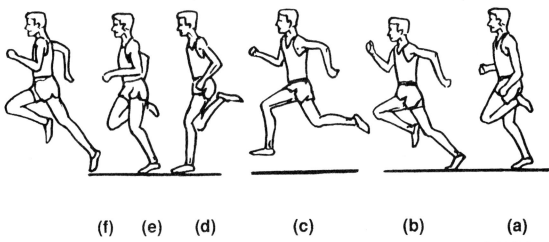

    (f)   **(e)**   **(d)**   **(c)**   **(b)**   **(a)**

Figure 8.1 Various positions of the body during the running cycle from (a) mid-support, (b) take-off, (c) flight, (d) touch-down, (e) mid-support and (f) take-off again. The action is depicted going from right to left

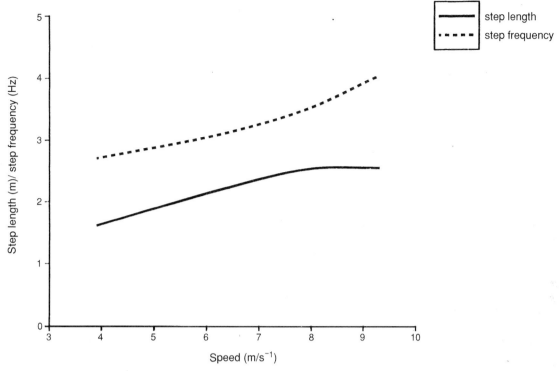

Figure 8.2 Changes in step length and step frequency as a function of running speed

step frequency, which rises more rapidly at higher speeds. As the step frequency increases, the cycle time reduces, but so too does the period of support. This reduces not only in absolute terms (reflecting the reduction in cycle time), but also as a proportion of the cycle time.

The physical effort required to propel the body forwards is produced during the support phase. If the time of this is reduced in both absolute and relative terms, then it can be appreciated that considerably more physical effort is required as speed increases. This is reflected in the average force generated at increasing speeds (see Table

8.4). The reduction in the oscillation of the centre of mass and the reduced flight time reflects the emphasis placed on driving forwards, rather than upwards, to increase running speed.

It might be expected that step length is related to body height and also sex, as females are generally shorter than males. Many studies have reported positive relationships (Dillman, 1975) supporting this idea, although others have been more equivocal (Williams, 1985).

Other descriptive aspects of the running action are to do with foot placement. In order to maintain balance, the support leg is adducted so that the foot

Table 8.1 Temporal changes in cycle time and support time for different speeds of running (from Luhtanen and Komi, 1978)

Speed (ms⁻¹)	Rise of step (mm)	Step length (cm)	Step frequency (Hz)	Cycle time (ms)	Flight time (ms)	Support time (ms)
3.9	109	1.6	2.7	380	180	200
6.4	86	2.2	3.1	320	180	140
8.0	70	2.5	3.5	280	160	120
9.3	67	2.5	4.0	230	130	100

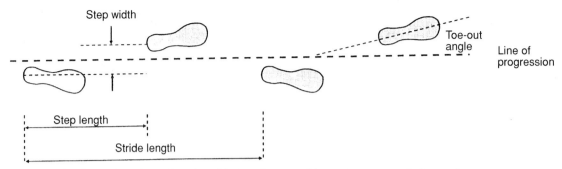

Figure 8.3 An illustration of step length, stride length, step width and toe-out angle in running

is placed underneath the body. However, it is not always placed exactly on the line of progression, and the distance between foot placements is referred to as the step width (Figure 8.3). In addition, the foot is placed on the ground in a position of abduction, giving foot placement a characteristic 'toe-out' angle which can typically be up to 10° (Cavanagh *et al.*, 1985; Williams, 1985).

The support phase begins at touch-down, when the foot makes first contact with the ground. The support leg is adducted and the foot is generally held in a supinated and dorsiflexed position, which means that the lateral heel of the foot makes first contact with the ground. Most people (around 80 per cent) run in this way, and are described as heel strikers. However, some runners have a tendency to plantar flex at touch-down, and this causes them to strike the ground first with the front of the foot. These runners are described as fore-foot strikers. An intermediate classification is mid-foot strikers, which describes those who make first contact with the lateral middle portion of the foot.

There are several factors that might cause people to run in these ways. Some runners have slightly shortened calf muscles, which leads to a natural plantar flexed ankle position, and so they will have a tendency to be a fore-foot striker. Others may have a muscle imbalance around the ankle joint leading to more pronounced ankle plantar flexion prior to touch-down. While rear-foot strikers are in the majority, it is found that, as running speed increases, there is a tendency to make first contact further towards the front of the foot, perhaps as a reflex mechanism to protect the body from the hard impact with the ground generated at higher speeds. Faster runners are more likely to be mid- or fore-foot strikers (Williams, 1985).

Kinematics of running

Running is a three-dimensional (3D) activity, but because it produces essentially linear motion, analyses have focused primarily on its two-dimensional (2D) characteristics. These characteristics have been expressed in the sagittal and frontal planes.

Sagittal plane kinematics

Most running analyses have focused on the angular changes associated with the lower limb segments and joints. Care must be taken in interpreting these angles, as their definitions frequently change from investigator to investigator. Typically, the angles for which data are given are the ankle and knee joints, and the thigh segments. The latter is chosen in preference to the hip joint because defining it is complicated by the difficulty of locating satisfactory standard landmarks on the trunk, and there has been little agreement in the literature between ranges of motion of the hip and thigh (Milliron and Cavanagh, 1990). These angles are also described in relation to the key temporal events in the running cycle – touch-down and take-off – and a typical graph is given in Figure 8.4.

These data show the range of motion of the joints, and also their relative phasing. It can be seen that the knee joint begins to flex before contact with the ground, providing an opportunity for the leg to absorb the shock of impact. The knee then extends, but begins to flex again just before take-off. The ankle joint usually plantar flexes at contact, resulting from heel strike, but is then quickly dorsiflexed. The subsequent dorsiflexion of the ankle joint reflects the movement of the body over the foot. The ankle is rapidly plantar flexed again during the drive off.

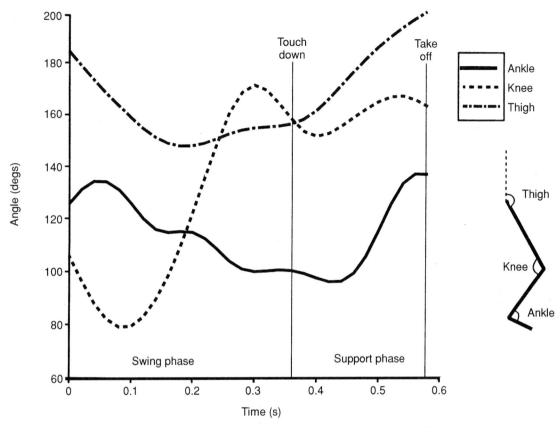

Figure 8.4 Typical angle time changes for the ankle, knee and thigh during running. The angular convention used is also illustrated

The hip begins in a position of flexion, but its direction of motion is one of extension and shows no further flexion in response to impact with the ground. It continues to extend during the shock absorption phase of support, and then extends more rapidly in the latter part of the support phase before flexing just before take-off. It can be seen then that each joint has its function. The knee provides shock absorption and contributes to the drive off, the hip drives the body over the support leg, and the ankle provides the support and the final drive.

The plantar flexion angle of the ankle joint increases with speed, reflecting the greater use of the ankle joint and lower leg muscles. The knee is flexed slightly at touch-down, and goes through a

Table 8.2 Angular ranges of motion (in degrees) at the ankle, knee and hip for different speeds of running (from Milliron and Cavanagh, 1990)

	Ankle		Knee			Thigh		
Running speed (ms⁻¹)	Dorsiflexion at TD	Plantar flexion at TO	Flexion at TD	Flexion post-impact	ROM	Maximum flexion	Maximum extension	ROM
3.4 slow	89	116	167	140	27	141	201	60
4.2 medium	88	121	164	140	23	139	203	64
5.0 fast	87	123	164	137	27	133	208	74

ROM = range of motion, TD = touch-down, TO = take-off

range of motion to absorb impact. However, this does not seem to be related to running speed, suggesting that other mechanisms for shock absorption must be used as speed increases. The smaller flexion angle of the thigh at higher speeds represents higher knee lift as running speed increases. The fairly constant extension angle is probably a reflection that the hip joint is at the limit of its range of motion.

The phase difference between joint angles is difficult to appreciate when presented as time histories. To overcome this, it is common to present angular changes as angle–angle diagrams, which allow the joint changes and their phasing during the whole cycle to be seen at a glance. This has particular significance for clinical applications of gait analysis. A typical angle–angle diagram is given in Figure 8.5 for the knee and thigh. Milliron and Cavanagh (1990) have demonstrated how these angular pictures can change dramatically as a function of uphill or downhill running on a treadmill.

Of equal importance, but less well researched, is the arm action. It has already been noted above that the arm action is contralaterally symmetrical with leg action, and has several functions. Good arm action leads to balanced running by countering the angular momentum produced by the legs. The arms are observed to rotate not only about the mediolateral axis of the trunk but also about its longitudinal axis. These two rotations help to balance the equal and opposite rotations produced by the legs. The arm action increases in its vigour as the running speed becomes faster, illustrating the importance of close coupling between arm and leg actions. The arm action also has one further benefit, in that the upward motion of the arms can be used to help lift the body off the ground. Hinrichs *et al.* (1987) have shown that this lift is small (about 2 per cent) but significant, and

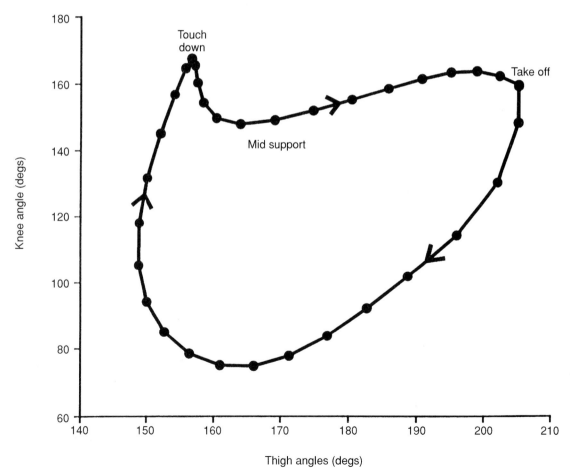

Figure 8.5 Typical angle–angle diagrams for the knee and thigh during running

happens because both arms are rising at the same time, even though one is moving forwards and upwards while the other is moving backwards and upwards. It is because of this opposition of movement that the arms are unable to provide any net contribution to forward drive.

Other observations in the running action which occur as a function of speed are the vigour, range of motion and degree of flexion at the knee and elbow joints. It has already been remarked that, as speed increases, the limbs go through a greater range of motion. In order to achieve this the limbs must be brought forwards more rapidly and, to do this, the limbs are flexed at the knee or elbow respectively. This flexing action serves to reduce their 'moment of inertia', and makes rotation about the hip and shoulder joints easier. Consequently, the limbs can be brought through more quickly, enabling them to travel further and producing a greater range of motion. This higher speed of movement also leads to a quicker recovery and a shorter cycle time, thus providing the basis for the increase in cycle frequency required at the higher speeds of running.

A characteristic of high speed running and sprinting is the high degree of flexion at the knee and the closeness of the foot to the buttock as the leg is brought through during recovery. As running has contralateral symmetry, the action of one limb can help the other. A vigorous and rapid arm action, through the principle of conservation of angular momentum, can help to drive the opposite leg in the same direction.

Williams *et al.* (1991) investigated the effects of fatigue on a range of 29 kinematic descriptors, the fatigue being induced by a 5000 m run. However, although they did find some small changes in stride length and hip and knee angles during the swing phase, all other variables investigated did not change significantly. It would appear that, in trained athletes, this fatiguing protocol was not sufficient to have an effect on their movement patterns.

Hamilton (1993) has found a kinematic approach useful in studying the effects of age on sprinting performance. She found, as expected, that sprinting speed reduced with age, but while it reduced gradually from the age of 30 to 70 years (8.9 to 7.0 ms⁻¹), it declined much more rapidly from 70 to 90 years (7.0 to 4.9 ms⁻¹). Other kinematic variables measured followed this trend. She concluded that men and women are less able to exert force with age, and that they have a decreased ability to move quickly through a full range of lower extremity motion.

Frontal plane kinematics

A study of movement in the frontal plane enables characteristics of rear-foot motion to be investigated. On contact with the ground, the foot is generally supinated. Immediately after contact, the foot is forced into a position of pronation. The range of motion and the extent of pronation have been of interest to researchers for some time because these characteristics have been thought to be associated with a variety of running injuries. While epidemiological studies have implicated excessive rear-foot motion in various running injuries, a specific cause and effect link remains elusive (Nigg *et al.*, 1995). Nevertheless there is a need to manage abnormal foot motion characteristics, and health care professionals (podiatrists, physiotherapists) have a major role to play.

Rear-foot motion is conventionally measured from a two-dimensional rear view of the lower leg. Figure 8.6 illustrates a typical position of the foot at touch-down and during a position of maximum pronation. The angle made by the lines on the shoe and the lower leg are used to indicate the angle of pronation. Strictly, this view gives the eversion angle of the foot, but as it is the major contributor to the pronation angle, the two are often used synonymously. The change in rear-foot angle with time is given in Figure 8.7. It can be seen that the greatest change takes place in the first part of the support phase. It can therefore be appreciated that the pronation of the foot at contact is a mechanism for shock absorption, and complements that of the knee described above. The angular changes are fairly accurately measured during the early part of

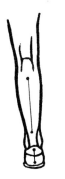 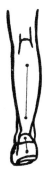

Touch-down   Maximum pronation

Figure 8.6 Typical position of the right foot and leg at touch-down (left diagram) and at maximum pronation (right diagram)

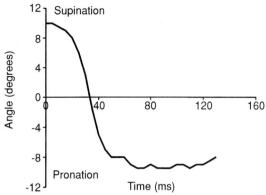

Figure 8.7 Typical rear-foot angle changes during the early part of the support phase, illustrating the rapid change from supination to pronation, after touch-down (time = 0). Take-off occurs at about 200 ms

the support phase but, due to a changing perspective from the two-dimensional view, the data become increasingly less accurate beyond about 50 per cent of the support phase.

Rear-foot changes have been studied in some detail. Edington *et al.* (1990) summarized data from a wide range of studies with most using running speeds between about 3.8–4.5 ms^{-1}, which constitutes a comfortable running speed for trained runners. The mean data for several footwear conditions are given in Table 8.3.

It can be seen from this survey that the running shoe has the effect of increasing the touch-down angle and, as a result, the total range of motion. There is little evidence to suggest that the shoe increases the angle of maximum pronation. Similarly, and contrary to popular belief, there is little evidence that the use of orthoses significantly reduces these angular measures. These results can be understood by remembering that the angular changes are generally very small, and are difficult to measure accurately. It is for this reason that new automatic three-dimensional methods of

measurement are being used to collect data accurately, quickly, and to test a variety of different situations.

Three-dimensional studies

The advent of rapid three-dimensional data collection systems has renewed interest in studying the kinematic characteristics of running. These systems have been available for some time, and have been applied extensively in the study of walking. In contrast, their application to running is still fairly new with only a small number of published studies. Most have been concerned with adequately defining the three-dimensional kinematics of rear-foot motion.

An early study of the three-dimensional motion of the ankle joint was reported by Taunton *et al.* (1985). This study used a mechanically linked triplanar goniometer to measure separately the angles of eversion, abduction and flexion at the ankle joint. They were able to identify differences as small as two degrees in the eversion angle when an orthosis was used. Gheluwe *et al.* (1995) investigated rear-foot movement using an optoelectronic system, and reported little difference between the pronation angle of the subtalar joint when calculated as a full 3D angle and the 2D inversion and eversion angle projected onto the frontal plane. Although this does not verify the accuracy of 2D data, it does confirm that the inversion–eversion angle used in 2D studies is a good predictor of pronation, as is assumed in 2D studies.

Mossley *et al.* (1996) used a video-based system to obtain data on the inversion–eversion, abduction–adduction and flexion–extension angles of the foot during running. Their analysis enabled these three angles to be quantified throughout the whole cycle, and not just the initial part of the support phase as is possible in 2D studies. They also reported that the change from inversion to

Table 8.3 Mean data from several studies for maximum pronation angle, touch-down angle and total range of motion, for different footwear conditions (from Edington *et al.*, 1990)

Activity	Touch-down supination angle (°)	Maximum pronation angle (°)	Total range of motion (°)
Bare foot	1.9	8.8	10.7
Running shoes	7.3	9.6	16.9
Running shoes with orthosis	6.3	9.5	15.8

eversion after touch-down occurred more gradually than indicated by 2D studies. It is likely that many more studies of this type will be conducted in the near future, giving a greater insight into the 3D nature of foot and ankle joint motion.

Kinetics of running

Progression during running is possible due to the generation of muscular force, which is applied against the ground. This force is generated in the muscles, acts around and across the joints and is transmitted to the ground in order to support the body during the support phase as well as to supply the necessary force for the drive-off into the next stride. The characteristics of the ground reaction force contain a wealth of information about how this action is conducted. It is possible, by using sophisticated biomechanical techniques, to estimate the forces acting through muscles and around joints. These data give a more detailed picture of how the running action takes place.

Ground reaction forces

The ground reaction force is measured by a force platform, which is capable of measuring forces along three orthogonal axes. The running action is performed so that the three measurement planes of

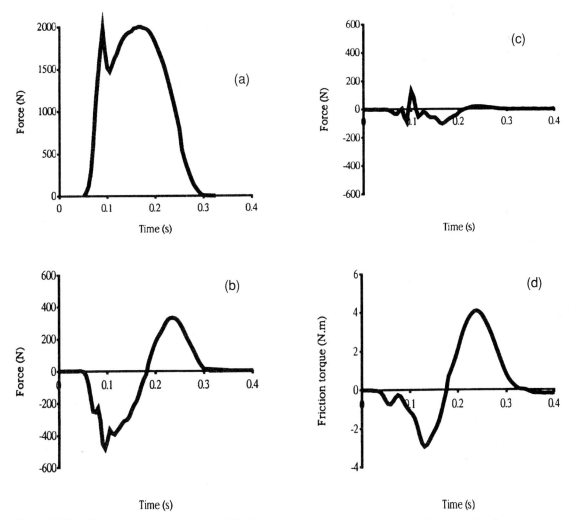

Figure 8.8 The three force components and friction torque for a typical runner who has a heel-strike technique. ((a) = vertical, (b) = anterior–posterior, (c) = medio–lateral, and (d) = friction torque (or free moment))

the force platform correspond to the vertical (longitudinal), anterior–posterior and medio–lateral axes of the body, and thus forces are reported which act on the body in these directions. A typical ground reaction force directed along each axis is given in Figure 8.8. It can be seen that the largest component is that of the vertical force, while the smallest is that of the medio–lateral force. Although it is conventional to represent the vertical force as positive, the sign of the other force curves is arbitrary and reflects the direction in which the subject is travelling over the force platform. These have to be interpreted in relation to the action as outlined below.

The vertical force component (Figure 8a) for a heel striker has two major peaks. The first peak is associated with initial contact at touch-down, and is often described as the impact peak. As the body undergoes controlled collapse to absorb the shock of impact, the force curve demonstrates a trough. This gives way to a second peak, which is produced by a combination of the loading of the body onto the ground and the drive into the next stride, and is termed the active or drive-off peak. This force curve is characterized by the magnitudes of each peak, their load rates, and the impulse (obtained by computing the area under the force time curve).

The anterior–posterior force component (Figure 8b) is characterized by a negative followed by a positive phase. The negative phase represents the braking force generated as the foot is stretched out in preparation for the touch-down, while the positive phase represents the propulsion force developed as the hip joint extends rapidly during the drive-off phase. Although there are changes in the initial negative part of the curve, these are associated with the absorption of shock, more readily seen in the vertical force curve above.

The medio–lateral force curve (Figure 8c) is the smallest of the three force components, and is also the most difficult to interpret. It has a predominantly negative phase followed by a positive phase. The general interpretation of these data is that, as the foot is brought inwards to the line of progression, a force is generated which slows the foot's motion. During the second half of the contact phase the foot, being angled outwards, has a propulsive element in the outwards medio–lateral direction, and therefore the interpretation is essentially the same as for the anterior–posterior force curves. McClay and Cavanagh (1994) have shown that, in exaggerated running, the medio–lateral force increases negatively if the foot crosses over the line of progression (to give a negative step width) but is positive if the foot is kept to the same side of the line of progression (to give a positive step width). There has been some speculation that the initial peak in the medio–lateral force curve may be related to the degree of pronation in rearfoot motion. There have been several investigations but none of them have established a clear link between these two variables, and Miller (1990) doubts that any such link in principle exists.

Another variable that can be measured by the force platform is the friction torque (or free moment) about the vertical axis (Figure 8d). This shows a characteristic negative phase during the early part of the contact, followed by a positive phase. The friction torque represents the twist applied by the foot to the ground, and this twist occurs due to rotation of the foot and leg as it is bought into position for heel strike. Again, during the drive-off phase, the leg is caused not only to be driven backwards and outwards, as described above, but also twists outwards as well. This is a most important characteristic of locomotion, but one that is rarely reported. Nigg (1986) has shown that the magnitude of the friction torque in running is about 4 Nm in each direction. Holden and Cavanagh (1991) investigated the relationship between the magnitude of friction torque and degree of pronation. They reduced the range of pronation of their subjects by making them wear shoes with a varus wedge, and increased it with a valgus wedge. They found that the friction torque produced by subjects in shoes with no wedge was about 6 Nm, largely agreeing with Nigg (1986), but was reduced to 3 Nm in the varus shoes and increased to 10 Nm in the valgus shoes. These data suggest that there is an important link between the degree of pronation and the twisting effect that acts on the foot and leg during the stance phase.

Running speed has been shown to affect ground reaction force variables. Nigg (1986) has found that the impact peak increased from 1100 N at 3.0 ms^{-1} to 1800 N at 6.0 ms^{-1}. Interestingly, he found that the magnitude of the drive-off peak (1800 N) did not change as a function of speed. With regard to the anterior–posterior component of force, Nigg reported that the propulsive force increased as running speed increased. It would appear that, in order to run faster, a greater force must be applied in the forward direction, and that the vertical force has a support function only. In contrast, Munro *et al.* (1987) reported increases in all ground reaction force variables with speed (Table 8.4). Their data would suggest that, to

Table 8.4 Changes in ground reaction force variables with speed (from Munro *et al.*, 1987)

Speed (ms⁻¹)	Mean force (BW)	Peak impact force (BW)	Drive off force (BW)	Load rate (BWs⁻¹)	Braking impulse (BWs⁻¹)	Propulsion impulse (BWs⁻¹)
3.0	1.40	1.57	2.51	77	−0.15	0.14
4.0	1.57	1.95	2.72	90	−0.21	0.21
5.0	1.70	2.32	2.83	199	−0.25	0.25

increase speed, runners need to increase both their vertical and horizontal forces.

Running style affects ground reaction force variables. Fore-foot strikers no longer exhibit an impact peak in the vertical direction. The force at impact continues to grow steadily, and merges with the loading and drive-off peak (peak 2 in Figure 8a). The impact peak load rate is considered as a measure of 'shock' applied to the body (Hennig *et al.*, 1993). Lees (1990) has obtained data on load rates for running at various speeds using heel strikers and fore-foot strikers. The load rate increased rapidly with speed, from $50\,\text{kNs}^{-1}$ at $2.0\,\text{ms}^{-1}$ to $300\,\text{kNs}^{-1}$ at $6.0\,\text{ms}^{-1}$. At these high load rates subjects chose to modify their running action and adopted a fore-foot strike style, which had the effect of reducing the load rate. The change to fore-foot striking was a mechanism for reducing the shock on the musculo-skeletal system at high running speeds. A reduction in shock can also be achieved by using suitably made running shoes with shock-absorbing material in the heel of the shoe. These are not as effective as the fore-foot as a shock reduction mechanism, but can be beneficial (Lees, 1990).

Body weight is another factor affecting the severity of the impact peak and its load rate. Frederick and Hagy (1986) reported that these two variables were significantly higher in heavier than in lighter individuals. Heavy individuals run the danger of 'bottoming out' in their running shoes, leading to the possibility of even higher impact forces.

Joint moments

The force data referred to above and the kinematic data discussed earlier may be combined to compute the net moments acting about each joint (Winter, 1990). The net joint moments are considered to reflect the general muscular effort generated about each joint. A typical pattern of net joint moments is given in Figure 8.9. After touch-down there is generally a positive (extension) moment acting around the knee and a positive (plantar flexion) moment acting around the ankle, which continue throughout the support phase. Some authors (e.g. Buzeck and Cavanagh, 1990; Czerniecki *et al.* 1991) report a small negative (dorsiflexion) moment around the ankle at the

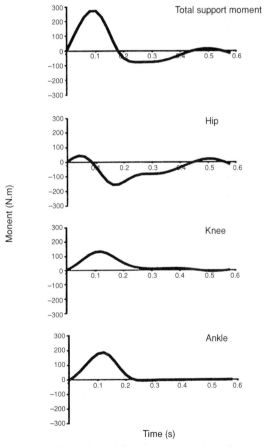

Figure 8.9 Typical net joint moments and total support moment for running from touch-down (time = 0) to take-off (time = 0.2 s) to touch-down again (time = 0.58 s). Extension moments at the hip, knee and ankle are positive

beginning of the touch-down phase, which resists forced plantar flexion at heel strike, and a small negative (flexion) moment around the knee at the end of the stance phase, which is probably an influence from the hip through the two joint muscles acting around both joints. The hip characteristically shows a positive (extension) moment at the beginning of the support phase, which then generally becomes a negative (flexion) moment. This has the effect of driving the body over the support leg in the early part of the stance phase but then slowing and reversing the backward angular rotation of the thigh in the latter stance phase. The flexion moment indicates that the hip musculature contributes little to the final drive into the flight phase. Ankle moments are typically reported to be between 150 and 200 Nm, knee moments between 200 and 250 Nm and hip extension and flexion moments between 50 and 150 Nm for each direction.

These data vary between subjects because individuals vary with regard to their preferred movement style. Some may use muscles of one joint more than another, giving rise to a subtly different movement pattern. In order to overcome this, Winter (1989) has used the total support moment to characterize the effort produced in the movement. This has been useful in the analysis of walking, and would appear to have similar benefits for the interpretation of data for running.

The power produced at the joints is computed from the net joint moment and the angular velocity of the joint. Typically, there is a power absorption at each joint at touch-down. The knee absorbs the most power (over 1000 W), indicating its role in shock absorption at touch-down. In the running action power is generated mainly at the hip and the ankle, which generate up to 1000 W each during drive-off, indicating the importance of the musculature about each of these joints. The knee tends to absorb power throughout the whole of the stance phase, again reflecting the fact that it is not a major contributor to the running action (Robertson, 1987).

It is of interest to know what forces act in muscles and across joints. These data can be used in a variety of ways to extend our knowledge of the operation of the musculoskeletal system, but a main stimulus is to obtain data which might be linked to injury in a cause-and-effect way. Although this goal has yet to be realized (Nigg and Bobbert, 1990), the approach is challenging to biomechanists. In order to obtain muscle and joint forces, a bioengineering approach is required. This uses the kinematic and kinetic data referred to above, but also requires a mathematical model of the lower limbs of the musculo-skeletal system. Harrison *et al.* (1986) implemented such a system and reported that, during running at $4.5 \, \text{ms}^{-1}$, muscle forces could be as high as seven times body weight in the gastrocnemius and 22 times body weight in the quadriceps, and that the maximum compressive forces across the knee could be as high as 33 times body weight. These extremely high forces around the knee explain why it is so frequently the site of injury in runners.

Clinical significance

Not only is running a popular activity in itself, but it is also a basis for performance in most sports. An increasing number of sports people are seeking medical advice and treatment for the injuries they sustain. A large number of these injuries are of the overuse type, and of these the vast majority are associated with some locomotor defect which occurs during running. A precursor to issuing medical advice and treatment is identification of the probable cause of injury. Although this can be a time-consuming process, the availability of dedicated gait labs and the need for more specialist advice means that an analysis of running to help in the diagnosis and treatment of running injuries is becoming commonplace. Many podiatrists and biomechanists already operate in this way.

Any assessment of running in relation to injury should be preceded by an activity history questionnaire, including recent training background, in order to identify training errors as a possible cause. Similarly, a skeletal alignment examination should be made to identify any alignment deficiencies (James and Jones, 1990). An inspection of the running footwear is invaluable in detecting certain problems. A visual inspection of the running style can be informative in identifying any immediate problems. Gait asymmetries are more noticeable during running and, if these are not visually obvious, a video recording might reveal differences in support time, step lengths or between left and right legs. Cavanagh *et al.* (1985) described an approach to the biomechanical profiling of runners that follows this general outline.

Kinematic analysis can be most useful for the investigation of rear foot motion. This technique, combined with the use of ground reaction forces, can give information about the severity of impact. Perry and LaFortune (1995) investigated both of these variables together and found that, if the range of pronation was restricted, there was an increase in the ground reaction force at impact. Interestingly, the reverse did not seem to apply. They speculated that if a patient was given an orthosis to relieve, for example, knee pain, the reduced range of pronation might actually lead to a worsening of the condition due to the higher forces generated. This very important interaction needs further careful investigation to ensure that the use of intervention techniques is appropriate for an individual.

Gait laboratories may be furnished with more sophisticated equipment than that used for clinical diagnosis. These allow the possibility for conducting original research projects that will in turn contribute to the development of expertise and to the process of injury assessment and treatment evaluation.

References

Buzeck, F. L. and Cavanagh, P. R. (1990). Stance phase knee and ankle kinematics and kinetics during level and downhill running. *Med. Sci. Sports Exer.*, **22**, 669–77.

Cavanagh, P. R., Andrew, G. C., Kram, R. *et al.* (1985). An approach to biomechanical profiling of elite distance runners. *Int. J. Sports Biomech.*, **1**, 36–62.

Czerniecki , J. M., Gitter, A and Munro, C. (1991). Joint moment and muscle power output characteristics of below knee amputees during running: the influence of energy storing prosthetic feet. *J. Biomech.*, **24**, 63–75.

Dillman, C. J. (1975). Kinematic analysis of running. *Exer. Sports Sci. Rev.*, **3**, 193–218.

Edington, C., Frederick, E. C. and Cavanagh, P. R. (1990). Rear-foot motion in distance running. In *Biomechanics of Distance Running* (P. R. Cavanagh, ed.). Human Kinetics.

Frederick, E. C. and Hagy, J. L. (1986). Factors affecting peak vertical ground reaction forces in running. *Int. J. Sports Biomech.*, **2**, 41–9.

Gheluwe, B. Van, Tielemans, R. and Roosen, P. (1995). The influence of heel counter rigidity on rear-foot motion during running. *J. Appl. Biomech.*, **11**, 47–67.

Hamilton, N. (1993). Changes in sprint stride kinematics with age in master's athletes. *J. Appl. Biomech.*, **9**, 15–26.

Harrison, R. N., Lees, A., McCullagh, P. and Rowe, W. B. (1986). A bioengineering analysis of human muscle and joint forces in the lower limb during running. *J. Sports Sci.*, **4**, 207–18.

Hennig, E. W., Milani, T. L. and Lafortune, M. A. (1993). Use of ground reaction force parameters in predicting peak tibial accelerations in running. *J. Appl. Biomech.*, **9**, 306–14.

Hinrichs, R. N., Cavanagh, P. R. and Williams, K. R. (1987). Upper extremity function in running 1: Centre of mass and propulsion considerations. *Int. J. Sport Biomech.*, **3**, 222–41.

Holden, J. P. and Cavanagh, P. R. (1991). The free moment of ground reaction in distance running and its change with pronation. *J. Biomech.*, **24**, 887–97.

James, S. L. and Jones, D. C. (1990). Biomechanical aspects of distance running injuries. In *Biomechanics of Distance Running* (P. R. Cavanagh, ed.). Human Kinetics.

Lees, A. (1990). The mechanical load on the body during sports and exercise. In *Synopsis of Sports Medicine and Sports Science*, Vol II. (K.M. Chan and F. H. Fu, eds.). The Chinese University.

Luhtanen, P. and Komi, P. V. (1978). Mechanical factors influencing running speed. In *Biomechanics VI-B* (E. Asmussen and K. Jorgensen, eds.). University Park Press.

McClay, I. S. and Cavanagh, P. R. (1994). Relationship between foot placement and mediolateral ground reaction forces during running. *Clin. Biomech.*, **9**, 117–23.

Miller, D. I. (1990) Ground reaction forces in distance running. In *Biomechanics of Distance Running* (P. R. Cavanagh, ed.). Human Kinetics.

Milliron, J. M. and Cavanagh, P. R. (1990). Sagittal plane kinematics of the lower extremity during distance running. In *Biomechanics of Distance Running* (P. R. Cavanagh, ed.). Human Kinetics.

Mossley, L. Smith, R., Hunt, A. and Grant, R. (1996). Three-dimensional kinematics of the rear-foot during the stance phase of walking in normal and young adult males. *Clin. Biomech.*, **11**, 39–45.

Munro, C. F., Miller, D. I. and Fuglevand, A. J. (1987). Ground reaction forces in running: A re-examination. *J. Biomech.*, **20**, 147–55.

Nigg, B. M. (editor) (1986). *Biomechanics of Running Shoes*. Human Kinetics.

Nigg. B. M. and Bobbert, M. (1990). On the potential of various approaches in load analysis to reduce the frequency of sports injuries. *J. Biomech.* **23 (suppl. 1)**, 3–12.

Nigg, B. M., Cole, G. K. and Bruggemann, G.-P. (1995). Impact forces during heel-toe running. *J. Appl. Biomech.*, **11**, 407–32.

Perry, S. D. and LaFortune, M. A. (1995). Influences of inversion/eversion of the foot upon impact loading during locomotion. *Clin. Biomech.*, **10**, 253–7.

Robertson, D. G. E. (1987). Functions of the leg muscles during the stance phase of running. In *Biomechanics X-B* (B. Jonsson, ed.), pp. 1021–7. Human Kinetics.

Taunton, J. E., Clement, D. B., Smart, G. W. *et al.* (1985). A triplanar electrogoniometer investigation of running mechanics in runners with compensatory overpronation. *Can. J. Appl. Sports Sci.*, **10**, 104–15.

Williams, K. R. (1985). Biomechanics of running. *Exer. Sports Sci. Rev.*, **13**, 389–441.

Williams, K. R., Snow, R. and Agruss, C. (1991). Changes in distance running kinematics with fatigue. *Int. J. Sport Biomech.*, **7**, 138–62.

Winter, D.A. (1990). *Biomechanics and Motor Control of Human Movement*, 2nd edn. Willey.

9 Jumping

A. C. Nicol

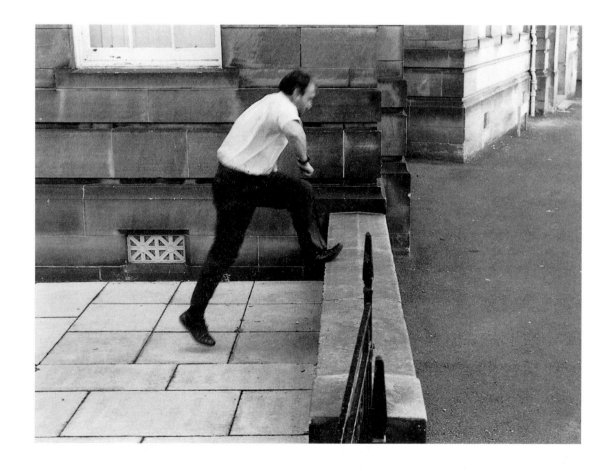

Introduction

During everyday activities it is sometimes necessary to reach higher for objects or to avoid obstacles by performing a jumping action. It is difficult to generate a specific definition of the action of jumping in order to cover both vertical jumps and horizontal leaps. Each of these activities will involve a period of time when the body is not in contact with the ground. To this end, jumping can be considered as a natural extension of running which, in turn, is a natural extension of locomotion.

While most of the research studies reported in the literature involved a sports viewpoint for the actions and training of athletes, this chapter will deal with the activity of jumping in an everyday context for human locomotion. The purpose is to build up a picture of the motion and forces involved in the action of jumping and then to lead into an analysis of possible muscle control and energy requirements for these activities. Vertical jumping actions will be covered first, and will be split into a vertical jump up with the return to the ground, followed by a drop landing which is equivalent to jumping off a chair or other high surface. The next section will deal with horizontal jumping, where an obstacle has to be cleared (e.g. wet ground or fragile materials on the floor).

Vertical jump

Much of the research into vertical jumping has concentrated on the training of athletes to maximize their performance, either in the high jump or in games such as volleyball and basketball. These jumps would normally require some aspect of pre-stretching of muscle structures in order to store elastic energy in the tendons. This type of action is usually not performed in everyday activities, and will therefore not be considered in this chapter.

Most studies involving jumping combine kinematic data (cine film or video) with force platform data (usually Kistler-type force platforms). These systems provide data on the motion of the segments of the body, and it is then possible to estimate the position of the whole body centre of mass. In addition, the ground reaction forces measured by the force platform will enable the calculation of moments at the ankle, knee and hip joint centres. Such information is useful for the estimation of muscular action and the eventual analysis of ligament and joint forces. In order to analyse a jump activity it is beneficial to begin with the description of the kinematics of the body segments.

For a vertical jump and landing sequence, the subject would usually begin in a vertical upright position and the jump activity would be initiated by a lowering of the centre of mass by hip and knee flexion. Figure 9.1 shows the sequence of events during this action, and it is possible for the hip centre to be lowered by 200 mm. The lower the centre of mass drops, the more distance is available for the push phase of the actual jump. As the body is accelerated upwards, the hips and knees extend with the generation of forces at the ground well in excess of 100 per cent body weight per foot (see Figure 9.2). Once the limbs are fully extended (including the ankle joint plantar flexion), the body lifts off and the flight phase commences.

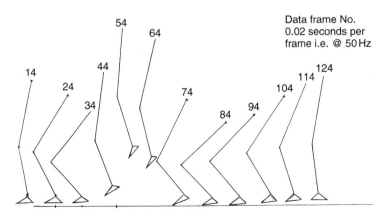

Figure 9.1 Stick diagram representation of the limb positions during jump up and down. The limb positions have been spread out from left to right, but the difference in time between each diagram is 0.2 s

Depending on the amount of work done by the muscles, the body will lose contact with the floor with a certain take-off velocity. This take-off velocity will be reduced by the action of gravitational acceleration ($9.81\,\mathrm{ms^{-2}}$), and a maximum height of the jump will be reached. Following this, the body will return to ground and the landing phase will be commenced. The initial strike of the foot on the floor will generate a very rapid rate of loading, and forces well in excess of 200 per cent of body weight will be experienced. The recovery of the body, once floor contact is made, means that the strike will be followed by a settling period until the subject becomes stationary in the upright vertical position.

Although it is possible to analyse the motion of the centre of mass of the body in terms of classical mechanics, one limitation of this procedure is that the location of the centre of mass at any one anatomical position is not fixed. As the hip and knee joints move, the centre of mass will move relative to the spine. As such, the classical mechanics assumption of a rigid body is not correct, and it would be necessary to investigate the position of each limb segment and to calculate a new position of the centre of mass for each sample of data. This is a specialized technique, and would be necessary for an accurate analysis for each individual within the population study.

For the purposes of this chapter, it is simpler to consider the motion of the trunk as being related closely to the motion of the centre of mass. To complement this, measurement of the vertical force between each foot and the ground gives the force applied in order to support the body under the action of gravity, to allow the body to lower in height, or to accelerate the body upwards in order to jump away from the ground. Such a record of force is shown in Figure 9.2, which shows the force on one foot. Total vertical force contributing to vertical acceleration of the body would, therefore, be double these values (assuming symmetrical distribution in the limbs). There are seven separate phases of this graph and these are as follows:

Phase 1: Area of the force graph below the line for half body weight (400 N) per foot means that the weight of the body is not being supported and that the body will accelerate downwards. At the end of this phase, the body will be moving with maximum downward velocity.

Phase 2: The second area is the deceleration of the downward velocity to stop the body at the lowest point prior to the jumping action. The lowest point of the centre of gravity motion occurs at the end of Phase 2, and the area enveloped by the curve shown hatched in areas 1 and 2 must be equal.

Phase 3: The large area and large forces above the half body weight line mean that the body will accelerate vertically upwards and, as such, area 3 is the main propulsive action for the jump activity.

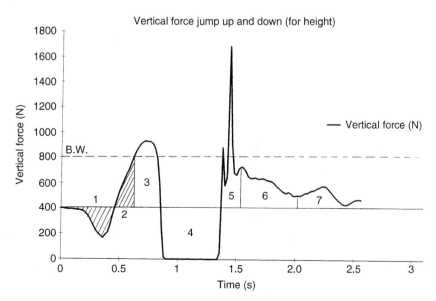

Figure 9.2 Vertical force applied to one foot during jump up and down

Once the force curve passes below half body weight, then there will be a small retardation to this upward acceleration before the end of Phase 3 at the instant of take-off.

Phase 4: When no force is applied to the floor, the body is not in contact and this is the flight phase. The duration of the flight phase is important since the body can be considered to be in free flight, and half the time of flight phase will be upward velocity and the second half will be the return to ground as downward velocity. It is therefore possible to calculate the height reached for the jump knowing the flight time and the value of gravitational acceleration as 9.81 ms^{-2}. **NB:** It is also possible to calculate the height reached by knowing the take-off velocity, which can be calculated using the area of stage 3. This area is the combination of force and time, which is the 'impulse' or change of momentum of the body. For the graph shown the flight time is 0.44 s, which would indicate a take-off velocity of 2.16 ms^{-1} and a height reached of 220 mm. Using the same graph, area 3 would produce an impulse of 203 Ns, which would give a take-off velocity of 2.5 ms^{-1}. It is usual to have a slight discrepancy between these two values because the motion of the human limb segments means that the assumption of a rigid body cannot be adhered to.

Phase 5: When the body lands on the ground, there is initial contact with the sole of the foot followed by a very rapid rise in force as the leg and the rest of the body decelerates rapidly from a downward velocity. Values of peak force well in excess of 2 × body weight are regularly obtained through each foot. The shape of Phase 5 is normally a sharp spike followed by a very rapid return to the end of the phase at some point around half body weight on each foot.

Phase 6: In order to recover height, the subject continues to apply a force in excess of half body weight per foot and the body accelerates upwards again.

Phase 7: This phase is the recovery to zero velocity, with the centre of mass usually coming close to the height for free standing and the force on each foot returning to half body weight (assuming symmetry of loading per foot).

The control of the landing is a very skilled process, and it is usual for non-athletic individuals to have extra phases as the fine control of the jump is finalized. Any force curve above the half body

weight line would indicate control of the mass upwards, whereas forces below the half body weight line would indicate 'overshoots', and would be required to allow the body to come back down to the centre of mass height. In the case of Figure 9.2 there is no 'overshoot'; in fact the forces continue to be greater than half body weight, indicating that the subject has not yet reached a steady position.

Much can be learned from this type of graph in terms of the motion of the body and, if kinematic data were also available, it would be possible to find the position of the force vector relative to the joints of the lower limb. Such a procedure is shown in Figure 9.3, where the stick diagram represents a subject at the lowest part of the pre-jumping activity (i.e. end of area 2 in Figure 9.2). If the vertical force of 924 N is applied at the foot, then the dotted line shows the 'line of action' of the force vector, which will pass through the centre of mass position provided no angular accelerations are incurred. Since the line of action does not pass through the ankle, knee or hip joint centres, the

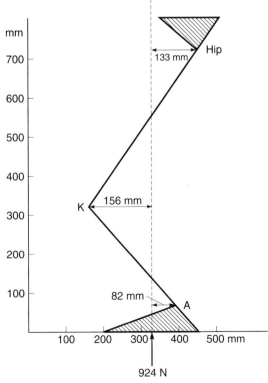

Figure 9.3 Limb position for the lowest height in the pre-jump phase of jump up and down. The vertical force of 924 N is applied at the mid-foot region

force will have an effect tending to flex/extend each of these joints. For example, the diagram would provide a leverage of 82, 156 and 133 mm at the ankle, knee and hip joints respectively. For a force of 924 N on each foot, this would infer moments of 75 Nm tending to dorsiflex the ankle, 152 Nm to flex the knee and 123 Nm to flex the hip.

Taking this procedure a step further, it is possible to calculate the moments at these joints throughout the whole sequence of the activity. Figure 9.4 shows a typical graph of hip, knee and ankle flexion/extension moments for a non-athletic male (age 46 years and mass 80 kg) jumping with arms by the side to obtain a reasonable height.

One point of note is that the landing phase generates very high rates of loading on to the force platform. Since the structure of the force platform will not be totally rigid, there will be a distortion of the top plate of the platform, as well as secondary distortions of the measurement devices and the base of the force platform.

Much work has been done to investigate the frequency response characteristics of such force platforms, and it is generally accepted that natural frequencies in excess of 500 Hz must be used for this type of study. If a force platform is used with a much lower natural frequency (e.g. 100 Hz) it is possible to generate transients of vibration of the elements of the force platform device, which will generate apparent upward forces that will be seen as negative forces applied to the foot. These transients are extremely difficult to isolate, and it is to be recommended that jump activities only be performed on force platforms with high natural frequencies.

To take the analysis one stage further, it is possible to combine the joint moments with the motion of the joints by multiplying moment with angular velocity. The units generated would be Nm and radians per second, which give a total unit of Nms^{-1} (a radian is unitless). This combined unit is the same quantity as power, and can be useful to indicate the contribution from muscles to the activity being studied. For the subject shown in Figure 9.4, the angular position of the limb can be used to calculate the angular velocity in radians per second. Combining these figures it is possible to generate the power, and the maximum power generated for the jump phase was calculated to be 1115 W at the knee and 350 W at the hip joint. It is not possible for human beings to generate this level of power continuously; therefore, there will be a combination of impulsive stored energy and impulsive muscle contraction. This type of research is covered by papers such at Watkins and Nicol (1986), Davies (1971) and Komi and Bosco (1978). The power values are very interesting (2000 W for the knee and 2400 W for the hip), but during landing the impact nature of the activity means that it is unlikely that the muscles can react quickly enough to generate a balance to the initial

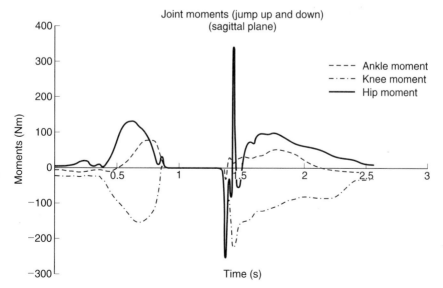

Figure 9.4 The flexion/extension moments at ankle, knee and hip joints during the jump up and down

high rate of loading. Denoth *et al.* (1984) have estimated that very little contribution from muscular contraction can be obtained in the first 30 ms of the landing.

In this connection, it is natural to consider how individual subjects and athletes can protect themselves from an overload situation during the high rate of loading in landing. This topic involves the question of style of landing, especially the motion of the limbs in terms of 'absorption' of the kinetics of the activity. Some work has been done in studying athletic adaptation for different surfaces and different heights of jump (see Panzer, 1988 and McNitt-Gray, 1993), and this is of great importance for understanding the athlete's ability to avoid injury. For non-athletes, Thompson and McKinley (1995) have investigated the importance of visual information for landing strategies and concluded that lack of vision would result in other factors (approach velocity, surface hardness, etc.) providing possible alternative input for pre-landing muscle control.

Another interesting parameter for the control of jumping is the effect of two-joint muscles, such as gastrocnemius, hamstrings and rectus femoris. If one muscle can contract and provide equilibrium conditions at two joints, it must be more efficient in physiological terms than having two muscles to contract and balance the two joints. Unfortunately, the layout of the three-dimensional muscular geometry will probably involve antagonism and 100 per cent efficiency will, therefore, be unobtainable.

Drop landing

In order to increase the height of a vertical jump, the training schedules of athletes will involve a drop from a height in order to 'springboard' up to a higher height of jump. The landing from a drop is intended to store energy in the elastic elements of the musculoskeletal system. While this action is beneficial for the training of athletes, the landing aspect is also an activity that may be involved in everyday life. The heights of drops can vary from 200 mm up to 900 mm and above (Bosco and Komi, 1978, 1989; Bedi *et al.*, 1987; Kerwin and Challis, 1985; Aura and Viitasalo, 1989).

For everyday activities, the drop landing can either involve a 'hard' landing (where the knees and hips do not 'absorb' the energy of the drop) or they can involve a soft landing (where knee and hip flexion occurs in order to take up the action of the landing). Figure 9.5 shows the graphs of force for hard and soft landings from a height of 235 mm.

It is readily noticeable that the time for the hard landing is approximately one-half of that for the soft landing. The motion of the body is controlled differently for the two activities and this is

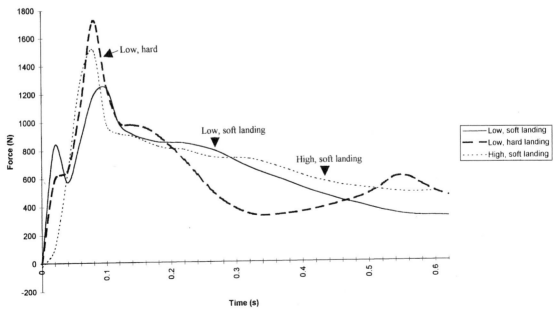

Figure 9.5 The vertical forces for landing from low and high heights

(a)

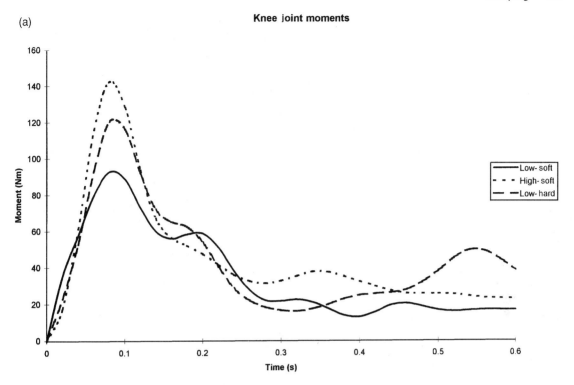

(b)

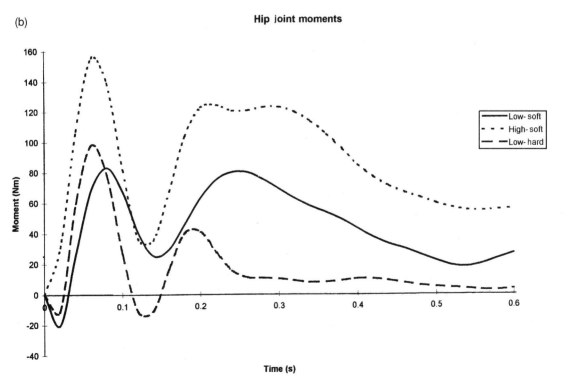

Figure 9.6 The flexion/extension moments at knee and hip joints for hard and soft landings from a low height, together with a soft landing from a large height (see text for details)

demonstrated in the values of flexion/extension moments at the hip and knee, where the hard landing generates knee moments around 120 Nm (see Figures 9.6a and b) compared to typical walking moments of 50–60 Nm.

When the drop landing height was increased to 600 mm, the forces and moments for a soft landing were also increased dramatically. The knee moment reached 150 Nm and the angle of knee flexion reached 120°. These data clearly show that the style of the landing will generate a large excursion of values for joint angle and joint moment, and the muscles will have to work accordingly. For large moments, it can be anticipated that the joint contact forces and ligament forces will also be large. For everyday activities it is necessary to anticipate the position of the ground when jumping down from a height, together with its consistency. If the ground

is hard concrete, it will be necessary to pre-empt the hardness of the landing by consciously landing with a large excursion of joint motion. On the other hand, if the ground is soft sand or mud, it will be possible to land with reasonably straight limbs and the ground will 'absorb' the energy by deformation and controlled force production. Unfortunately it is not always possible to pre-empt the landing phase and, for emergency landing, it is likely that very high loadings will be imposed on the structures of the limb.

Horizontal jumping

The previous sections have isolated the jumping activity only in terms of considering vertical force production. Since human life involves

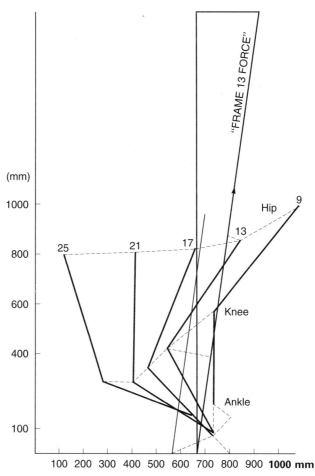

Figure 9.7 The stick diagram representation for the limb positions during landing from a large horizontal jump

three-dimensional environments, it would have been possible to look at horizontal forces applied to the foot during these 'vertical' jumping activities. Since the vertical jumps would generate very small horizontal components of jump, it is convenient to assume that these would be zero. For horizontal jumping, the horizontal force production will be a major component of the loadings onto the human limb. Various research papers have been published on the take-off forces in long-jump since the regulations for long jump mean that the foot has to hit a toe board, and this would be convenient for the correct placing of a force platform (see Hay *et al.*, 1977).

For a study of everyday horizontal jumping, the type of activities involved would include stepping over objects, hopping over obstructions and jumping over gaps and puddles to clear territory upon which the subject would not wish to step. In these circumstances it would be useful to investigate the forces and motion of the take-off and landing phases of the activity. To this end, data were collected specially for two distances of horizontal jump, the first being 0.925 m and the second being a running horizontal jump of 1.85 m. These distances correspond to 0.5 and 1.0 times the jumping subject's height.

During take-off the subject must generate an upward force to propel the body upwards, and the flight time will be critical for the distance covered.

The second parameter of importance is the take-off horizontal velocity, and the combination of horizontal velocity and flight time will dictate the distance travelled before landing. This therefore means that the subject must also produce a large horizontal force to propel the body with large horizontal take-off velocity. For the large leap (Figures 9.7 and 9.8) the body was travelling forward and, at take-off, generated a vertical force on the leg of approximately 1800 N, which corresponds to 2.5 × body weight. At the point of take off, the body's forward velocity was approximately 4 ms^{-1}. At the same time, a peak horizontal force of 250 N was also recorded. The knee and hip extended from a position of 50° flexion, and generated knee moments greater than 100 Nm and hip moments of approximately 200 Nm. These loadings are very high, and indicate the stressful nature of a one-legged jump take-off for a horizontal leap.

The landing forces for this leap were approximately 2.5 × body weight vertically and about 0.5 × body weight horizontally. As can be expected, the knee joint is a critical structure in accommodating the forces on landing on one leg, and very large moments of around 300 Nm were experienced (see Figure 9.9). Although these large moments are only applied for around a tenth of a second, the rate of loading on the structures at the knee, such as cruciate ligaments and patella tendon, can be excessive.

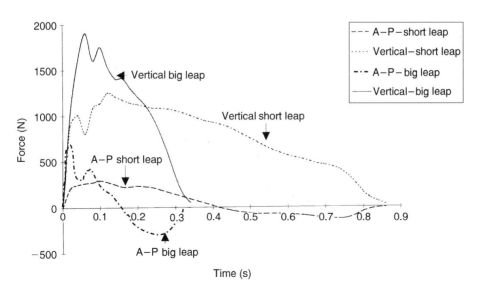

Figure 9.8 The vertical and horizontal anterior–posterior forces during the landing of a large leap (one body height length) and a short leap (half body length)

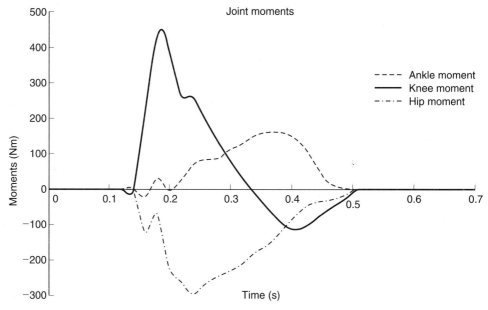

Figure 9.9 The flexion/extension moments at ankle, knee and hip joints for landing from a large horizontal leap

Discussion

Jumping is an activity that can be very complex in terms of the co-ordination of the joints of the lower limb and in the production of large ground reaction forces in both the vertical and horizontal directions. Research into the loading of internal structures, such as knee ligaments and joint cartilage, has mainly concentrated on walking activities for rehabilitation purposes. Unfortunately, jump activities cannot be analysed fully with the rather basic analytical methods used for walking. The rate of loading will necessitate non-linear modelling of soft tissues, and the short time duration of the events means that mathematical procedures used for joint force optimization are liable to become unstable.

It is therefore logical to compare the 'external' loading for jumping with that for walking, so that an indication can be obtained of the relative proportion of moments, muscle tensions and joint contact forces. This chapter has dealt with jumping as an activity that is used during everyday life, but the fully-trained competitive athlete would exceed the values reported herein by a large margin. It is not surprising that serious long-term injuries are common, and a better understanding of the mechanics of jumping should help athletes and coaches to train more safely. For clinical personnel involved in the treatment of athletes and non-athletes, it is vital that the severity of the jump activity is appreciated before a structured programme of rehabilitation can be implemented efficiently.

References

Aura, O. and Viitasalo, J. T. (1989). Biomechanical characteristics of jumping. *Int. J. Sport Biomech.*, **5**, 89–98.

Bedi, J. F., Cresswell, A. G., Engel, T. J. and Nicol, S. M. (1987). Increase in jumping height associated with maximal effort vertical depth jumps. *Res. Q. Exer. Sport.*, **58(1)**, 11–15.

Bosco, C. and Komi, P. V., (1978). Utilization of elastic energy in jumping and its relation to skeletal muscle fibre composition in man. In *Biomechanics VIA Proc. VI Int. Cong. Biomech.* (E. Asmussen and K. Jörgensen, eds.). University Press, Baltimore.

Bosco, C. and Komi, P. V. (1980). Influence of aging on the behaviour of leg extensor muscles. *Eur. J. Appl. Physiol.*, **45**, 209–19.

Davies, C. T. M. (1971). Human power output in exercise of short duration in relation to body size and composition. *Ergonomics*, **14**, 245–56.

Denoth, J., Gruber, K., Keppler, M. and Ruder, H. (1984). Forces and torques during sports activities with high accelerations: *164 Proc. Eur. Soc. Biomech.*, Switzerland.

Hay, J. G., Wilson, B. D. and Dapena, J. (1977). A computational technique to determine the angular momentum of the human body. *J. Biomech.*, **10**, 269–77.

Kerwin, D. G. and Challis, J. H. (1985). Muscle elasticity – an examination of calculation procedures. *Sports Sci.*, **3**, 248–9.

Komi, P. V. and Bosco, C. (1978). Utilization of elastic energy and its relation to skeletal muscle fibre composition in man. *Biomechanics* Vol. 2A, pp. 79–85. University Park Press, Baltimore.

McNitt-Gray, J. (1993). Kinetics of the lower extremities during drop landings from three heights. *Biomechanics*, **26**, 1037–46.

Panzer, V. P. (1988). Lower extremity loads in landings of elite gymnasts. In *Biomechanics* (G. de. Groot, A. P. Hollander, P. A. Huijing and G. J. van Ingen Schenau, eds.), pp. 724–34. Free University Press.

Thompson, H. W. and McKinley, P. A. (1995). Landing from a jump: the role of vision when landing from known and unknown heights. *Neuroreport*, **6**, 581–4.

Watkins, J. and Nicol, A. C. (1986). Biomechanics analysis of the leg action in a round of flic-flac. In *Sports Science* (J. Watkins, T. Reilly and L. Burwitz, eds.), pp. 162–7. SPON.

10 Reaching, pointing and using two hands together*

P. van Vliet

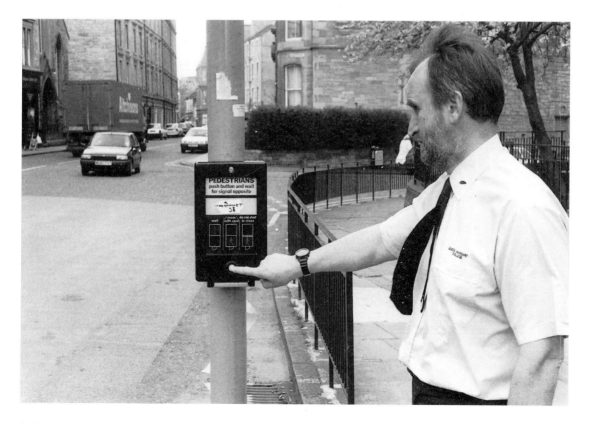

* The author would like to gratefully acknowledge Ailie Turton for her helpful comments on this chapter.

Introduction

Research on reaching to grasp an object has emerged largely in the last 12 years, and has been driven primarily by questions of motor control. The development of two- and three-dimensional motion analysis systems during this period has allowed the kinematics of reaching to be studied in detail. Reaching movements require substantial analysis because they vary considerably according to the purpose of each particular movement. The kinematics depend on factors such as the goal of a task (for example, to drink from a cup or move an object), on characteristics of the object itself (such as size, weight and shape) and on the location of the object to be grasped in relation to the body. Most investigations of reaching so far have dealt with reaching for objects in front of the body, although of course in everyday life reaching occurs in many different directions. This chapter will examine the literature on reaching and related activities.

A kinematic description of reaching for an object

Because reaching varies according to the demands of a particular situation, each reaching task needs to be analysed specifically. For example, grasping a cup on a table in front of the body, when the starting position is with the hand palm down on the knee, requires the following anatomical movements (Carr and Shepherd, 1987):

shoulder forward flexion
shoulder external rotation
protraction and lateral rotation of the scapula
elbow flexion then extension
supination of the forearm
wrist extension and radial deviation
abduction and opposition at the carpometacarpophalangeal joint of the thumb
extension of the metacarpophalangeal joints of the fingers with the interphalangeal joints in some flexion, and
conjunct rotation of the fingers towards the thumb.

Some of these components will change when the cup is located at the side of the body, for example, or when the cup is exchanged for a pencil. A dramatic example of how the goal of a task determines movement components is provided by Rosenbaum and Jorgensen (1992). Their subjects were required to grasp a small horizontal cylinder, resting on two supports, and to stand it up on either one end or the other.

Depending on which end the cylinder was to stand, subjects chose either a supinated or pronated grasp. Despite these variations some key features about reaching have been identified in the literature, and these will now be described. Typically, the literature has considered reaching as two components: transport of the hand to the object, and opening and closing of the hand to grasp.

Transport of the hand to the object

Displacement
Jeannerod (1981, 1984) provides one of the earliest detailed descriptions of reaching for objects in front of the body. His studies, using two-dimensional co-ordinates obtained from a video camera positioned at the side of the subject, track the position of the wrist during reaching under a variety of conditions. These include grasping different three-dimensional objects, with or without vision, during the reach. Figure 10.1a shows the path of the wrist during the movement.

Velocity
Figure 10.1b demonstrates a typical velocity profile for the wrist during reaching. It is asymmetric, with velocity increasing quickly at first to a peak, followed by a longer phase of decreasing velocity. This pattern is typical of reaching and other aimed movements. It was observed as early as 1899 by Woodworth, who was the first to identify two phases in slow, aimed movements. He observed subjects drawing a pencil backwards and forwards between lines on a piece of paper attached to a rotating drum. Initially there was a fast phase, as the hand moved towards the line, followed by a slower phase, where the pencil could be guided more accurately to the target. The initial high velocity phase in reaching has been described as ballistic, and the slower phase is supposed to represent a period where visual feedback is used to ensure an accurate grasp of the object (Jeannerod, 1981, 1984; Marteniuk *et al.*, 1987, 1990).

Smyth and colleagues (1988) give an example of the two-phase structure of aimed movements that you can try yourself. Hold your arm out straight to one side, then move it fairly quickly so that you touch the tip of your nose with your index finger. There is a fast phase, followed by a slow phase just before you touch your nose.

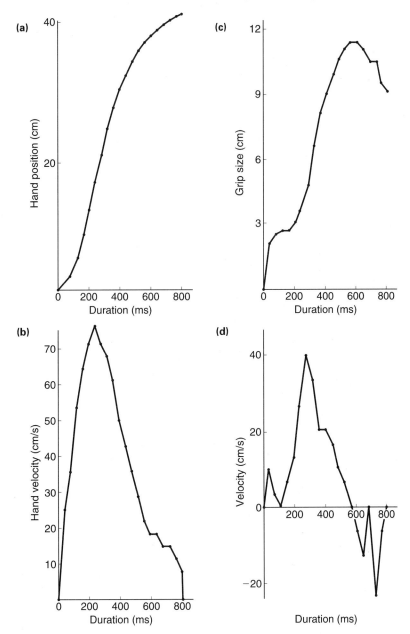

Figure 10.1 Position and velocity profiles of the two components of a reaching movement as a function of time (Jeannerod, 1984; reprinted with permission of the Helen Dwight Reid Educational Foundation, published by Heldref Publications, Washington)

Jeannerod observed a particular period of low velocity when the hand was near the target, as shown in Figure 10.1b. For the most part, his findings have been corroborated by later studies using three-dimensional motion analysis systems (e.g. Marteniuk *et al.*, 1987, 1990; Castiello *et al.*, 1993).

Usually there is just one asymmetric bell-shaped velocity profile in aimed arm movements, but this is not always the case. Wing and Miller (1984) examined the velocity profiles of subjects whose task was to slide a small plastic sensor over a horizontal surface in order to move a dot on an oscilloscope in front of them into a target area. They reported a large initial peak velocity, followed by a variable number of smaller velocity peaks.

The peak velocity for reaching movements usually occurs before 50 per cent of the movement duration. The studies discussed here involved distances which could easily be achieved without excessive movement of the trunk. Movement duration is usually defined as the time at which the object is grasped minus the time at which the movement started.

Kinematic parameters such as peak velocity are typically presented as absolute values and/ or as 'normalized' values, i.e. expressed as a percentage of the total movement duration. The position of the peak velocity in the movement varies with different tasks, and has been reported as between 32 and 35 per cent (van Vliet *et al.*, 1995a) for movements performed at a brisk pace, and 38 and 42 per cent (Gentilucci *et al.*, 1991) for movements performed at a natural speed. The actual time taken to achieve peak velocity has been reported as 240–264 ms by Gentilucci *et al.* (1991), and 350–375 ms by Castiello *et al.* (1993), where subjects moved at natural speeds. The size of the peak velocity depends on the speed requirements of the task and the distance to be covered. An example of peak velocity values in an experiment where subjects were asked to reach a distance of 20 cm at a natural speed was between 646 and 744 mms^{-1} (Gentilucci *et al.*, 1991). In a further example, where subjects were asked to reach to a distance requiring 10° less than maximum elbow extension (between 26 and 45 cm from the start position for these subjects) at a brisk pace, peak velocity was between 550 and 650 mms^{-1} (van Vliet *et al.*, 1995a). Average velocities in these experiments were 329–479 mms^{-1} (Gentilucci *et al.*, 1991) and 277–314 mms^{-1} (van Vliet *et al.*, 1995a) respectively. Movement duration will also vary according to the speed and distance required. It has been reported as between 775 and 829 ms (Castiello *et al.*, 1993) for a distance of 35 cm and 870–950 ms in the study by van Vliet *et al.* (1995a).

Hand aperture

Typically, the hand will open and close once on the approach to an object. Figure 10.1c illustrates the opening and closing of the hand with respect to time. The maximum aperture tends to occur in the second half of the movement. Castiello *et al.* (1993) reported that this occurred at 54–62 per cent, Jeannerod (1984) at 74–81 per cent and Gentilucci *et al.* (1991) at 59–72 per cent of the movement duration. The size of the maximum aperture depends on the size of the object to be grasped, but the hand opens much wider than the actual diameter of the object. Castiello *et al.* (1993) reported maximum apertures of between 5.8 and 5.9 cm for an object 2 cm in diameter, and 11.3–12 cm for an object with a diameter of 7.5 cm.

The contribution of thumb and index finger to the hand aperture during the approach to an object has been examined by Wing and Fraser (1983). It was observed that the index finger rather than the thumb was responsible for closing the hand as it approached the object, and it was proposed that the stability of the thumb has a role in guiding the transport of the hand to the object.

Central nervous system control of reaching

Co-ordinative structures for reaching

Among the numerous questions of motor control that scientists are currently attempting to solve is the problem of controlling 'degrees of freedom', first posed by Bernstein in (1967). The movement possibilities for the upper limb are numerous, and present a complex control problem for the central nervous system. The magnitude of the problem is illustrated by Tuller *et al.* (1982), who draw attention to the potential number of movement units to be controlled in an arm movement. If the individual muscles controlling the shoulder, elbow and wrist joints were considered as individual movement units to be controlled, the motor plan would require 26 values to be specified at each point in time. If individual muscle motor units were considered in the same way, they estimate at least 2600 values would need to be specified.

How can these degrees of freedom be reduced to a more manageable number? Bernstein suggested that movement units be linked together into co-ordinative structures, where a group of muscles is constrained to act as a single unit. The definition of a co-ordinative structure has broadened to include not just muscles, but other ways of linking parts of movements together.

Jeannerod (1981, 1984) proposed such a co-ordinative structure for the control of reaching. In his studies, he observed that the transport and grasp phases were linked together at key temporal events. At the beginning of the movement, subjects opened their hand at the same time as starting to move the hand towards the object. Also, during the movement, there was a significant correlation between the time at which the maximum grasp aperture was reached and the time of the low velocity phase he observed in the transport. Although the time at which maximum aperture occurred was different for each reaching movement, varying between 74 and 81 per cent, it was consistently linked to the start of the low velocity phase. Furthermore, this correlation was present whether or not subjects had vision of the object during the reach. This latter observation has been investigated since by Gentilucci *et al.* (1991), who could not identify this clear link between the two phases. They did, however, observe the low velocity point at about 70 per cent of movement duration, and observed that the hand closure was initiated during the deceleration phase.

Since Jeannerod's suggestion of a co-ordinative structure for reaching, there have been several investigations into how interdependent these two components of reaching are. The approach taken in these experiments has been to manipulate one component and examine the effect on the other component. Haggard and Wing (1991) delivered mechanical perturbations to the arm during reaching, and recorded a concomitant decrease in hand aperture in response to the perturbation after which the hand would resume opening to grasp the object. Paulignan *et al.* (1991) arranged three pieces of dowel in front of the subject, illuminated the central one and asked subjects to grasp the illuminated dowel. On some trials, the illuminated dowel changed soon after the subject started to move so that the left or right dowel was illuminated instead. These 'perturbations' of hand transport caused the hand aperture to open and close an extra time during the movement, as in the mechanical perturbation study. Changes to transport, therefore, affect changes in grasp, implying interdependence between the two components.

The grasp component was manipulated by Marteniuk *et al.* (1987), who compared reaching for different sized discs. Subjects were right-handed, and movement was from right to left across the body rather than forward in the sagittal plane. For smaller discs the peak velocity occurred earlier in the movement, allowing for a longer deceleration phase. Paulignan *et al.* (1991) also manipulated the size of the object to be grasped to

see the effect on the transport component. The method was to mount a narrow dowel in the centre of a wide dowel and illuminate either one for the subjects to grasp, sometimes changing the illuminated dowel after the movement had begun. As expected, the grasp became wider or narrower according to the change in size of the dowel, and the transport of the hand was also interrupted, causing the peak deceleration to occur later in the trial if the size of the dowel was changed. Thus, changes occur to the transport component in response to different grasp requirements, and the two phases therefore do seem to be coupled.

Role of vision

Jeannerod (1984) describes two visuomotor control channels for reaching. The transport component reflects 'determination by the visual system of the co-ordinates of a point in body-centred space', and the grasp component reflects 'visual computation of shape, size, and weight of the object'. His experiments, where subjects were deprived of vision of the object to be grasped after their movement had started, show that vision of the object before reaching enables the position of the object and the maximum aperture necessary for the grasp to be programmed **prior to** the movement. The role of visual feedback during the movement, according to Jeannerod, is to increase **precision** of the grasp.

A relevant question here is, how quickly can a person respond to visual feedback when performing arm movements? Keele and Posner (1968) found that it takes about 200 ms to use vision to correct aiming movements. They trained subjects to move a stylus from one position to another in different amounts of time, and sometimes turned off the room lights unpredictably as soon as the movement began. Visual feedback only affected accuracy of the movement when movements took about 200 ms or more. In certain situations, visual response time has been found to be as quick as 120 ms (Zelaznik *et al.*, 1983).

Absence of vision and having insufficient time to process visual information can cause compensations in reaching. Wing *et al.* (1986) reported that, when subjects had their eyes closed during reaching or when they reached fast, the maximum aperture was greater than with eyes open or when reaching at normal speed. In both the blind and the fast reaching, the transport components were less accurate than in normal speed reaching. It was proposed that opening the hand wider might have been an error-compensating adjustment that was used for reduced visual feedback.

Fitts' law

Various attempts have been made to represent mathematically the process by which parameters of aimed movements are specified. In 1954 Fitts attempted to do this, and this has led to considerable research since. One of his experiments (Fitts, 1954) involved subjects moving a stylus as quickly as possible from one target to another. The width of the targets, as well as the distance between them, was varied. For a given target width (i.e. size of target), movement duration increased with movement distance. Also, for a given distance between targets, movement duration increased when target width decreased. He therefore identified a 'speed – accuracy trade-off' in these aimed movements.

Fitts concluded that the speed, distance and accuracy of a movement made under visual control are linked by the following relationship:

$$MT = a + b \log_2 2A/W$$

where MT = movement time, A = distance, W = target width, and a and b are empirical constants. This equation has become known as 'Fitts' Law', and has been investigated by others (e.g. Crossman and Goodeve, 1983; Schmidt *et al.*, 1979), who have produced modified versions of it.

Effects of different tasks on reaching

The findings described regarding the effects of reaching different distances and for different sized objects demonstrate that the formation of these movements is specific to the task being performed. In addition, studies on normal subjects have indicated that the functional goal of a reaching task is important in terms of how the movement is planned and executed. Accuracy requirements and the end goal of a task affect the kinematics of reaching. A study by Marteniuk *et al.* (1987) demonstrated this very well. Grasping a fragile object (a light bulb) was compared with grasping a soft resilient object (a tennis ball). Peak velocity (expressed as a percentage of movement duration) occurred earlier in the trajectory when more precision was required, allowing for a longer deceleration phase. Different tasks performed with the same object were also compared by Marteniuk *et al.* (1987). A disc was grasped, either to throw it into a large box or to place it in a tight fitting well. The peak velocity occurred earlier in the more precise fitting task. Thus the proportion of time spent in each phase can vary according to the task. Another example is described by van Vliet (1993), who compared subjects reaching to move an upright mug with those reaching in order to move the mug while turning it over. Subjects opened their hands wider to grasp the mug in the turning task.

Motor programmes

The identification of elementary components of reaching movements, whose control is largely of central origin, lends support to the idea of the existence of motor programmes. Keele's (1968) definition of a motor programme, which has become widely accepted, is 'a set of muscle commands that are structured before a movement sequence begins, and that allows the entire sequence to be carried out'. The existence of separate grasp and transport phases that are temporally linked can be seen as one example of such a motor programme. Another is what has been described as the triphasic EMG pattern of muscle activation in flexion–extension movements of the arm. This was first identified by Wachholder and Altenburger (1926), who recorded agonist and antagonist muscle activity in normal subjects during flexion–extension movements of the arm. The triphasic pattern they observed can be described as follows: 'during movements performed at a moderate speed the initial burst of activity of the agonist muscle was followed by a burst of activity of the antagonist, appearing during the movement itself; finally a second burst of activity of the agonist was observed at the end of the movement' (Jeannerod, 1988). The same alternating pattern was also observed for fast movements. Others have confirmed Wachholder and Altenburger's findings (Terzuolo *et al.*, 1973; Angel, 1974; Hallet *et al.*, 1975). The exact function of the antagonist burst is still under investigation, but it has been suggested that it represents a central 'braking' strategy to help achieve accuracy of movement. The triphasic pattern is thought to be centrally programmed, as it has been observed in subjects with peripheral deafferentation of the moving segments (Hallet *et al.*, 1975). It is probable that the presence of the pattern depends on 'the inertial properties of the limb to be moved and on the task to be achieved' (Jeannerod, 1988). It is not clear whether the pattern occurs similarly in more complex arm movements, such as natural goal-directed reaching movements.

Neuronal populations for reaching

Progress is being made in identifying areas of the brain which control different aspects of reaching movements. There is support for the existence of separate transport and grasp components from Kuypers (1973), who states that damage to pyramidal tract fibres results in impairments of fine finger movements, whereas damage to the extrapyramidal tract causes impairments of gross arm movements, including transport of the hand towards an object. A common methodology in this area of neuroscience is to record the firing of individual neurons in the motor cortex while particular movements are performed. The studies are usually conducted with monkeys, who are trained to do certain tasks. Single neuron recordings from inferior area six in the monkey have shown that there are two sets of neurons separately coding the transport and grasp components of reaching (Gentilucci *et al.*, 1988; Rizzolatti *et al.*, 1988). One set of neurons responds to the specific spatial location of an object. The other responds to vision of objects if the object size is appropriate for the type of grasp controlled by the particular neurons, and become active during particular types of grasping movements. These findings support Jeannerod's hypothesis that two visuomotor channels exist for reaching; one influenced by the location of the object and the other influenced by the characteristics of the object which determine the grasp to be used. There is also evidence that different **types** of grasp are subserved by different populations of neurons. Muir and Lemon (1983) have identified a sub-population of pyramidal tract neurons in monkeys which are principally active during pincer grasp, where just the thumb and index finger are used, and relatively inactive during a power grasp, where all fingers are used together.

Studies by Evarts (1981) showed that neurons in the motor cortex are active to different degrees according to the amount of **force** in the required movement and its direction. Rather than individual neurons firing specifically for a particular direction, the discharge rates of the different neurons varied, each direction having a cell that fired most vigorously for it. Georgopoulos *et al.* (1986) have hypothesized that the **direction** in which the arm moves represents the weighted sum of the directions signalled by neurons in the motor cortex. The resultant direction is that with the largest weighted sum.

Pointing movements

In accordance with Fitts' Law, the kinematics of pointing vary depending upon the size of the target to be pointed at. With smaller targets, movement durations are longer and peak and average velocity values are smaller. A longer deceleration phase is present with smaller targets (Gentilucci *et al.*, 1991; Mackenzie *et al.*, 1987).

In comparisons of grasping and pointing, it is apparent that the same response to increased accuracy requirements occurs in both cases (Gentilucci *et al.*, 1991). Marteniuk *et al.* (1987) however, found that the deceleration phase was longer for grasping than pointing when the same distance and same size target was used. They suggested that this could be because the impact with the object is used to decelerate the hand in pointing, so the same careful approach to the object was not required. This idea is supported by the results of Teasdale and Schmidt (1991). Their experiment required subjects to move a stylus attached to a handle from a start position to a target, and asked them to hit the target with varying amounts of impact, and in varying movement times. The deceleration phase was longer for small impact movements than large impact ones. It was concluded that the duration of the deceleration could be a consequence of the implied impact constraints of the task. In support of this, Worringham (1987), in his unpublished doctoral dissertation *Spatial variability and impact force in aiming movements*, has shown that impact forces decrease linearly with decreased target size.

Using two hands together

Questions of motor control have also led to some interesting findings on bimanual movements. These have mainly been to do with the idea that the two arms may be controlled by a single mechanism (i.e. a co-ordinative structure), rather than being controlled completely independently of each other. Kelso *et al.* (1979) observed subjects pointing to two targets at once, where one target was further away from the starting point and narrower than the other. According to Fitts' Law, an increased movement duration would be expected for the more difficult task. However, both movements had approximately equal movement durations, implying that the two arms were constrained by a single mechanism.

Jeannerod's study (1984) included observations of a bimanual movement, involving reaching for a small bottle with one hand and removing a plug at the top with the other. Complete data from only seven movements from two subjects were available for analysis. He observed that the two movements began at the same time and, like Kelso *et al.* (1979), that the movement durations were the same despite the different level of difficulty of the two movements. Other kinematic features of the two arms were also the same, including the time at which peak velocity occurred (which was the same in five out of the seven movements), the size of the peak velocity, and the time at which the maximum aperture occurred (which was less than 80 ms different for the two hands in all seven movements).

A very similar bimanual movement was studied by Castiello *et al.* (1993). The task was to grasp a cylinder with one hand and open the lid of the cylinder, using a pull tab, with the other. Forty movements were performed by each of six subjects. Movement durations were again similar for the two arms. However, the precision task had a longer deceleration phase, with the peak velocity occurring earlier in the movement. The movement duration tended towards that of the more precise task. These authors concluded that the central control of the two arms was similar, but that the kinematic parameters are individual to each arm.

Homologous tasks were also studied by Castiello *et al.* (1993), where both hands either grasped large or small cylinders. Significant correlations were found between the times of peak velocity, maximum aperture, peak acceleration and peak deceleration of the two arms. This observation, plus that of Kelso *et al.* (1979), implies that, for homologous pointing or grasping tasks, a single central mechanism is employed to control the two arms. In terms of understanding everyday movements the findings on non-homologous movements are probably more valuable, as homologous tasks are rarer than non-homologous ones.

Reaching in stroke patients

Reaching tasks in the neurologically impaired have not been investigated to the same extent as in individuals with intact neurological systems. Much of the work carried out has concerned people with stroke, so these studies will be reviewed here as an example of how neurological impairments can affect reaching. The studies that have been done on

stroke subjects demonstrate that they are able to change kinematic aspects of the movement towards a more normal pattern as they recover, and show the differences between the reaching of stroke and normal subjects. Van Vliet *et al.* (1995b) examined the ability of stroke subjects to adjust their reaching according to different task constraints. The eight subjects had scores of between three and five on the arm section of the Rivermead Motor Assessment (Lincoln and Leadbitter, 1979), so were not yet very skilled at reaching. When asked to drink from a cup filled with water the stroke subjects performed the movement in a shorter time than when they were required to move in the same way, demonstrating some ability to adjust their movement for task constraints. The same subjects were measured again three to four weeks later (van Vliet *et al.*, 1995b). They showed a greater peak velocity in the drinking task compared to the moving task, so still demonstrated an adjustment for task constraints. During this time, average velocity of movement increased and the variability of where the peak

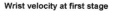

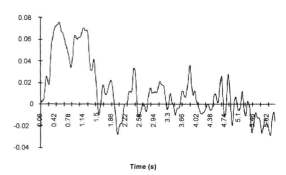

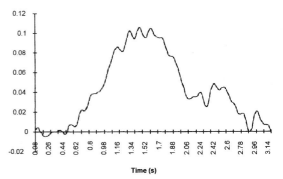

Figure 10.2 Wrist velocities at the two stages of recovery, 3 and 4 weeks apart

velocity occurred within the movement decreased. Some subjects showed an improvement in the smoothness of the movement, in that there were fewer velocity peaks (see Figure 10.2). This was also found by Trombly (1993) in a study of five subjects with stroke, where measurements were made over a period of 10 weeks. The presence of several velocity peaks suggest that stroke subjects are using a more corrective mode of control, with feedback being instrumental in guiding the hand to the object, compared to normal subjects, whose reaching appears to rely more on specification of movement parameters prior to the beginning of the movement with visual feedback being used only for fine tuning. Trombly also observed an increase in the amplitude of peak velocity, a decrease in movement duration and a more normal time to peak velocity over the 10 weeks. Lough and Wing (1984) also reported an increase in the amplitude of peak velocity of the hand and a decrease in movement duration over time in the arm movements of stroke subjects. Wing *et al.* (1990) found an increase in the peak angular velocity of the elbow over time.

In a study of compensatory movements used by stroke patients it was found that, initially, stroke subjects use a lot of trunk flexion to help transport the hand to the object (Turton, 1991). Reaching movements were recorded by a video camera positioned above the table, and electrogoniometers were attached to the hand to measure hand opening. Figure 10.3 shows this finding for the seven stroke subjects examined. Shoulder intrusion was defined as 'how much the shoulder moves towards the object ... during the movement' (Turton, 1991). The amount of this trunk flexion decreased as the ability to flex the shoulder improved. Although some stroke subjects were often unable to open the hand sufficiently to grasp an object such as a cup, some (who had sufficient grasp aperture) compensated for potential inaccuracies of grasp by opening the hand wider than necessary (Turton, 1991). This is the same strategy as that used by the unimpaired people who reached at fast speeds in Wing *et al.*'s study (1986). In general descriptive terms, Carr and Shepherd (1987) list this and other ways in which people with stroke typically compensate for their decreased ability to perform components of upper limb movements. These include:

excessive shoulder girdle elevation and lateral flexion of the trunk to compensate for poor shoulder forward flexion and abduction

excessive elbow flexion, internal rotation of the shoulder and pronation of the forearm

flexion of the wrist

difficulty extending and flexing the metacarpophalangeal joints with the interphalangeal joints in some flexion and

excessive extension of the fingers and thumb on release of an object.

Differences from normal reaching

Reaching in stroke subjects is slower than that of normal subjects. Slowing down the movement would allow more time to use visual and kinaesthetic feedback. In van Vliet *et al.*'s study (1995b), stroke subjects moved shorter distances than normal subjects but took longer. Their mean movement durations were between 4.64 and 5.98 s, compared to normal subjects' 0.87–0.95 s. Mean peak velocity was between 126 and 145 mms^{-1}, compared to normal subjects' 550–650 mms^{-1}. Van Vliet *et al.* (1995b) and Trombly (1993) report values for the position of peak velocity within the 50 per cent of the movement duration, which is similar to normal. Stroke subjects' reaching is more variable than that of normal subjects. In van Vliet *et al.*'s study (1995b), movement duration, peak velocity, average velocity and the time at which peak velocity occurred in the movement were significantly more variable in stroke subjects.

Muscle activity

Lough and Wing (1984) conducted a case study of one stroke subject with left-sided hemiplegia

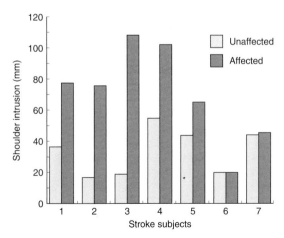

Figure 10.3 Mean shoulder intrusion for subjects' unaffected and affected reaching (Turton, 1991)

where measurements were made with the subject's arm resting on a horizontal support attached to the wheelchair in which the shoulder and elbow could be moved. Only adduction/abduction of the shoulder and extension/flexion of the elbow could be performed in this support. One of the movements required of subjects was to adduct the shoulder while extending the elbow. It was observed that, over time, the trajectory followed by the hand in this movement became more direct. The initial movements deviated to the right, which the authors suggested reflected compensation for shoulder adduction by elbow extension, or over-compensation for elbow extension by shoulder adduction. It was suggested that this showed an inability to co-ordinate inter-joint activity. Trombly (1993) compared stroke subjects' abilities to reach three different locations in front of the body. One location required shoulder adduction with elbow extension, another required moving directly forward, and the other, shoulder abduction with elbow extension. As peak velocity of the hand increased over time, the anterior deltoid became more active relative to the pectoralis major when performing these tasks.

Lough (1987) measured the activity of biceps and triceps while stroke subjects used their arms to slide a cradle along a track between target points. There was a persistence of biceps activity during extension, which the author saw as a failure in the normally flexible control of antagonist function. Sahrmann and Norton (1977), however, also examined flexion/extension movements of the elbow, and found no evidence that antagonist flexor activity interfered with agonist extensor activity. Instead, muscle activity in the antagonist was characterized by decreased and prolonged activation. Wing *et al.* (1990) examined flexion and extension movements of the elbow using the same apparatus as Lough (1987). They found no evidence that elbow flexion recovered consistently better or faster than elbow extension.

Future research needs

This chapter has focused mainly on kinematic information about reaching, which stems from questions about how the central nervous system controls arm movement. It is generally accepted that this methodology provides an informative window into the nature of central nervous system control. Other methods, though, including studies of muscle activity can also be revealing. One of the

problems with this latter approach is that a particular movement can be achieved by using a number of different combinations of muscle activity. The overall goal, as we have seen, can also influence the actual movement chosen. This means that the findings of electromyography studies can be accepted for the particular context in which the movement was performed, but one should be wary of generalizing the findings to other situations. Also, the results of these studies are confined to knowledge about the muscles that were monitored. Other muscles, not being monitored, may well have an important role in the performance of a task.

For clinicians trying to analyse and retrain arm movements, however, the information available on muscle activity involved in simple joint movements in anatomy and physiology texts is frustratingly insufficient when considering the interaction of muscle activity in task-oriented movements. For this reason it would be helpful to see more studies of muscle activity such as the Basmajian and Deluca (1985) analysis of holding a glass, though this information should be used carefully by clinicians.

Most research on reaching has focused on reaching to grasp objects in front of the body. Everyday life, however, frequently involves reaching for objects above the head, on the floor and beside and behind the body. The three-dimensional motion analysis systems now available should enable more research on these tasks. It is perhaps therapists, rather than motor control scientists, who would be more interested in the results of these kinematic analyses, so it may be up to therapists to conduct these studies. Arm movements are enabled partly by the postural adjustments made prior to and during a task. Postural adjustments for reaching have been studied (e.g. Crosbie *et al.*, 1995), but not extensively as yet and more research is needed. There is considerable information on the development of reaching in children, which it has not been possible to describe here. One of the main contributors in this area has been von Hofsten (1979). Lastly, upper limb movements in disabled populations need to be further examined to improve our understanding of abnormal upper limb movement. Hypotheses can then be generated about the best ways to restoring improved function to disabled people, and then tested. This science-based process should provide a better basis for formulating ideas on treatment than has been possible in the past.

References

Angel, R. W. (1974). Electromyography during voluntary movement. The two-burst pattern. *Electroencephalogr. Clin. Neurophysiol.*, **36**, 493–8.

Basmajian, J. V. and Deluca, C. J. (1985). *Muscles Alive: Their Functions Revealed by Electromyography*. Williams & Wilkins.

Bernstein, N. (1967). *The Co-ordination and Regulation of movements*. Pergamon Press.

Carr, J. H. and Shepherd, R. B. (1987). *A Motor Relearning Programme for Stroke*. 2nd edn. Heinemann Physiotherapy.

Castiello, U., Bennett, K. M. B. and Stelmach, G. E. (1993). The bilateral reach to grasp movement. *Behav. Brain. Res.*, **56**, 43–57.

Crosbie, J., Shepherd, R. B. and Squire, T. J. (1995). Postural and voluntary movement during reaching in sitting: the role of the lower limbs. *J. Hum. Move. Stud.*, **28**, 103–26.

Crossman, E. R. F. W. and Goodeve, P. J. (1963/1983). Feedback control of limb-movement and Fitts' Law. *Q. J. Exp. Psychol.*, **35A**, 251–78.

Evarts, E. V. (1981). Role of motor cortex in voluntary movements in primates. In *Handbook of Physiology* (V. B. Brooks, ed.). American Physiological Society.

Fitts, P. M. (1954). The information capacity of the human motor system in controlling the amplitude of movement. *J. Exp. Psychol.*, **47**, 381–91.

Gentilucci, M., Fogassi, L., Luppino, G. *et al.* (1988). Functional organization of inferior area 6 in the macaque monkey. I. Somatotopy and control of proximal movements. *Exp. Brain Res.*, **71**, 475–90.

Gentilucci, M., Castiello, U., Corradini, M. L. *et al.* (1991). Influence of different types of grasping on the transport component of prehension movements. *Neuropsychologica*, **29(5)**, 361–78.

Georgopoulous, A. P., Schwartz, A. B. and Kettner, R. E. (1986). Neuronal population coding of movement direction. *Science*, **233**, 1416–19.

Haggard, P. and Wing, A. M. (1991). Remote responses to perturbation in human prehension. *Neurosci. Lett.*, **122**, 103–8.

Hallett, M., Shahani, B. T. and Young, R. R. (1975). EMG analysis of stereotyped voluntary movements in man. *J. Neurol. Neurosurg. Psychiatry*, **38**, 1154–62.

Jeannerod, M. (1981). Intersegmental co-ordination during reaching at natural visual objects. In *Attention and Performance* (J. Long and A. Baddeley, eds.), pp. 153–68. Erlbaum.

Jeannerod, M. (1984). The timing of natural prehension movements. *J. Mot. Behav.*, **16**, 235–4.

Jeannerod, M. (1988). *The Neural and Behavioural Organization of Goal-Directed Movements*. Clarendon Press.

Keele, S. W. (1968). Movement control in skilled motor performance. *Psychol. Bull.*, **70**, 387–404.

Keele, S. W. and Posner, M. I. (1968). Processing of visual feedback in rapid movements. *J. Exp. Psychol.*, **77**, 155–8.

Kelso, J. A. S., Southard, D. L. and Goodman, D. (1979). On the co-ordination of two-handed movements. *J. Exp. Psychol.: Hum. Percept. Perf.*, **5**, 229–38.

Kuypers, H. G. (1973). The anatomical organization of the descending pathways and their contributions to motor control especially in primates. In *New Developments in Electromyography and Clinical Neurophysiology* (Vol. 3) (J. E. Desmedt, ed.). Karger.

Lincoln, N. B. and Leadbitter, D. (1979). Assessment of motor function in stroke patients. *Physiotherapy*, **65**, 48–51.

Lough, S. (1987). Visual control of arm movement in the stroke patient. *Int. J. Rehab. Res.*, **10(4)** (suppl. 5), 113–19.

Lough, S. and Wing, A. M. (1984). Measurement of recovery of function in the hemiparetic upper limb following stroke: A preliminary report. *Hum. Move. Sci.*, **3**, 247–56.

MacKenzie, C. L., Marteniuk, R. G., Dugas, C. *et al.* (1987). Three-dimensional movement trajectories in Fitts' Law: Implications for control. *Q. J. Exp. Psychol.*, **39**, 629–47.

Marteniuk, R. G., Jeannerod, M., Athenes, S. and Dugas, C. (1987). Constraints on human arm movement trajectories. *Can. J. Psychol.*, **41(3)**, 365–78.

Marteniuk, R. G., Leavitt, J. L., Mackenzie, C. L. and Athenes, S. (1990). Functional relationships between grasp and transport components in a prehension task. *Hum. Move. Sci.*, **9**, 149–76.

Muir, R. B. and Lemon, R. N. (1983). Corticospinal neurons with a special role in precision grip. *Brain Res.*, **261**, 312–16.

Paulignan, Y., MacKenzie, C., Marteniuk, R. and Jeannerod, M., (1991). Selective perturbation of visual input during prehension movements. *Exp. Brain Res.*, **87**, 407.

Rizzolatti, G., Camarda, R., Fogassi, G. *et al.* (1988). Functional organization of inferior area 6 in the macaque monkey. II. Area F5 and the control of distal movements. *Exp. Brain Res.*, **71**, 491–507.

Rosenbaum, D. R. and Jorgensen, M. J. (1992). Planning macroscopic aspects of manual control. *Hum. Move. Sci.*, **11**, 61–9.

Sahrmann, S. A. and Norton, B. J. (1977). The relationship of voluntary movement to spasticity in the upper motor neuron syndrome. *Ann. Neurol.*, **2**, 460–5.

Schmidt, R. A., Hawkins, B., Franck, J. S. and Quinn, J. T. (1979). Motor-output variability: a theory for the accuracy of rapid motor acts. *Psychol. Rev.*, **86**, 415–51.

Smyth, M. M., Morris, P. E., Levy, P. and Ellis, A. W. (1988). *Cognition in Action*. Lawrence Erlbaum.

Teasdale, N. and Schmidt, R. A. (1991). Deceleration requirements and the control of pointing movements. *J. Motor Behav.*, **23(2)**, 131–8.

Terzuolo, C. A., Soechting, J. F. and Viviani P. (1973). Studies on the control of some simple motor tasks. I. Relations between parameters of movements and EMG activity. *Brain Res.*, **58**, 212–16.

Trombly, C. A. (1993). Observations of improvement of reaching in five subjects with left hemiparesis. *J. Neurol. Neurosurg. Psychiatr.*, **56**, 40–45.

Tuller, B., Turvey, M. T. and Fitch, H. L. (1982). The Bernstein perspective: II. The concept of muscle linkage or co-ordinative structure. In *Human Motor Behaviour: An Introduction* (J. A. Scott Kelso, ed.), pp.253–70. Lea and Febiger.

Turton, A. (1991). *Recovery of Co-ordination of Arm and Hand Movements following Stroke*. MSc thesis. Polytechnic of East London.

van Vliet, P. (1993). An investigation of the task specificity of reaching: implications for retraining. *Physiother. Theory Pract.*, **9,** 69–76.

van Vliet, P., Kerwin, D. G., Sheridan, M. and Fentem, P. (1995a). The influence of goals on the kinematics of reaching following stroke. *Neurol. Rep.*, **19(1),** 11–16.

van Vliet, P., Kerwin, D. G., Sheridan, M. and Fentem, P. (1995b). A study of reaching in stroke patients. In *Physiotherapy in Stroke Management* (M. A. Harrison, ed.). Churchill Livingstone.

von Hofsten, C. (1979). Development of visually-directed reaching: the approach phase. *J. Hum. Move. Stud.*, **5,** 160–178.

Wachholder, K. and Altenburger, H. (1926). Beitrage zur Physiologie der willkurlichen Bewegung. X Mitteilung. Einzelbewegungen. *Pflugers Arch. Ges. Physiol.*, **214,** 642–61.

Wing, A. M. and Fraser, C. (1983). The contribution of the thumb to reaching movements. *Q. J. Exp. Psychol.*, **35A,** 297–309.

Wing, A. M. and Miller, E. (1984). Research note: peak velocity timing invariance. *Psych. Res.*, 46, 121–7.

Wing, A. M., Turton, A. and Fraser, C. (1986). Grasp size and accuracy of approach in reaching. *J. Mot. Behav.*, **18,** 245–60.

Wing, A. M., Lough, S., Turton, A. *et al.* (1990). Recovery of elbow function in voluntary positioning of the hand following hemiplegia due to stroke. *J. Neurol. Neurosurg. Psychiat.*, **53,** 126–34.

Woodworth, R. S. (1899). The accuracy of voluntary movements. *Psychol. Rev. Monogr.* (suppl. 3).

Zelaznik, H. N., Hawkins, B. and Kisselburg, K. (1983). Rapid visual feedback procesing in single-aiming movements. *J. Mot. Behav.*, **15,** 217–36.

11 Hand function

V. A. Blair

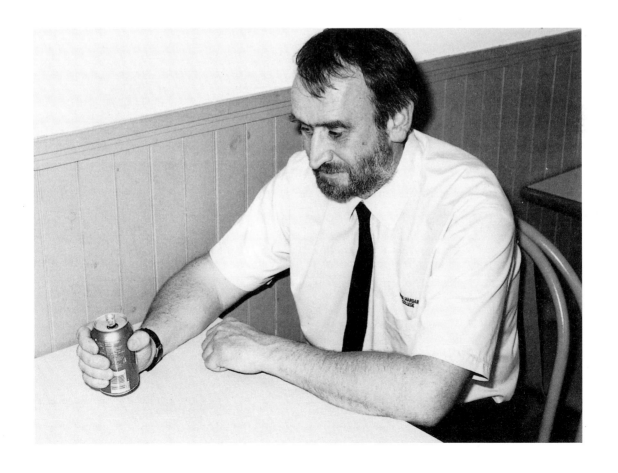

Introduction

Much of the current literature on hand function tends to concentrate on hand strength. This is probably because the assessment of hand strength is one of the easier aspects of hand function to actually measure objectively. Therefore, the majority of the work reviewed in this chapter will focus on the assessment of hand function in relation to grip strength. However, it is useful first to remind ourselves that the hand is a very complex structure capable of the performance of not only a multitude of motor tasks but also of relaying sensory information about the temperature, the shape and texture of objects to the brain.

The hand does not function in isolation, and is dependent on the integrity of the shoulder and elbow complexes to allow the appropriate positioning of the hand in space to complete the desired task. The motor and sensory tasks performed by the hand are all geared to the body's overall functioning in terms of performing the activities of daily living (ADL) that are necessary for survival. There are a vast array of scales for assessing ADL, too many to review in a single chapter, and therefore this chapter will review those most commonly used in the assessment of the upper limb and which necessitate detailed assessment of hand function. In clinical practice hand function is not assessed in complete isolation from the remainder of the upper limb; therefore it is important to be able to appreciate the multiplicity of hand function in relation to ADL.

Measurement of upper limb function

Several measurement tools have been developed specifically for examining functional ability of the upper limb including hand function (Carroll, 1965; Jebsen *et al.*, 1969; Aniansson *et al.*, 1980; Lundgren-Lindquist and Sperling, 1983; Desrosiers *et al.*, 1993). In recent years, the majority of these assessments have been designed to assess upper limb function in elderly subjects. This reflects the increase in the elderly population globally and the resulting demands on rehabilitation services to attempt to preserve an individual's independence in ADL for as long as possible. To achieve this it is necessary to accurately assess upper limb function, and several different methods have been recommended.

The upper extremity function test

Carroll (1965) was one of the first authors to attempt to develop a quantitative test of upper extremity function. The upper extremity function test (UEFT) consisted of 33 tests scored on a scale of 0–3 (Figure 11.1). The test was designed to measure hand and arm function in activities that would simulate normal everyday activities of daily living. It was developed to be a simple and quick assessment, which could be administered by doctors and technicians in a busy outpatient setting. Carroll assumed that the complex upper limb movements used in ADL could be reduced to patterns of grasp, pinch and grip in the hand, pronation and supination of the forearm, flexion and extension of the elbow and elevation of the arm.

To determine the content of the upper extremity function test, preliminary assessments of function were conducted on 200 upper limb conditions ranging from traumatic conditions to arthritic and neurological impairments. Carroll did attempt to consider the repeatability and validity of the upper limb function test, and compared the results obtained using it with those of a standard hand activity ADL test. However, he fails to give any details of what this standard test was, and gives no details as to the value of the correlation coefficients obtained. He attempted to establish the repeatability of the assessment using serial measurements of 30 upper limbs at one-monthly intervals. Within these 30 assessments, pathologies varied from 7 normal subjects to 23 chronically impaired subjects. Identical scores were obtained at the re-test session in the normal subjects. Re-test results for the subjects with impaired upper limbs were more variable – one result was identical, there was a difference of one point in five cases, two points in five cases, three points in seven cases, five points in two cases, and six, seven and eight points in one case each.

Carroll also attempted to consider inter-observer errors in the application of the upper extremity test. Two experienced observers independently assessed 48 upper limbs. Identical scores were obtained in 22 of the assessments, 10 differed by one point, four by two points, five by three points, four by four points and three by five points.

Despite a lack of detail regarding the repeatability and reliability of the upper extremity function test, Carroll is still acknowledged as contributing greatly to the quest to find objective measures of upper extremity function. Carroll concluded that

Basic function	Score

Grasp:
  1. Block 4"
  2. Block 3"
  3. Block 2"
  4. Block 1"	

Grip:
  5. Pipe 1 3/4"
  6. Pipe 3/4"	

Lateral prehension: 7. Slate 1 x 5/8 x 4"	

Pinch:
  8. Ball, repeat with ballbearings of different sizes:
  9. Index finger and thumb
 10. Middle finger and thumb
 11. Small finger and thumb
 12. Ring finger and thumb
 13. Index finger and thumb
 14. Middle finger and thumb
 15. Small finger and thumb	

Placing: Basin placed over nail Iron onto shelf	
Supination and pronation: Pour water from jug to glass Pour water from glass to glass Place hand behind head Place hand on top of head Hand to mouth	
Write name	
Total:	

Scoring system: 3 = performs test normally; 2 = completes test but takes abnormally long time to complete; 1 = performs test partially; 0 = can perform no part of the test.

Figure 11.1 Upper extremity function test

the upper extremity function test was 'reasonably well' correlated with a standard ADL test, gave consistent results when repeated in chronically impaired limbs and that there was 'close agreement' between scores obtained by different observers.

Carroll conducted tests using the upper limb function test on 79 elderly nursing-home patients, and found 120 abnormal extremities within this population. From these extensive tests he proposed that an increase of 10 points represented a significant improvement in what the patient could do with the hand in ADL activities, and that a decrease of 10 points represented a significant reduction in hand function. Unfortunately there are no figures provided in the literature to substantiate these claims. He concluded that this study had shown 'sufficient reliability and consistency' to measure improvement and deterioration in upper limb function when the test was performed serially.

Rather than trying to quantify hand function in terms of scores, many of the assessments reviewed have involved timed tests. The Jebsen hand function test (Jebsen *et al.*, 1969, cited in Jette, 1985) is a method of assessing hand function based on the amount of time taken to complete a series of hand functions normally used in the performance of ADL. The functions assessed included writing, card turning, picking up small objects, simulated feeding, stacking draughts, picking up large light objects and picking up large heavy objects (Figure 11.2). In Jebsen's original study, normative data on the amount of time taken to perform the upper limb tasks were established for two age groups – 20–59 year olds and 60–94 year olds. In 1973, Taylor *et al.* established normative data, using the Jebsen hand function test, for children and adolescents from 6 to 19 years of age. Increased time taken to perform the test was indicative of decreased hand function.

In 1992, Hackel *et al.* used the Jebsen hand function test to investigate whether hand function declined with age. In Jebsen's original study in 1969, the results of all the elderly subjects aged from 60–94 years were grouped together to form the norm. Hackel *et al.* divided their test populations into smaller subgroups of 60–69 years, 70–79 years and 80–89 years, and found that there was a significant positive correlation between hand function and age and that a more accurate assessment of hand function could be ascertained if the subject was assessed in relation to the appropriate normative data of that particular subgroup.

In Sweden, two major studies have been conducted to evaluate functional activity in 70-year-old men and women (Aniansson *et al.*, 1980) and in 79-year-old men and women (Lundgren-Lindquist and Sperling, 1983). Studies were conducted to test mobility, reach, muscular co-ordination and manual ability (which included handling electrical plugs, changing a light bulb and manipulating keys in locks). The ability to prepare food and feed were considered of vital importance in being able to live independently. In particular, the ability to open jars, bottles and food packaging was tested. A

Activity
Hygiene and dressing activities: 1. Grasping opposite ear lobe with arm in front of head 2. Grasping opposite ear lobe with hand behind head 3. Fitting hand between buttock and seat 4. Placing finger tips at opposite big toe
Pronation and supination tests: 5. Pouring water from a jug to glass 6. Pouring water from one glass to another and back again
Reach: 7. Lift a glass and a 1 kg packet onto shelves of height 180, 160, 140 cm
Manual ability: 8. Pulling out and inserting a key in a lock 9. Pulling out and inserting a plug in a socket 10. Unscrewing and screwing an electric light bulb 11. Inserting coins in a slot 12. Dialling numbers on a telephone

Figure 11.3 Activities used to assess upper limb function in 70-year-old men and women in Sweden (Aniansson *et al.*, 1980)

Activity
Co-ordination (using peg board)
Ability to open jars and bottles with different sized tops

Figure 11.4 In a subsequent study by Lundgren-Lindquist and Sperling (1983), the following tests were added to those in Figure 11.3

Activity
1. Writing
2. Card turning
3. Picking up small objects
4. Simulated feeding
5. Stacking draughts/counters
6. Picking up large light objects
7. Picking up large heavy objects

Figure 11.2 Jebsen hand function test

surprisingly high number of subjects had difficulty opening foodstuffs, for example 87 per cent of women and 31 per cent of men in the 79-year-old age group were not able to open a jar with a smooth lid. The activities tested in these two studies are summarized in Figures 11.3 and 11.4. In addition to recording the time taken to complete the tasks Aniansson *et al.* (1980) also used a subjective scale by which the observer graded the subject's ability to perform the task in terms of 'without difficulty', 'with some difficulty' and 'not able to carry out task'.

TEMPA

A Canadian team of occupational therapists has recently developed another assessment of upper limb function in elderly patients. Desrosiers *et al.* (1993) named the assessment the TEMPA (Test Évaluant les Membres supérieurs des Personnes Agées); the test involves nine tasks related to ADL (Figure 11.5). The ability to perform the tasks is assessed in terms of the speed of execution of the task, a functional rating that corresponds to the assistance needed to complete the task, and a task analysis that notes any difficulties encountered performing the task.

Activity
1. Pick up and move jar
2. Open jar and take spoonful of coffee
3. Pour water from jug into glass
4. Open a lock and take the top off a pill box
5. Write and affix postage stamp
6. Put on scarf
7. Shuffle and deal cards
8. Use coins
9. Pick up and move small objects

Figure 11.5 Upper extremity function test for the elderly (TEMPA)

Desrosiers *et al.* determined the test–re-test and the inter-rater reliability of the TEMPA on a sample of 29 subjects aged 62–82 years with various degrees of upper limb dysfunction and varying degrees of functional ability. An initial assessment was conducted by one observer. Three to seven days later, the same observer reassessed the subject in the presence of a second observer. Each observer assessed the subject independently. Intraclass correlation coefficients ranged from moderate to high (0.70–1.0), demonstrating temporal stability and good agreement between different observers.

Desrosiers also considered the construct validity of TEMPA by assuming that upper limb function should relate directly to functional autonomy in ADL. Herbert *et al.* (1988) measured functional autonomy using the Functional Autonomy Measurement System (SMAF), which consists of five functional areas – ADL, mobility, communication, mental function and instrumental ADL. Each of these items is scored on a scale of 0–3, 0 being autonomy in task and 3 being totally dependent. The validity of SMAF has been established by comparing the SMAF scores with the time required for nursing care, and correlation coefficients of TEMPA compared to SMAF scores for personal care were high (Spearman's rho 0.74). TEMPA would appear to provide a valid and reliable measurement of upper limb function in an elderly population.

Problems associated with the measurement of hand and upper limb function

Reviews of ADL assessment by Jette (1985), Feinstein *et al.* (1986) and Eakin (1989a) have highlighted some of the problems associated with the assessment of function. The main problems are summarized in the following sections.

Lack of evidence of validity and reliability

One of the principal problems in the past with the assessments that are currently being used is that few were tested for reliability and validity. From the current literature it is apparent that efforts are now being made to rectify this problem. Only those methods that have been tested, or are in the process of being tested, have been referenced in this review.

Liang and Jette (1981) reviewed 12 scales used in the assessment of rheumatoid arthritis (RA).

They suggested that, for the accurate assessment of function, scales should demonstrate the following five criteria:

1. The instrument used should permit quantification
2. The instrument used should be shown to be a valid measure
3. The measure should be reliable
4. Data collection procedures should be standardized
5. The instrument should be able to distinguish changes in the condition being assessed.

Of the 12 assessments reviewed, none completely fulfilled all five criteria. It was found than none of the instruments were able to detect subtle changes in the patient's condition, and less than half of the scales had been tested for validity and reliability.

On completion of the review, Liang and Jette (1981) suggested that future work on the assessment of function should address the problems that they had highlighted; in particular, efforts should be made to validate functional assessment techniques. It was also noted that some forms of arthritis, especially juvenile arthritis and the spondylarthropathies, have unique functional problems, and although standardization of functional assessment is desirable, these conditions may necessitate the development of assessment techniques designed specifically for these conditions.

The diversity of scales and indexes

These can be grouped under three headings:

1. *Functions assessed.* Scales currently used cover a wide range of different functions, and have been developed to assess different medical conditions at different stages of the recovery process. In addition, certain scales are applicable to only one environment whereas others allow assessment of either in- or out-patients.
2. *Method of scoring function.* Different scales have different methods of scoring the same function. For example, some scales use a three-point and some a four-point scale, while others use descriptions rather than numbers to quantify functional ability.
3. *Mode of administration.* There is debate as to whether the mode of administration affects the reliability of the assessment; that is, should an interview, a questionnaire or observation be used to assess function?

The diversity of scales means that, if a subject was measured using two different methods, little (if any) comparison can be made between the resulting scores.

Operational procedures

There seems to be confusion as to whether independence in a function should be defined as including the use of aids and adaptive equipment or not. Some scales define independence in an activity as 'the ability to perform the function without the help of another person or use of adaptive equipment', whereas others allow the use of equipment 'providing the patient does not need human assistance'. Dunt *et al.* (1980) highlighted the importance of specifying the circumstances under which the ADL assessment is made, particularly in the use of aids or personal assistance. Due to this vagueness in definitions, Eakin (1989b) questions whether different ADL scales are actually measuring the same thing, and whether the results of different scales are comparable.

Other factors affecting functional measurement

The physical and mental condition of the patients will affect how they perform the activities. For example, pain, stiffness and joint deformity all affect the ability of a rheumatoid patient to perform ADL. In addition, the motivation of patients will contribute to their willingness to participate in the test.

Sheikh *et al.* (1979) also highlighted that there is sometimes a difference between what patients can do and what they actually do, and claimed that there are subtle differences between what the patient **wants** to perform, **needs** to perform, **can** perform and actually **does** perform. The situation is further complicated because these variables may alter from day to day, or indeed hour to hour.

Another major influence is the environment in which the functions are performed. For example, a test performed in the simulated home environment of an occupational therapy department may give a very different picture of the patient's ability to that in the real home environment. This may occur simply because the equipment and general layout (including the heights of work surfaces, etc.) will influence how the patient functions.

Summary of hand and upper limb measurement methods

There are many different methods of measuring upper limb and hand function and, from the studies performed, there does not appear to be one preferred method. Due to the lack of standardization both in the activities assessed and the methods used to quantify function, the uses of functional assessment are seriously compromised. Comparisons cannot be made, as it is questionable whether different scales are measuring the same thing.

Difficulties arise in the measurement of hand function because it is the product of a multiplicity of factors, many of which, such as the personality and the motivation of the patient, are intangible.

Although many authors have recognized the need for standardization, problems arise because some functional problems are peculiar to certain medical conditions. Scales may therefore still need to be 'customized' for the problems in function to be identified and rectified, and it may be necessary to maintain an array of scales and indexes.

Assessment of grip strength

As stated at the beginning of this chapter, the vast majority of published material on the assessment of hand function relates to the assessment of hand strength and, in particular, to grip strength. Grip strength is crucial for the performance of ADL. With the exception of locomotor activities, grip is used in almost every ADL, from when we awaken in the morning until we retire to bed at night; for example:

in washing, personal hygiene and dressing
at breakfast – preparing and eating food
at work – the hand is used in manual and office tasks, in driving, etc.
at lunch – in preparing and eating food
at home and in recreation – in DIY, sport, gardening, etc.
at night – washing, personal hygiene, undressing.

Despite the wide variety of tasks which we do with our hands, the majority of these tasks involve only two basic types of grip pattern. Napier (1956) identified these patterns as (1) the **power grip** and (2) the **precision grip**.

The power grip involves holding an object between the partially flexed fingers against the counter-pressure supplied by the palm, the thenar eminance and the distal segment of the thumb. As the name suggests, it is used when full strength is required.

Lehmkuhl and Smith (1983) further subdivide the power grip. The **cylindrical grasp** is where the entire palmar surface of the hand folds around a cylindrical object – for example, holding a can of juice, a hammer, a squash/tennis racket, etc. The

hook grasp is used when carrying a suitcase or briefcase, where digits two to five are used as a hook and the thumb usually remains inactive. When grasping a round object such as a ball, an apple or an orange, a **spheric grasp** may be used. This is where all the digits adhere to the surface of the object being held.

When a more accurate or delicate grip is required, the precision grip is used. It involves holding the object between the palmar or lateral aspect of the fingers and opposing thumb. Again, there are different classifications of precision grip. The **tip precision grip** is where the tip of the thumb is used against one of the other fingers to lift up a small object; for example, when picking up a bead, tack, coin, etc. The **lateral prehension grip** may be used when holding a thin object, such a key or piece of paper, when the object is held between the thumb and the lateral side of the index finger. For writing and picking up small objects, the **palmar prehension grip** is used; the thumb opposes one or more of the other digits and the object is held by the palmar surfaces of the distal phalanges of the digits involved in the grip (see Figure 11.6).

The following review of literature considers the many different uses of grip strength, the methods used to assess it and the factors that affect these measurements. The vast majority of the work published on grip strength considers the power grip.

The use of grip strength measurements

Grip strength is not merely a measure of hand strength or indeed limited to the assessment of the upper limb. It has many different clinical applications; for instance, it has been used as an indicator of total body strength, and as such is used in fitness testing (Balogun *et al.*, 1990, 1991a, 1991b, 1991c; Newman *et al.*, 1984). Spiegal *et al.* (1987) demonstrated that grip strength was a useful indicator of functional ability in serial measurements of rheumatoid patients. Grip strength has also been used to evaluate the effectiveness of drug treatment in relieving morning stiffness in rheumatoid patients (Myers *et al.*, 1980).

Due to its wide range of clinical applications many different methods have been devised to assess grip strength, depending on the purpose of the grip strength test and the type of subject tested.

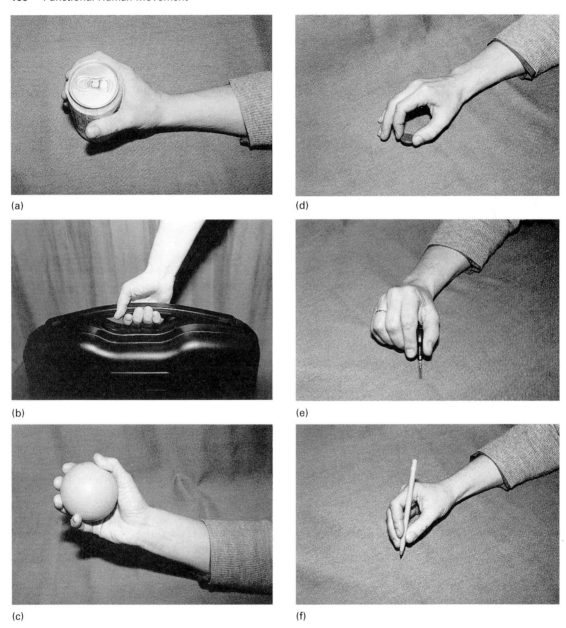

Figure 11.6 Examples of different types of grip: (a) the cylindrical grasp; (b) the hook grasp; (c) aspheric grasp; (d) the tip precision grip; (e) the lateral pretension grip; (f) the palmar prehension grip

Methods used to assess grip strength

Although the majority of methods reviewed used objective measures of grip strength, one group of investigators, Downie *et al.* (1978), did attempt to compare both subjective and objective measures of grip strength.

Subjective assessment of grip strength: the visual analogue scale

Downie *et al.* (1978) assessed grip strength by comparing actual grip strength, measured using a sphygmomanometer, with subjects' estimate of their grip strength marked on a 9 cm visual analogue scale (VAS). The extremes of the scale were marked as 30 mmHg (the pre-inflated pressure of the sphygmomanometer cuff) and 300 mmHg (the maximal pressure capable of being recorded by the sphygmomanometer). The subjects were also asked to describe their grip strength using a verbal scale of very weak, weak, normal and strong. In addition to the subjects' subjective assessment of their grip strength, an estimate of their strength was also made by a medically trained observer who estimated their grip based on how tightly the subject could grip three of the observer's fingers. The observer graded the strength (in mmHg) against the descriptive scale above. Three observers worked independently to gather the data – one performing the sphygmomanometer test, one conducting the subjective test of how the patients graded their grip strength, and one estimating grip strength as the subjects squeezed three fingers. Ninety-three rheumatoid patients and seven healthy subjects participated in the project.

The results suggested that the medical observer's estimate of the subjects' grip strength was superior to that of the patients; i.e. there was a positive correlation between estimated and actual grip strengths. The lack of correlation between the patients' estimation and actual strength suggested that the VAS was not the most appropriate method of assessing grip strength. Downie *et al.* (1978) suggested that the VAS may show more meaningful results if used as a serial measure, where patients would compare their present strength to a previous score rather than to an estimate of the actual strength. Little detail is given about the subjects used; in particular, their age and their level of comprehension are not recorded. It would be interesting to know if the VAS in another format would have given the same results. For example, the subjects might have found it easier to estimate their grip strength had the descriptions of grip strength been written on the visual analogue scale rather than the sphygmomanometer values at the extremes. It is doubtful whether 30 mmHg or 300 mmHg were meaningful measurements to lay people.

Objective measures of grip strength

Many different instruments have been designed for the objective measurement of grip strength, from the simple adaptation of blood pressure equipment, the sphygmomanometer (Downie *et al.*, 1978; Kowanko *et al.*, 1982), to devices specifically designed to measure a particular aspect of hand function. An *et al.* (1980) designed a set of strain

gauged instruments to measure, for example, pinch, grasp and lateral deviation strength of the intrinsic muscles of the fingers, and the universal meter to measure functional strength of the fingers and thumb. The Jamar dynamometer is the strain gauged system which has gained most clinical acceptance, and has been used regularly used in patient studies (Mathiowetz *et al.*, 1985a, 1985b, 1990).

There are many devices commercially available for the assessment of grip strength, and it would be impossible to review them all. A summary of some of the devices used is shown in Table 11.1, and a brief description of three of those most commonly used in clinical practice follows.

The vigorometer
The vigorometer consists of an air-filled bulb connected to a pressure gauge. Three different sizes of bulb are available; a small bulb is used when testing pinch grip, and the medium and large bulbs are used for the assessment of power grip. When the bulb is squeezed in the hand, the change in pressure is read from the dial on the pressure gauge.

The Jamar dynamometer
The Jamar dynamometer is a strain gauged system. It is constructed of two steel bars, which are linked together. To measure grip strength, the subject is instructed to attempt to squeeze the two bars together. As the subject squeezes the bars they bend, causing a change in resistance of the strain gauges, and there is a corresponding change in voltage output. The output is directly proportional to the force exerted on the bars.

The sphygmomanometer and modified sphygmomanometer
The standard equipment used for the measurement of blood pressure is often used for the measurement of grip strength and, indeed, for the assessment of strength of a number of muscle groups (Helewa *et al.*, 1981). Its widespread availability in the clinical setting, cheapness and ease of application have made it a popular method of assessment with clinicians both in the hospital and domiciliary settings. Originally it was used with little or no modifications – simply a standard Davis bag attached to a mercury manometer – but, more recently, the modified sphygmomanometer (MS)

Table 11.1 Methods used to measure grip strength

Author	Instrument used	Units	Number of trials	Measurement used for analysis	Testing position
An *et al.* (1980)	strain gauges	Newtons			
Balogun *et al.* (1991a)	Harpenden dynamometer	kg	2	maximum	four positions
Balogun *et al.* (1991b)	Harpenden dynamometer	kgf	2	maximum	standing: full elbow extension
Balogun *et al.* (1991c)	Harpenden dynamometer MS	kgf mmHg	2	maximum	standing: full elbow extension
Downie *et al.* (1978)	VAS MS	9 cm scale mmHg	3	mean of second and third trial	arm unsupported: elbow angle not specified
Fransson and Winkel (1991)	strain gauged pliers	Newtons	7	mean	standing
Fraser and Benten (1983)	vigorometer	lb/in^2	1		sitting: 90° elbow flexion
Gilbert and Knowlton (1983)	load cell	Newtons	2	mean	sitting: full elbow extension
Goldman *et al.* (1991)	Jamar	kgf	3	mean	not specified
Jarit (1991)	Jamar	kgf	3	maximum	sitting: 90° elbow flexion
Kellor *et al.* (1971)	Jamar	lb	2	maximum	subjects could adopt any elbow position
Lunde *et al.* (1971)	Kny-sheer dynamometer	lb	1		from head level to full extension
Lusardi and Bohannon (1991)	Jamar MS	kg mmHg	2	mean	sitting: 90° elbow flexion
Mathiowetz *et al.* (1985a)	Jamar	lb	3	mean	sitting: 90° elbow flexion
Mathiowetz *et al.* (1985b)	Jamar	not specified	3	mean	sitting: 90° elbow flexion
Mathiowetz *et al.* (1990)	Jamar	lb	3	mean	sitting: 90° elbow flexion
Marion and Niebuhr (1992)	Jamar	lb	6	maximal	sitting: 90° elbow flexion
Newman *et al.* (1984)	strain gauge system	Newtons	2	mean maximum	elbow position not specified
Shiffman (1992)	Jamar	lb	3	mean	sitting: 90° elbow flexion
Solgaard *et al.* (1984)	vigorometer My-gripper steel spring dynamometer	Newtons	5	mean	sitting: 90° elbow flexion
Somadeepti *et al.* (1990)	Jamar	lb	3	mean	not specified
Spiegel *et al.* (1987)	sphygmomanometer	mmHg	3	mean	not specified
Teraoka (1979)	Smedley dynamometer	kg	2	maximum	full elbow extension in sitting, lying and standing
Unsworth *et al.* (1990)	inflatable cuffs	mmHg	3	maximum	not specified

has become commonly used. In the MS, the Davis bag is folded into four equal parts with the remainder of the cuff wrapped around it and taped into place. It is smaller and easier to grip than the standard cuff.

Studies of the reproducibility and validity of the vigorometer, Jamar dynamometer and modified sphygmomanometer

Several studies have been performed to evaluate the performance of grip strength measurement tools in the clinical setting. Mathiowetz (1985c) stresses that, for grip strength data to be meaningful, it must be measured in a reliable and valid way. With such an array of methods and protocols, it is not surprising to learn that the validity and reliability of grip strength measurement devices using any one protocol has, until recently, received scant attention.

The vigorometer
Solgaard *et al.* (1984) investigated the validity of the vigorometer by loading it in a universal testing machine and comparing its output to that of the My-Gripper and a steel spring dynamometer. Both the My-gripper and the vigorometer with the medium balloon gave very precise measurements when tested for linearity throughout the range of applied loads, 50–500 N, but the steel spring dynamometer and the vigorometer with the small and large balloons attached tended to give lower than expected outputs for larger forces. Each instrument was loaded five times, and its reproducibility established by comparing the variation coefficients. The vigorometer with the medium balloon and the My-gripper showed the least variation between repeated measurements. Solgaard investigated whether the precision of the instruments was affected by the grip strength of the individual. One hundred healthy subjects aged between 20 and 87 years performed five repeats of grip strength tests on each hand, using each of the instruments. It was found that the My-gripper had higher precision than the other instruments when measuring weaker subjects, and that the vigorometer with medium balloon had the highest precision of the three instruments when measuring stronger subjects, with a coefficient of variation of around 6 per cent. From this study, Solgaard concluded that the vigorometer was an acceptable, reliable and precise method of measuring grip strength.

The Jamar dynamometer
Mathiowetz *et al.* (1985a) describes the determination of the calibration accuracy as one method of determining an instrument's validity. Fess (1987) tested each of the five handle positions of the Jamar dynamometer by applying known loads at each of the positions, and considered calibration coefficients of 0.9994 to be acceptable.

Using this method, Mathiowetz *et al.* (1984) found the Jamar dynamometer to have a calibration accuracy of ±3 per cent. In 1987, Flood-Joy and Mathiowetz investigated the inter-instrument reliability of the Jamar dynamometer by calibrating three different instruments and comparing the calibration results. They did not find a significant difference in the calibration accuracy of the three devices.

Following calibration of the Jamar dynamometer, Flood-Joy and Mathiowetz (1987) considered the reliability and validity of grip strength evaluations in the clinical setting by measuring the strength of 27 female occupational therapy students aged 20–39 years. They conducted a series of tests to determine the inter-rater reliability, and to compare the test–re-test reliability for one, two and three trial tests, and the reliability of using the highest score as the outcome measure. All of the tests were conducted using the second handle position of the Jamar dynamometer. At the first testing session, two observers were present and independently recorded the grip strength. Subjects were then re-tested a week later by one of the examiners.

Mathiowetz found the inter-rater reliability to be high, with a correlation coefficient of 0.97 or above for all of the tests, and concluded that, when two experienced observers followed a standardized protocol, they could obtain similar measurements of grip strength. When considering the test–re-test reliability of different numbers of trials, it was found that the mean of the three trials was most consistent, having a correlation coefficient of 0.80 and above. On average, the lowest correlation was found when only one trial was used as a measurement of grip strength.

The sphygmomanometer and modified sphygmomanometer
Balogun *et al.* (1991c) investigated the validity and reproducibility of the modified sphygmomanometer (MS) by conducting a test–re-test experiment. In the first test, the validity of the MS was investigated by comparing the grip strength recorded against a 'gold standard', which was the

strength of the same subject tested using the Harpenden dynamometer. The results confirmed that the MS was a valid method of measuring grip strength, as it was shown to be positively related (r = 0.841, $p > 0.00001$) to the corresponding measurements taken with the Harpenden dynamometer.

The reproducibility of the MS was determined by performing a second measurement of grip strength test, using the MS, twenty-four hours after the original test. Both sets of tests were performed on 34 healthy volunteers aged between 16 and 28 years. Results showed that grip strength measured using the MS was highly reproducible in the twenty-four hour interval between the first and subsequent tests. Based on these results, Balogun concluded that the MS was a valid and reliable method of measuring grip strength.

The effect of measuring grip strength with different instrumentation

Table 11.1 shows that one of the biggest problems with the assessment of grip strength has been the lack of standardization in terms of both the instrumentation used and the testing protocol adopted. It is extremely difficult to compare results when two completely different measurement devices have been used, and results must be interpreted with extreme caution. If two different measurement tools have been used, then two different hand configurations will have been employed during the production of grip and therefore different muscles will have been tested.

Even with the same instrument, care is needed to use the same protocol each time the subject is tested if results are to be comparable. Goldman *et al.* (1991) investigated the difference in grip strength at the five handle positions of the Jamar dynamometer. Maximum grip strength was produced at the second and third handle positions, with a reduction in grip strength in the remaining three positions.

A similar situation occurs using the vigorometer; that is, it is necessary to use the same size of balloon for all tests on the same subject. Fraser and Benten (1983) found that men aged 30–39 years produced a mean grip strength of 17 lb/in^2 measured with the large bulb, whereas the same men produced a mean grip of 21.5 lb/in^2 when measured using the medium balloon.

Fransson and Winkel (1991) investigated the effect of grip span and grip type on hand strength

using a pair of pliers instrumented with strain gauges. The highest resultant force at the jaws of the pliers was obtained at a handle separation of 50–60 mm for women and between 55–65 mm for men. For wider handle separations, the resultant force reduced by 10 per cent.

It can therefore be seen that hand configuration must be standardized to obtain meaningful serial measures of hand grip strength.

Another problem associated with using different devices is that results cannot be compared directly, as different devices tend to use different units of measurement. Therefore, conversion factors need to be used before one can begin to compare the results. As mentioned previously, Balogun *et al.* (1991c) compared results obtained from the Harpenden dynamometer to those obtained from the same subject using a MS, and used linear and multiple regression equations to convert the MS output in mmHg to the kgf units measured by the dynamometer. The aim of this study was to validate the MS.

Lusardi and Bohannon (1991) performed a study specifically to compare grip strength measured with a modified sphygmomanometer and that measured using a Jamar dynamometer. Thirty-four healthy females aged 19–64 years participated in the study. Grip strength measurements of the subject's dominant hand were made using a Jamar dynamometer, MS pre-inflated to 20 mmHg and MS pre-inflated to 30 mmHg. Two measurements were taken using each instrument, and the order of testing was randomly assigned. The measurements obtained from the three instruments varied in comparability, with good comparability between the two MSs (r = 0.836) and lesser comparability between the Jamar and each of the MSs (r = 0.417 and r = 0.509 respectively).

The lack of direct comparability may well have been anticipated as the instruments use different transmission mediums to measure grip strength, and different hand configurations are used during the tests. The MS measures pressure produced within the sphygmomanometer cuff, while the Jamar dynamometer is measuring force exerted on the handle. The different hand configuration used during the production of grip will produce different joint and muscle mechanics, which will affect hand strength. Lusardi and Bohannon (1991) stated that 'there was no clear indication that initial starting pressure influenced grip strength results'. This is in direct contrast to the work of Unsworth *et al.* (1990), who found that initial starting pressure in the cuff did give significantly different results

($p < 0.05$) when testing both in a materials testing machine and with rheumatoid patients.

Normative data

There have been several studies using various instruments attempting to produce normative data for grip strength. Fraser and Benten (1983) used the vigorometer to assess the grip strength of 120 healthy subjects aged from 20 to 79 years. This study highlighted the need for consistency in the size of bulb used with the vigorometer for repeated tests. Subjects repeated the grip strength test using both the large- and medium-sized bulbs, and results varied depending on the bulb size.

Lunde *et al.* (1972) measured the grip strength of 57 college women using the Kny-Sheer dynamometer. In addition to establishing norms, Lunde is one of the few investigators to attempt to perform longitudinal studies of grip strength in either normal subjects or patients affected by a particular condition. Nine subjects were tested annually for three years, and 32 subjects were tested over two years. It was found that there was no significant difference in grip strength over the duration of the tests. The results are based on a very small sample population and the age of the subjects was not specified, so it is questionable as to whether a similar longitudinal study would have shown the same results in an older population. The results, therefore, may not be applicable to all normal subjects of different ages.

Few studies, apart from Newman *et al.* (1984), have considered the need for normative data of grip strength for healthy children. Newman conducted grip strength tests on 1417 healthy school-children using a strain gauged dynamometer system. This system is not commercially available and, therefore, the findings of this study cannot be repeated with another population of schoolchildren to investigate whether the results are repeatable and applicable to all children in a particular age group or just to those children tested.

The Jamar dynamometer has been used in several studies in an attempt to establish grip strength norms. Kellor *et al.* (1971) tested the grip strength of 250 men and women and also tested pinch grip strength and hand dexterity using a peg board test. Mathiowetz (1985a) also used the Jamar dynamometer to measure the grip strength of 310 male and 328 female adults; he, too, measured pinch. Despite the fact that both studies used the same instrumentation and similar age groups (subjects aged between 20 and 90 years), a

direct comparison still cannot be made for several reasons resulting from a lack of standardized testing procedures. Kellor *et al.* (1971) did not specify a standard position for the test; subjects were allowed to rest their arm on the tabletop if they wished, and were able to position the elbow in either flexion or extension. Mathiowetz (1985a), however, had a standardized procedure with all subjects seated with the elbow flexed to ninety degrees during the test. As will be discussed in the next section, grip strength may be influenced by body posture, elbow position or by both. Another discrepancy between the two studies existed in the Jamar handle position used for the test – Mathiowetz states that the second handle position was used for all subjects, whilst Kellor does not specify which handle position was used or whether or not it was adjusted to suit the individual.

Measurements used to represent grip strength

The above two studies also differed in the measurements considered to be most representative of a subject's grip strength. Kellor *et al.* (1971) took two measurements and recorded the highest value, whereas Mathiowetz (1985a) took three measurements and used the mean values in his analysis. It can be seen from Table 11.1 that there is no set procedure as to how many measurements should be taken, and whether the mean or maximal values best portray a subject's grip strength. Newman *et al.* (1984) uses neither the mean nor the maximum but the 'mean maximum', which was the mean of four tests, two with each hand, and the 'mean peak', the mean of the highest value for each of the four tests. A problem arises because a single trial may not be a true reflection of the strength the subject is capable of – it often takes a practice trial for the patient to know exactly what is required, and yet too many practice runs may cause learning or fatigue to influence results.

Mathiowetz (1990) recommends that the average of three trials be used, claiming that this method resulted in improved test–re-test reliability compared to that achieved with one trial or the best of two trials. Mathiowetz (1990) investigated whether practice or fatigue effects influenced grip strength when the mean of three trials was used. Forty-nine healthy subjects and forty-nine rehabilitation patients aged 17–81 years participated in the study, and the scores of three successive trials of each hand were recorded with 15 second inter-trial rest periods. Of all the subjects tested, four had significant differences between trials; only one of the four was from the rehabilitation group. Fatigue was thought to be the most likely cause of the difference between trials, as the scores were gradually decreasing. It was also noted that, in all four subjects, the differences occurred in the latter half of the test and it was therefore possible that it may have been due to the cumulative effect of the multiple trials. For the majority of subjects in both groups the three-trial method had minimal effect on the grip strength recorded, and the effect on the two groups of subjects was not significantly different. Mathiowetz therefore recommended that this procedure was suitable for use with both healthy subjects and patients.

Effect of body posture and elbow position

There are differing views as to the effect of body posture and elbow position on grip strength.

Teraoka (1979) conducted the most extensive study of the effect of posture on grip strength by testing 9543 subjects aged 15–55 years in three positions – standing, sitting and supine lying. In all three positions, the elbow was maintained in full extension. A significant difference was found in grip strength depending on body posture. Grip strength in standing was found to be significantly greater than in sitting, which was found to be significantly greater than in supine lying.

More recently, Balogun *et al.* (1991a) studied the effect of both body posture and elbow position on grip strength. The grip strength of 61 subjects (26 male and 35 female) aged 16–28 years was tested in four positions – sitting with the elbow in 90° of flexion, sitting with the elbow in full extension, standing with the elbow in 90° of flexion and standing with the elbow in full extension. Results revealed that there was a significant difference in grip strength measured with the subject seated with the elbow at 90° of flexion and when standing with the elbow in full extension. In agreement with Teraoka (1979) there was an increase in grip strength from sitting to standing, and Balogun was also able to identify an increase from elbow flexion to extension.

Mathiowetz (1985b) considered the effect of elbow position, but not body posture, on the grip strength of 29 women aged 20–34 years. All tests were conducted with the subject seated. Tests were performed on both hands, and were repeated with the elbow in full extension and 90° of flexion. In contrast to Balogun *et al.* (1991a), it was found that the women's grip strength was significantly stronger in both hands with the elbow in the flexed rather than extended position.

The position of the wrist during grip strength tests has also been investigated by Kraft (1972), who found no significant difference in grip strength when the wrist was in neutral, 15 or 30° of extension. However, grip strength was found to be significantly lower when the wrist was flexed to 15°. Pryce (1980) confirmed that lower grip strengths were recorded when the wrist was in 15° of flexion, and similar results were found with ulnar deviation of 30°.

Lamoreaux and Hoffer (1995) evaluated the effect of wrist deviation on grip and pinch strength. Strength was measured with the wrist in neutral and maximal ulnar and maximal radial deviation. It was found that the effect on pinch grip was not significant, but grip strength was significantly reduced ($p < 0.0001$).

From Table 11.1 it can be seen that some studies used the elbow-flexed position, some the extended position and others did not specify the elbow position. The inconsistency in the testing position of the subjects makes comparison between studies questionable. In a bid to allow comparisons to be made, The American Society of Hand Therapists (1981) advocated that all patients be tested in a standard position. It is recommended that the subject be seated with the shoulder adducted and neutrally rotated, elbow flexed to 90°, forearm in neutral position, and the wrist between 0 and 30° of extension and 0 to 15° of ulnar deviation. Mathiowetz *et al.* (1985b) supports the elbow-flexed position for testing; however, Balogun *et al.* (1991a) found this position gave the lowest grip strength. Despite this, Balogun did not suggest dismissing the suggestions made by the American Society of Hand Therapists, as it is recognized that there is a need for a standardized testing position and without it data cannot be compared with norms if different protocols have been used.

Summary of methods used to measure grip strength

It can be seen that there is much debate and little consistency concerning the instruments used and the protocols employed in the assessment of grip strength. The studies discussed have shown that different instruments produce different measures of grip strength due to different measurement media, and that different muscle and joint mechanics are involved when different hand configurations were used to grip the different instruments.

The work reviewed also highlighted that, even when the same instrument was used, discrepancies still existed in the methods implemented. The work of Fraser and Benten (1983) described how using different sizes of bulb with the vigorometer influenced grip strength results.

The comparison of the works of Mathiowetz (1990) and Kellor *et al.* (1971), who both used the Jamar dynamometer, showed how difficult it was to draw any comparisons in the work because of the different protocols used in each study.

Unsworth *et al.* (1990) demonstrated that using inflatable cuffs at different starting pressures influenced grip strength results.

Because of the inconsistencies in the assessment techniques used to date, it is debatable whether 'norms' for grip strength exist for any of the instruments reviewed. These norms may only be applicable to similar subjects measured in exactly the same way using the same instrument and the same testing protocol. It is clear, however, that there is a complete lack of standardization in testing procedures used to measure grip strength.

Factors affecting grip strength

Despite the lack of consensus on the instrumentation and testing protocols used, several factors have been shown to influence grip strength regardless of the instrument or technique used. Table 11.2 summarizes the authors and the different instruments and populations used in identifying these factors.

Physical characteristics of the subject

Sex
From Table 11.2 it is clear that several authors have found a relationship between the sex of the subject and grip strength. Despite the limitations previously described in the normative data available, it was found that men were generally stronger than women. The normative data for men and women cover a wide range of possible grip strengths and, in isolated cases, some women are stronger than some men.

Measurement of grip strength of healthy adults using the vigorometer, the Jamar dynamometer and the MS all reported greater grip strength in men compared to women. Fraser and Benten (1983), using the vigorometer, found men significantly stronger than women. Kellor *et al.* (1971), using the Jamar dynamometer, confirmed that men had a more powerful grip strength than women and that this superiority was maintained throughout adult life. In addition, Kellor *et al.* (1971) investigated hand dexterity by performing timed peg board tests, and it was found women were more dextrous than men.

Balogun *et al.* (1991a) found that males had higher grip strength than women at all testing postures and elbow joint angles. The grip strength of children showed a similar pattern to adults. Newman *et al.* (1984) tested 1417 children aged 5–18 years and found that, at all ages, boys had greater grip strength than girls.

Age
Studies on the effect of age on grip strength suggest a curvilinear relationship, i.e. increasing up to about the age of 20 years, peaking somewhere between 19 and 50 years and then gradually declining. Table 11.2 summarizes the results of several authors who found a relationship between grip strength and age.

Newman *et al.* (1984) attempted to establish norms for the 5–18 years age group. As mentioned previously, boys were stronger than girls at all ages. The grip strength of girls increased, almost linearly, up to the age of 13 years, after which the mean grip strength tended to remain constant. Boys tended to show an approximately linear increase throughout the age group studied.

Balogun *et al.* (1991b) measured the grip strength of 960 healthy subjects aged 7–84 years and found that grip strength was positively related to age up to the third decade of life. Thereafter, grip strength was inversely related to age. It was found that grip strength increased with chronological age for both sexes, but tended to peak at different ages. The grip strength of males peaked between 30 and 39 years and in women it was found to peak between 20 and 29 years, after which there was a gradual decline in both sexes.

Mathiowetz *et al.* (1985a) attempted to establish clinical norms in the 20–75 years age group. As with Balogun *et al.* (1991b) the peak grip strength was recorded between 25 and 39 years, but Mathiowetz does not stipulate if the peak occurred at different ages for each of the sexes.

Teraoka (1979) tested the largest population, 9543 healthy male and female subjects, but only considered the effect of age up to 55 years. Grip strength was found to be related to age, sex and body position. It depended on body posture in both sexes and in all age groups. There was an increase in grip strength in male subjects between the ages

Table 11.2 Factors affecting grip strength

Author	Instrument	Population	Sex	Age	Height/weight	Hand dominance
An et al. (1980)	strain gauges					
Balogun et al. (1991a)	Harpenden dynamometer	(F = 26, M = 35), healthy 16–28 years	M > F	positive correlation	positive correlation	dominant only tested
Balogun et al. (1991b)	Harpenden dynamometer	(F = 480, M = 480), healthy 7–84 years	M > F	positive correlation up to 3rd decade; thereafter a negative correlation	positive correlation	R > L
Balogun et al. (1991c)	Harpenden dynamometer MS	(F = 6, M = 31), healthy 16–28 years				R only tested
Downie et al. (1978)	VAS	7 healthy				
	MS	93 rheumatoid				
Fransson and Winkel (1991)	strain gauged pliers	(F = 8, M = 8), healthy 18–60 years	M > F			R only tested
Fraser and Benten (1983)	vigorometer	(F = 60, M = 60), healthy 20–80 years	M > F	increase to 30 years, then deterioration with age, especially after 50 years		no significant difference between R and L
Gilbert and Knowlton (1984)	load cell	(F = 16, M = 20), healthy 20–26 years	M > F			dominant only
Goldman et al. (1991)	Jamar	(F = 16, M = 10), healthy 23–29 years (F = 11, M = 10), hand patients 23–84 years				both hands tested injured less than non-injured
Jarit (1991)	Jamar	44 controls, 44 baseball players				non-dominant 89.78% of dominant in baseball players; 86.75% in control group

Study	Instrument	Sample	Sex	Age	Height/weight	Side/dominance
Kellor et al. (1971)	Jamar	(F = 126, M = 126), healthy 18–84 years	M > F	negative correlation		R > L
Lunde et al. (1971)	Kny-sheer dynamometer	F = 57, healthy			positively correlated with height and weight	dominant hand 13% stronger than non-dominant
Lusardi and Bohannon (1991)	Jamar MS	F = 34, healthy 19–64 years				
Mathiowetz et al. (1985a)	Jamar	(F = 328, M = 310), healthy 20–94 years	M > F	peaked 25–39 years, gradual decline		R > L
Mathiowetz et al. (1985b)	Jamar	F = 29, healthy 20–34 years				R > L
Mathiowetz et al. (1990)	Jamar	49 controls, 49 rehabilitation patients				
Marion and Niebuhr (1992)	Jamar	F = 30, healthy 21–45 years				R only tested
Newman et al. (1984)	strain gauged system	1417 healthy children, 5–18 years	M > F	boys – linear increase. Girls increase to 13, then plateau	positive correlation with height and weight	dominant hand >strength
Shiffman (1992)	Jamar	(F = 20, M = 20), healthy 24–87 years		negative correlation with age		R > L
Solgaard et al. (1984)	vigorometer My-gripper steel spring dynamometer	(F = 55, M = 45), healthy 20–87 years		negative correlation with age	positive correlation with height and weight	dominant > non-dominant
Somadeepti et al. (1990)	Jamar	(F = 30, M = 30), unilaterally injured, mean age 28 years	M > F			
Spiegal et al. (1987)	sphygmomanometer	92 rhematoid patients, mean age 58 years				R and L measured, results not specified
Teraoka (1979)	Smedley dynamometer	9543, healthy 15–55 years	M > F	negative correlation with age		R > L
Unsworth et al. (1990)	inflatable cuffs					

of 15 and 18 years for both the left and right hands, and this increase continued to about 30 years of age. There was then a general decline to 55 years, the maximum age Teraoka considered. In the female population, grip strength increased between 15 and 20 years of age in both the left and right hands and this increase continued until about the age of 35 years, after which (similarly to the male population) there was a gradual decline to the age of 55 years.

Most studies have considered the effect of aging only in terms of hand strength; few have considered the effect of aging on hand function. However, Shiffman (1992) investigated the effect of aging on functional performance in subjects aged 24–87 years. Grip strength was measured using the Jamar dynamometer. In addition, the activities of pouring milk into a cup and removing money from a wallet were analysed from video recordings of the actions. It was found that there were statistically significant differences with age in grip strength, prehension patterns and time taken to perform tasks. Hand function tended to remain stable until the age of 65 and thereafter there was a deterioration in functional ability, subjects taking significantly longer times to complete tasks.

Longitudinal studies are needed to investigate the effect of grip strength with age, as the majority of studies have only considered grip strength at one moment in time. Spiegel *et al.* (1987) did re-test after a one-year absence, but as only rheumatoid patients were considered, there was no control group to consider the normal aging process. Lunde *et al.* (1972) did repeat tests on nine college woman annually for three years, but no significant difference was found between tests in that age group – a more elderly population may well have shown a different pattern.

Height and body weight
Several authors identified in Table 11.2 have reported a positive correlation between grip strength and body weight, and also between grip strength and height.

Balogun *et al.* (1991b) considered grip strength as a function of age, height, body weight and Quetelet index to determine the viability of using the physical characteristics of the subject to predict grip strength. The Quetelet index is a measure of weight adjusted for height, and is an objective measure of body adiposity. Balogun measured grip strength and the physical characteristics of 960 subjects aged 7–84 years. Using linear, multiple and stepwise regressions, grip strength was found to be positively related to body weight and height for all groups, and positively related to the Quetelet index during the first two decades of life. It was also noted that grip strength could be reliably predicted from a subject's age, weight, height and Quetelet index. Results indicated that over 80 per cent of the total variance in grip strength of both sexes was attributable to body weight, with height contributing less than 1 per cent for males and 2 per cent for females. For both male and female subjects the Quetelet index and age contributed less than 1 per cent to the prediction of grip strength. By investigating such a wide age group, Balogun was able to identify that body weight in adolescents and young adults was found to be the most viable predictor of grip strength but that, in the older age groups, age was the most viable predictor of grip strength. It was recommended that normative data of grip strength should be based both on body weight and age rather than age alone.

Hand dominance
The effect of hand dominance on grip strength has important clinical implications. In the assessment and treatment of hand injuries it is common clinical practice to assess the unaffected hand and base the aim of treatment on achieving the same strength in the affected hand, assuming there to be no significant difference between the two. The effect of hand dominance has been difficult to establish, as many studies do not specify whether the dominant or non-dominant hand was tested. In addition, because the majority of people tend to be right-handed, there are few studies with enough left-handed people to enable statistical analysis to be performed on the data.

The problem of different measures used in the analysis of the results again limits comparisons between studies. Of those authors who specified hand dominance, Fraser and Benten (1983) and Mathiowetz (1985a) found no significant differences in grip strength between the right and left hands; by contrast, Lunde *et al.* (1972) found the dominant hand to be 13 per cent stronger than the non-dominant.

Jarit (1991) looked specifically at the effect of hand dominance on the grip strength of college baseball players. Using the Jamar dynamometer, the grip strength of 44 baseball players and 44 controls was measured. The aim of the study was to determine whether the normal grip strength ratio of dominant to the non-dominant hand in college baseball players was significantly greater than that of the control group. The result indicated that there was no significant difference in the dominant and non-dominant hand grip strength ratios of baseball players compared to the normal control group. In the control group the non-dominant hand was 86.75 per cent as strong as the dominant hand, and in the baseball players' group the non-dominant hand was 89.78 per cent as strong as the dominant hand.

Fraser and Benten (1983) found a significant difference between the grip strength of the right and left hands in female subjects, but not in male subjects, when tested using the vigorometer. All of the subjects tested were right hand dominant. They also identified a possible link between occupation and grip strength, as many of the male subjects used their left hand in a power grip to stabilize objects while performing fine skilled movements with their right hands. To investigate this further, Fraser and Benten (1983) conducted tests on 22 right-handed male stonemasons, carvers, joiners and wood machinists. It was found that 13 had stronger grip in the left hand compared to the right.

Fraser and Benten therefore concluded that, when using the uninjured hand as a reference for recovery, it is necessary to consider the patient's occupation and, in particular, the function of both hands when determining whether the patient has achieved full recovery of grip strength.

Sincerity of effort

The level of the subjects' motivation will affect their willingness to exert maximal effort during the test procedures. Several studies have developed ways of distinguishing sincere efforts from fake efforts. Gilbert and Knowlton (1983) and Somadeepti *et al.* (1990) used the plots of the force–time characteristics of the grip strength test to identify sincere and fake efforts. Both the fake and sincere force–time curves showed an initial build up of force. This plateaued at a level close to maximum force in cases of sincere effort; however, for fake trials there was often an initial spike followed by a gradual decline in the magnitude of force.

Warm-up prior to testing

Marion and Niebuhr (1992) found that subjects had increased grip strength following submaximal trials prior to maximal grip strength trials. The grip strength of 33 women was measured using the Jamar dynamometer; all handle positions were tested. Prior to maximal effort, the 15 subjects performed six submaximal trials. The remaining 15 subjects performed six maximal efforts, followed by six submaximal efforts. For maximal tests the subjects were instructed to squeeze the handle as hard as possible, and for submaximal tests they were instructed to apply approximately 50 per cent of their maximal effort. Results showed that higher grip strength was recorded in the group who had performed a warm-up prior to exerting maximal effort. This result was repeated at each of the handle positions.

In a second set of experiments, the same procedure was repeated but using only the second Jamar handle position. Again it was shown that subjects exerted a greater maximal grip strength after a warm-up period. It had been hypothesized that the maximal grip strength would occur at the end of the six trials, but this hypothesis was not supported. Instead, it was found that the effect of warm-up was the same across all trials.

Physical impairment

All of the aforementioned factors influence grip strength in healthy subjects. In addition to these, other factors will influence grip strength in subjects suffering upper limb impairments. Pain, stiffness and joint deformity all affect the grip strength of rheumatoid arthritic patients. The problem of assessing grip strength in the rheumatoid patient is further complicated by the fact that the condition of the patient can vary, not only from day to day but, due to morning stiffness, from hour to hour.

Kowanko *et al.* (1982) addressed this problem by conducting a study in which the subjects performed domiciliary self-measurement of their grip strength using a sphygmomanometer. Measurements were repeated at 0800, 1100, 1300, 1500, 2000 and 2300 hours. The patients' subjective experiences of pain and stiffness were assessed using horizontal integer scales numbered 0 (no pain or stiffness) to 10 (worst possible pain and stiffness). There was no significant difference in grip strength taken at the same time of day on different days, but there were significant variations when grip strengths were compared for different times of the day. The variation in the day was thought to be due to the circadian variations in symptoms experienced by RA patients. Grip strength was found to be lowest in the earliest part of the day. Negative correlations were found between the subjects' subjective experiences of pain and stiffness and magnitude grip strength. Kowanko *et al.* (1982) argues that for rheumatoid patients, where symptoms vary so much, serial measurements provide a much clearer picture of their condition rather than a single measurement taken at a hospital clinic appointment, which may not truly reflect the patients' condition.

The measurement of pinch grip

As mentioned earlier, most of the literature pertaining to grip strength refers to power rather than pinch grip. Literature available on the measurement of pinch grip suffers from many of the same criticisms of power strength measurement, i.e. there is lack of standardization in the measurement devices used, the positioning of the subject during measurement and the protocol used, and a lack of information concerning the validity, calibration accuracy and repeatability of the measurements obtained.

The most common devices used to measure pinch strength are the B&L Engineering pinch gauge (Mathiowetz *et al.*, 1985a, 1985b; Mathiowetz, 1990) and the vigorometer (Oberg et al., 1994). Mathiowetz *et al.* (1985a) attempted to provide normative data for both power grip and pinch grip in a sample of 310 male and 328 female subjects aged between 20 and 94 years, and recommended the use of the B&L Engineering pinch meter, having established its accuracy to be of the order of ±1 per cent. The factors discussed that affect power grip strength have also been shown to influence the measurement of pinch grip strength.

From the review of current literature, it can be seen that there are major discrepancies in the methods used to measure grip strength. It may seem surprising that such little standardization has occurred when grip strength measurements are used in so many clinical applications.

Summary of limitations

There is no standard instrument and no accepted standard protocol employed (despite the recommendations of the American Society of Hand Therapists, 1981) to measure grip strength. In addition, there is no standard measurement (i.e. mean or maximum values) used to represent grip strength. Until these issues are addressed, little comparison can be made between studies and grip strength norms cannot be established.

References

American Society of Hand Therapists (1981). *Clinical Assessment Recommendations*. ASHT Garner.

An, K., Chao, E. Y. S. and Askew, L. J. (1980). Hand strength measurement instruments. *Arch. Phys. Med. Rehabil.*, **61**, 366–8.

Aniansson, A., Rundgren, A. and Sperling, L. (1980). Evaluation of functional capacity in activities of daily living in 70-year-old men and women. *Scand. J. Rehab. Med.*, **12**, 145–54.

Balogun, J. H., Akomolafe, C. T. and Amusa, L. O. (1990). Reproducibility and criterion-related validity of the modified sphygomanometer for isometric grip strength. *Physiother. Can.*, **42(6)**, 290–95.

Balogun, J. A., Akomolafe, C. T. and Amusa, L. O. (1991a). Grip strength: effects of testing posture and elbow position. *Arch. Phys. Med. Rehabil.*, **72**, 280–83.

Balogun, J. A., Akinloye, A. A. and Adenlola, A. (1991b). Grip strength as a function of age, height, body weight and Quetelet index. *Physiother. Theory Prac.*, **7**, 111–19.

Balogun, J. A., Akomolafe, C. T. and Amusa, L. O. (1991c). Reproducibility and criterion related validity of the modified sphygmomanometer for isometric testing of grip strength. *Physiother. Can.*, **42(6)**, 290–95.

Carroll, D. (1965). A quantitative test of upper extremity function. *J. Chron. Dis.*, **18**, 479–91.

Desrosiers, J., Hebert, R., Dutil, E. and Bravo, G. (1993). Development and reliability of an upper extremity function test for the elderly: the TEMPA. *Can. J. Occup. Ther.*, **60(1)**, 9–16.

Downie, W. W., Leatham, P. A., Rhind, V. M. *et al.* (1978). The visual analogue scale in the assessment of grip strength. *Ann. Rheum. Dis.*, **37**, 382–4.

Dunt, D. R., Kaufert, J. M., Corkhill, R. *et al.* (1980). A technique for precisely measuring activities of daily living. *Comm. Med.*, **2**, 120–25.

Eakin, P. (1989a). Assessments of activities of daily living: a critical review. *Br. J. Occup. Ther.*, **52(1)**, 11–15.

Eakin, P. (1989b). Problems with assessments of activities of daily living. *Br. J. Occup. Ther.*, **52(2)**, 50–54.

Feinstein, A. R., Josephy, B. R. and Wells, C. K. (1986). Scientific and clinical problems in indexes of functional disability. *Ann. Intern. Med.*, **105(3)**, 413–20.

Fess, E. E. (1987). The need for reliability and validity in hand assessment measurements. *J. Hand Surg.*, **11A(5)**, 621–3.

Flood-Joy, M. and Mathiowetz, V. (1987). Grip strength measurement: comparison of three Jamar dynamometers. *Occup. Ther. J. Res.*, **7**, 490–97.

Fransson, C. and Winkel, J. (1991). Hand strength: the influence of grip span and grip type. *Ergonomics*, **34(7)**, 881–92.

Fraser, C. and Benten, J. (1983). A study of adult hand strength. *Occup. Ther.*, October, 296–9.

Gilbert, J. C. and Knowlton, R. G. (1983). Simple method to determine sincerity of effort during a maximal isometric test for grip strength. *Am. J. Phys. Med.*, **62(3)**, 135–44.

Goldman, S., Calahan, T. D. and An, K. (1991). The injured

upper extremity and the Jamar five-handle position grip test. *Am. J. Phys. Med. Rehabil.*, **70(6)**, 306–8.

Hackel, M. E., Wolfe, G. A., Bang, S. M. and Canfield, J. S. (1992). Changes in hand function in adult aging as determined by the Jebsen test of hand function. *Phys. Ther.*, **72(5)**, 49–53.

Helewa, A.,Goldsmith, C. H. and Smythe, H. A. (1981). The modified sphygmomanometer – an instrument to measure muscle strength: a validation study. *J. Chron. Dis.*, **34**, 353–61.

Herbert, R., Carrier, R. and Bilodeau, A. (1988). The functional autonomy measurement system (SMAF): description and validation of an instrument for the measurement of handicaps. *Age and Aging*, **17**, 293–302.

Jarit, P. (1991). Dominant hand to non-dominant hand grip strength ratios of college baseball players. *J. Hand Ther.*, July – September, 123–6.

Jebsen, R. H, Taylor, N. and Trieschmann, R. B. (1969). An objective and standardized test for hand function. *Arch. Phys. Med. Rehabil.*, **50**, 311–19.

Jette, A. M. (1985). State of the art in functional status assessment. In *Measurement in Physical Therapy* (J. M. Rothstein, ed.), pp. 137–68. Churchill Livingstone.

Kellor, M., Frost, J., Silberberg, N. *et al.* (1971). Hand strength and dexterity. *Am. J. Occup Ther.*, **25(2)**, 77–83.

Kowanko, I. C., Knapp, M. S., Pownall, R. and Swannell A. J. (1982). Domiciliary self-measurement in rheumatoid arthritis and the demonstration of circadian rhythmicity. *Ann. Rheum. Dis.*, **41**, 453–5.

Kraft, G. and Destels, P. (1972). Position of function of the wrist. *Arch. Phys. Med. Rehabil.*, **53**, 272.

Lamoreaux, L. and Hoffer, M. M. (1995). The effect of wrist deviation on grip and pinch strength. *Clin. Orth. Rel. Res.*, **314**, 152–55.

Lehmkuhl, L. D. and Smith, L. K. (1983). *Brunnstrom's Clinical Kiesiology* (4th edn.) F. A. Davis Company.

Liang, M. H. and Jette A.M. (1981). Measuring functional ability in chronic arthritis: a critical review. *Arth. Rheum.*, **24(1)**, 80–86.

Lunde, B. K., Brewer, W. D. and Gargia, P. A. (1972). Grip strength of college women. *Arch. Phys. Med. Rehabil.*, **53**, 491–3.

Lundgren-Linquist, B. and Sperling, L. (1983). Functional status in 79-year-olds. *Scand. J. Rehab. Med.*, **15**, 117–23.

Lusardi, M. M. and Bohannon, R. W. (1991). Hand grip strength: comparability measurements obtained with the Jamar dynamometer and a modified sphygmomanometer. *J. Hand Ther.*, July – September, 117–22.

Marion, B. and Niebuhr, B. R. (1992). Effect of warm-up prior to maximal grip contractions. *J. Hand Ther.*, July – September, 143–6.

Mathiowetz, V., Weber, K., Volland, G. and Kashman, N. (1984). Reliability and validity of grip and pinch strength evaluations. *J. Hand Surg.*, **9A**, 69–74.

Mathiowetz, V., Kashman, N., Volland, G. *et al.* (1985a). Grip and pinch strength: normative data for adults. *Arch. Phys. Med. Rehabil.*, **66**, 69–74.

Mathiowetz, V., Rennells, C. and Donahoe, L. (1985b). Effect of elbow position on grip and key pinch strength. *J. Hand Surg.*, **10A(5)**, 694–6.

Mathiowetz, V. (1990). Effects of three trials on grip and pinch strength measurements. *J. Hand Ther.*, October – December, 195–8.

Myers, D. B., Grennan, D. M. and Palmer, D. G. (1980). Hand grip function in patients with rheumatoid arthritis. *Arch. Phys. Med. Rehabil.*, **61**, 369–73.

Napier, J. R. (1956). The prehensile movements of the human hand. *J. Bone Jt. Surg.*, **38**, 902–13.

Nelson, J. K, Yoon, S. H. and Nelson, K. R. (1991). A field-test for upper body strength and endurance. *Res. Q. Exer. Sport*, **62(4)**, 436–41.

Newman, D. G., Pearn, J., Barnes, A. *et al.* (1984). Norms for hand grip strength. *Arch. Dis. Child.*, **59**, 453–9.

Oberg, T., Oberg, U. and Karsznia, A. (1994). Handgrip and fingerpinch strength. *Physiother. Theory Prac.*, **10**, 27–34.

Pryce, J. C. (1980). The wrist position between neutral and ulnar deviation that facilitates the maximum power grip strength. *J. Biomech.*, **13**, 505.

Sheik, H. K., Smith, D. S., Meade, T. W. *et al.* (1979). Repeatability and validity of modified activities of daily living (ADL) index in studies of chronic disability. *Int. Rehab. Med.*, **1(2)**, 51–8.

Shiffman, L. M. (1992). Effects of aging on adult hand function. *Am. J. Occup. Ther.*, **46(9)**, 785–92.

Solgaard, S., Kristiansen, B. and Jensen, J. S. (1984). Evaluation of instruments for measuring grip strength. *Acta Orthop. Scand.*, **55**, 569–72.

Somadeepti, N. C., Smith, G., Nelson, R. C. and Sadoff, A. M. (1990). Assessing sincerity of effort in maximal grip strength tests. *Am. J. Phys. Med. Rehabil.*, **69(3)**, 148–53.

Spiegel, J. S., Leake, B., Spiegel, T. M. *et al.* (1987). What are we measuring? *Arth. Rheum.*, **31(6)**, 721–7.

Taylor, N., Shand, P. L. and Jebsen, R. H. (1973). Evaluation of hand function in children. *Arch. Phys. Med. Rehabil.*, **54**, 129–35.

Teraoka, T. (1979). Studies on the peculiarity of grip strength in relation to body positions and aging. *Kobe J. Med. Sci.*, **25**, 1–17.

Unsworth, A., Haslock, I., Vasandakhumar, V. and Stamp, J. (1990). A laboratory and clinical study of pneumatic grip strength devices. *J. Rheumatol.*, **29**, 440–44.

12 Orofacial function in speech

W. J. Hardcastle

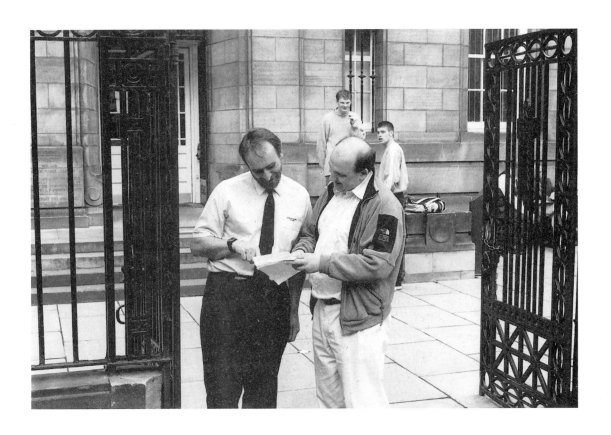

Introduction

The process of speaking involves the complex interaction of a number of different physiological structures. These include the brain, respiratory system, larynx, tongue, lips, jaw, velum and pharynx. Apart from their function in speech production, all these structures are involved in other life-supporting activities such as breathing, chewing and swallowing food and, in the case of the vocal folds within the larynx, preventing foreign bodies from passing into the lungs. All the structures vary considerably in the range, rate and direction of movement, and all need to be co-ordinated both temporally and spatially for the purpose of speech production. There are estimated to be at least 60 different muscles involved in the production of even a single word, and these muscles vary considerably in both type and patterns of innervation. It is not surprising therefore that one of the central challenges in speech science is how to account for the control of these many different degrees of freedom in producing the desired goal: a meaningful speech utterance.

The degrees of freedom problem is not unique to speech production, but applies also to other types of human activity such as those discussed elsewhere in this volume. The problem for speech control is that not only are so many structures to be managed moving in such a variety of manners, but that the whole process is constrained by the need to produce speech that has to be understood by the listener. This means that the speech production system has to adapt, among other things, to a changing communication environment; for example speaking over the telephone or in the presence of loud ambient noise.

Speech production should thus be viewed in terms of its involvement in a speaker–listener communication interaction. The processes involved in such an interaction can be illustrated schematically in terms of the so-called 'speech chain' (see Figure 12.1).

An intention to speak is formulated in the brain of the speaker, probably in the frontal lobe area of the left cortical hemisphere. The intention is coded in terms of what has been called a neurolinguistic plan, which lays the 'blueprint' for the utterance.

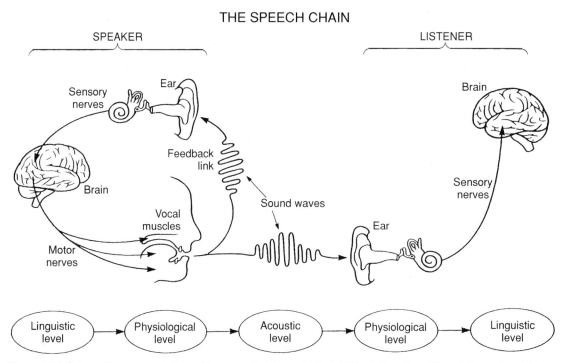

Figure 12.1 Schematic representation of the so-called 'speech chain', illustrating the different forms in which a spoken message exists in its progress from the brain of the speaker to the brain of the listener (from Denes and Pinson, 1993)

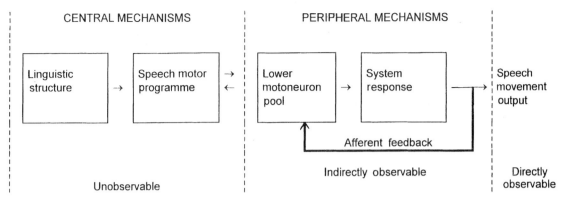

Figure 12.2 Schematic diagram showing the degree of accessibility to investigation of various central and peripheral processes of speech motor control (from Abbs, 1996)

This is in turn translated into motor commands to various different muscles and muscle groups supplying the organs of speech. Under the influence of these motor commands the speech structures move, and an audible acoustic signal is produced that passes through the airways to impinge on the ear of both the speaker and listener. Different parts of this process are more accessible than others. Figure 12.2 (from Abbs, 1996) illustrates the degrees of accessibility to observation of some of the main functions as far as the speaker is concerned.

In this chapter we will be focusing on the peripheral and relatively observable motor part of the chain, the movement of the various organs of speech themselves.

Physiological subsystems for speech production

The structures involved at the peripheral end of speech production can conveniently be grouped in terms of three systems – the respiratory, laryngeal and supralaryngeal systems. Each system has a unique role to play in speech production and, in many ways, the motor and sensory characteristics of each are quite different. In his intensive survey of the mechanisms of speech motor execution and control, Abbs (1996) points to the different biomechanical constraints operating throughout the systems, resulting in different control mechanisms. For example, the control of pitch by the relatively slow moving tuning of tension in the vocal folds within the larynx is quite different from the ballistic-type gestures of the tongue tip in producing an alveolar stop sound such as /t/ in 'atom'

(Abbs, 1996). Sensory motor control will vary also throughout the systems; the distribution of sensory receptor organs is unequal and probably reflects the different roles the three systems play in speech production.

The main structures involved in the production of speech are illustrated schematically in Figure 12.3. Figure 12.4 is a more detailed diagram of the head and neck region showing a mid-sagittal section view, which is the view traditionally used by phoneticians to describe the articulation of speech organs. It is based on a lateral X-ray image similar to those that provided much of the early data on the movements and postures of organs such as the tongue and velum in relation to fixed points of the skull. It should be remembered that there is also an important cross-sectional coronal dimension to the structures, which is often neglected in traditional descriptions. The main characteristics of each of the three physiological systems, the respiratory, laryngeal and supralaryngeal systems, will now be described briefly. Although the emphasis of this chapter is on supralaryngeal structures in the mouth and nose, for a full understanding of orofacial function it is important to consider also how these structures interact with the other main systems for the purposes of speech production.

The respiratory system

The respiratory system, comprising the lungs, diaphragm, thoracic cartilages and trachea, produces the outgoing flow of air that is necessary for the production of most speech sounds. The flow is caused by compression of the volume of the air in the lungs by a combination of muscular forces and

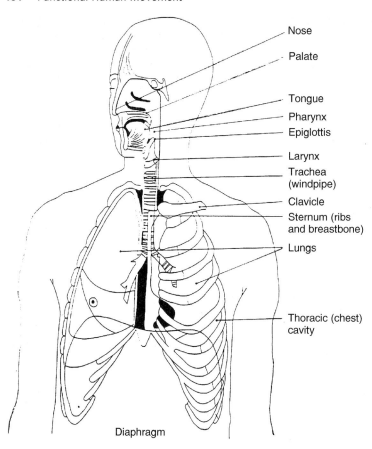

Nose

Palate

Tongue

Pharynx

Epiglottis

Larynx

Trachea (windpipe)

Clavicle

Sternum (ribs and breastbone)

Lungs

Thoracic (chest) cavity

Diaphragm

Figure 12.3 Highly schematic diagram of the main structures involved in the production of speech. This diagram shows the general orientation of the three main physiological systems involved in speech production; the respiratory system (trachea, lungs, thoracic cavity), the laryngeal system (larynx, consisting of the laryngeal cartilages, vocal folds; epiglottis), and the supralaryngeal system (articulatory organs such as the lips, tongue, jaw (mandible), pharynx, hard and soft palate) (from Crystal, 1997)

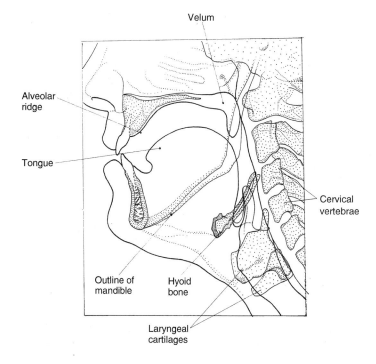

Velum

Alveolar ridge

Tongue

Outline of mandible

Hyoid bone

Cervical vertebrae

Laryngeal cartilages

Figure 12.4 Diagram of head and neck region based on a lateral sagittal X-ray image showing the main supralaryngeal structures involved in speech production (drawing courtesy of Janet Beck)

the elastic recoil force exerted by the cartilages of the rib cage. As Kent *et al.* (1996) point out (following Hixon *et al.*, 1976), the abdominal muscles are thought by some also to be actively involved in the expiratory phase of respiratory activity. The system aims generally to produce a steady air pressure of 5–10 cm H_2O for most speech purposes, but can generate higher pressures depending on the demand (e.g. loud speech). Small transient fluctuations in the pressure associated with some speech sounds such as oral plosives (the initial sounds in words like 'tea, pea', etc.) also take place.

The respiratory cycle is also precisely timed for the requirements of speech production. The inspiratory period is very short, and is timed to occur usually at major syntactic or prosodic boundaries (e.g. between clauses or sentences), with the expiratory phase prolonged for at least eight times the duration of the inspiratory phase. There is some evidence that the planning of a speech utterance is reflected in the respiratory cycle (Perkell, 1997).

Laryngeal system

Figure 12.4 shows the laryngeal structure positioned at the top of the trachea or windpipe, the tube that channels air to and from the lungs. The laryngeal structure itself consists of a number of cartilages, ligaments and muscles enclosing the vocal folds, which can be likened to an adjustable biological valve modifying the air stream from the lungs. Special muscles within the larynx alter the tension of the vocal folds, their length and the area of opening between them. These alterations determine whether the vocal folds are firmly closed (as happens, for example, during swallowing, coughing or during production of a so-called glottal stop as in the Cockney pronunciation of 'butter' as [bʌʔə]), wide apart (as in quiet breathing), or approximated to be set in vibration under appropriate conditions of muscle tension, stiffness and an air pressure difference above and below the folds.

According to the generally accepted source-filter theory of speech sound production, the vibrating vocal folds create a source of excitation of the whole vocal tract (the air passages above the level of the larynx) under particular aerodynamic and biomechanical conditions. Changing configurations of the structures above the level of the larynx within the mouth and nose cavities alter the resonating characteristics of the airways and result in perceptually different speech sounds such as the

vowels [i] (as in 'see') [ɔ] (as in 'saw'), etc. Most vowel sounds are 'voiced'; that is, the vocal folds vibrate during their production. Other sounds, such as consonants (e.g. the first sound in the word 'see'), may be produced either voiced or voiceless – i.e. with or without accompanying vocal fold vibration. The voiced/voiceless distinction is important linguistically as it signals a difference in meaning for words in many different languages (e.g. the difference between 'Sue' with a voiceless fricative [s] and 'zoo' with a voiced fricative [z]). Apart from controlling the voiced/voiceless distinction, the vocal folds have a number of other important linguistic functions. For example, changing longitudinal muscle tension within the vocal folds can change the pitch of the voice and various tension configurations can signal changes in phonation type (determining whether the voice sounds harsh, creaky, breathy, etc).

The vocal folds themselves are complex structures, and their composition has been the subject of a great deal of detailed investigation. For the purpose of the present discussion it is important to understand the factors influencing vibration of the folds, as these factors offer the key to the co-ordination of the laryngeal with the supralaryngeal and respiratory systems. The generally accepted myoelastic-aerodynamic model explains how vocal fold vibration occurs. During each individual cycle of vibration, the folds are approximated with appropriate muscle tension. Air pressure builds up below the approximated folds until eventually they are forced apart in the lower region first. As the air passes through the opening in the folds the velocity increases, and this effect, coupled with the inherent elastic properties of the folds, causes them to snap back together again. The cycle repeats itself as long as the muscular tension is appropriate and air continues to flow through from the lungs. If airflow is relatively inhibited, for example if there is a change to the flow in the mouth (as when the lips are brought together) and the nasal cavity is blocked off by the velum (see Figure 12.4) then, under normal circumstances, vocal fold vibration will be inhibited. That is why most obstruent sounds (i.e. those sounds involving a major obstruction to the airflow in the oral cavity) tend to be voiceless among the languages of the world.

Supralaryngeal system

Above the level of the larynx, the airflow from the lungs may be further modified by a number of structures within the nose and mouth cavities.

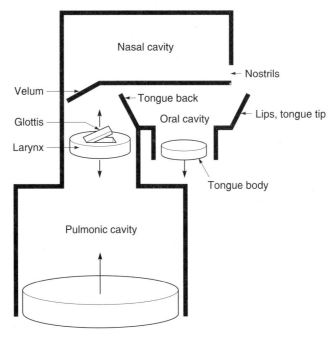

Figure 12.5 Schematic diagram representing the speech production system as a series of valves, pistons and cylinders. The velum, lips, tongue tip and tongue back are shown as adjustable valves. The pulmonic system, tongue body and larynx can all operate as pistons. The laryngeal structure contains the glottis (space between the vocal folds) represented as an internal valve (from Ohala, 1983)

Moveable, flexible structures, such as the tongue and lips, are capable of a variety of different shapes and configurations that alter the resonating characteristics of the airspace. They can also serve as the source of the sound, such as in the production of, for example, a fricative sound such as [s] in 'saw', where a local turbulent air stream and associated acoustic 'hissing' noise is created by the tongue tip in close proximity to the hard palate and upper front teeth. The aerodynamic characteristics of these supralaryngeal structures can be illustrated as in Figure 12.5, where the system is represented as a series of valves, pistons and air cylinders. The diagram is a useful way of conceptualizing the various functions of speech organs, at least as far as their roles in modifying the airflow is concerned.

The speech organs within the oral tract are particularly well adapted to the task of producing speech sounds. The tongue is a relatively large, flexible structure, with many of the physical characteristics of a fluid-filled sac, and it is able to assume a wide variety of different shapes and configurations. It has been described by some as a muscular hydrostat, a muscular structure devoid of bony or cartilaginous skeleton (Kier and Smith, 1985), sharing many of the same characteristics as an elephant's trunk or the tentacles of an octopus.

Four main 'extrinsic' muscles move the main bulk of the tongue about the oral cavity, while smaller fast-acting 'intrinsic' muscles are mainly responsible for changing the internal shape of the tongue. Interactions between the intrinsic and extrinsic muscle systems enable the tongue to achieve the wide range of precisely controlled configurations necessary for the production of many speech sounds. For example, the fricative [s] requires for its successful production a narrow channel formed by a groove in the most anterior part of the tongue (the so called tip/blade region) against the upper palate and front incisor teeth, while at the same time maintaining an airtight seal along the lateral margins of the tongue and the side gums. For many descriptive purposes it is convenient to divide the tongue into two independently controllable functional systems – a tip/blade system and a tongue body system (Hardcastle, 1976). The relative independence of these two systems can be illustrated by the configuration required for production of a retroflex stop (such as occurs in many Indian languages), where the tip and blade of the tongue are curled up and back to contact the postalveolar region of the palate, or in the production of the word medial [kt] consonant sequence in a word such as 'tractor', where the tongue body makes full contact with the junction between the hard and soft palates at the same time as the tip and blade are raised to contact the alveolar region of the palate.

The acoustic consequences of tongue movements within the oral region have been studied in depth, and a number of theoretical models of articulatory/acoustic relationships are now available (Stevens, 1997). One such theory is the so-called quantal theory, which proposes that there are certain so-called critical regions of the vocal tract where small articulatory adjustments, say by the tongue in contact with the palate, can have relatively large acoustic consequences (Stevens, 1989). As Kent *et al.* (1996) point out, these regions pose a problem for articulatory control because they demand a high degree of articulatory precision to achieve a specific result. In terms of control theory, strategies may be employed so that these 'critical' regions are avoided as favoured places of articulation.

Also within the oral cavity is the soft palate or velum, a muscular flap that can be likened to a biological valve separating the mouth region from the nose (see Figure 12.5). When raised and retracted by the levator and tensor palatini muscles it seals off the air passage into the nose, and when lowered it enables air from the lungs to pass into both mouth and nose cavities. The latter condition exists during production of so-called nasal sounds such as [m], [n], etc. The soft palate is mechanically linked to the tongue via the palatoglossus muscle (anterior faucal pillars), and there does seem to be a clear relationship between the position of the tongue and degree of elevation of the velum (low vowels such as [a] are associated with a more lowered velum).

The velum determines the degree of acoustic coupling between oral and nasal cavities, which is the key to perceptual impressions of nasality in the voice.

The lips and lower jaw (mandible) are other important supralaryngeal speech organs. The lips are capable of a wide variety of different shapes and configurations, due largely to the particular anatomical arrangement of the facial muscles (Seikel *et al.*, 1997). Closing the lips is important for the production of so-called bilabial sounds (such as [b] in 'but'), and forward movement with a rounded configuration may occur in some people's production of the vowel sound in the word 'cool'. Reciprocal activity takes place between lips and jaw for the closing and opening movements that take place when producing the [b] sound in the word 'above'; as the lips close, the mandible is raised from a relatively open position for the first vowel, then at the release of the [b] the lips are opened while the mandible is lowered. There is also reciprocal activity between the lower and the upper lip during the bilabial closing gesture.

Speech production

Speech production is characterized by co-ordination of the three physiological systems: the respiratory, laryngeal and supralaryngeal. The complexity of such co-ordination can be illustrated by considering the main activities of the speech organs during production of the word 'schooner' (phonetically [skunə]) (see Table 12.1). For ease of description, the activities of the various structures are time aligned to a phonetic transcription along the top of the Table, where phonetic symbols are placed in a linear sequence. The description is based on quantitative data from two instrumental techniques, electromagnetic articulography (EMA), tracking vertical and horizontal movements of the lips, mandible and various points on the surface of the tongue, and electropalatography (EPG), recording the location of tongue contact on the hard palate. The techniques are discussed in more detail in the final section of this chapter. In the instrumental record of the word (Figure 12.6) the EMA and EPG data are synchronized, with the acoustic signal represented as a waveform along the top of the figure.

The parametric articulatory description in Table 12.1 and the articulatory kinematic records in Figure 12.6 exemplify some important aspects of speech production. First, there is no clear one-to-one correspondence between speech segments as represented by the transcription symbols and particular configurations of the speech organs. If there were, this would greatly simplify the motor control problem for speech production. A model could, for example, postulate a stored set of entities such as phonemes (/s/, /k/, /u/, etc.) each with a characteristic set of articulatory configurations that

Table 12.1 Main activities of the speech organs during the production of the word 'schooner'

	s	k	u	n	ə
Tongue tip/blade	Raised to alveolar ridge with grooved configuration	Lowered to lower teeth during the velar closure for [k]	Maintains lowered position	Raised for the oral closure at the alveolar ridge	Lowered to neutral position then raised briefly for the tap [r]
Tongue body	Forward upward movement	Raised and bunched back making closure at junction between hard and soft palates then lowered	Lowered slightly from retracted raised position but maintaining stiffness	Lowered to neutral position	Lowered
Lips	Begin to protrude in anticipation of [u]	Rounding and protrusion maintained	Rounding increased	Returns to neutral lip position	Neutral position maintained
Mandible	Raised along with tongue body movement	Raised position maintained	Kept raised	Kept raised then lowered slightly	Lowered slightly to aid release of tongue tip/blade, then kept lowered
Velum	Raised to close off nasal cavity	Raised position kept	Begins to lower during the vowel in anticipation of the [n]	Lowered	Begins to be raised for vowel
Vocal folds	Apart allowing air to pass through	Stay wide apart during closure	Begin to approximate and vibrate soon after the release of the stop closure	Vibrating	Vibrating
Respiratory system	Provides air pressure to create turbulence for fricative	Air pressure, build up during closure phase of stop	Maintaining transglottal pressure difference for voicing	Maintaining pressure difference	Maintaining pressure difference

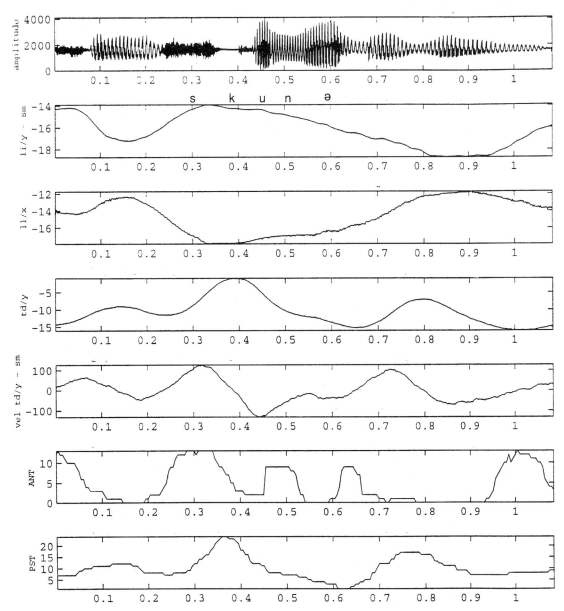

Figure 12.6 Computer printout of instrumental records of the sentence 'say schooner again', spoken by a speaker of Scottish English. The top trace shows the speech waveform, which is used for segmenting and labelling the speech signal. The next four traces show kinematic details from the Carstens electromagnetic articulograph (see final section of this chapter). The EMA traces are from the top: vertical up–down movement of the jaw; horizontal front–back movement of the lower lip (negative = forward); vertical up–down movement of the tongue dorsum; velocity of tongue dorsum movement. The lower two traces show information from electropalatography; total tongue palate contacts activated in the anterior region of the palate (ANT trace) and total number activated in the posterior region of the palate (PST trace)

could be selected at will by the system for production of a speech utterance. However, although there appears to be some evidence from tongue slip data for the phoneme as having some reality as a production unit (Shattuck-Hufnagel,

1987), the relationship between individual phonemes and particular movements of speech organs is far from clear. In fact some recent theories of speech production, for example Fowler (1980), question the separation of linguistic forms such as phonemes from their physical manifestations. One of the problems is the concept of co-articulation, the simultaneous movement of different articulations or different parts of the same articulator. One consequence of this is that a phoneme will vary considerably in its production, depending on the environment in which it occurs (e.g. which sounds precede and follow it.) An example is the forward movement of the lips in Table 12.1, which begins at the onset of the [s] (see also the EMA trace in Figure 12.6.) Here the lip movement is in fact anticipating the production of the rounded vowel [u], which occurs later in the word. This type of anticipatory co-articulation is prevalent in normal connected speech, and many theories have been proposed to account for the phenomenon (Kent and Minifie, 1977; Weismer, 1988).

The traces in Figure 12.6 and the commentary in Table 12.1 exemplify another characteristic of speech movements; the fact that movement trajectories tend to be smooth, with sliding contacts along fixed structures such as the hard palate and teeth, rather than movements straight up to and abruptly away from target positions. For example, the tongue body is gradually raised during the [s] to reach its maximum displacement during the closure for the [k] stop (see Figure 12.6). The maximum velocity for this gesture occurs about midway through the raising. The release of the closure is represented by a lowering of the displacement curve (in Figure 12.6) and an associated decrease in posterior palate contact (as shown by the post-EPG totals display). Another feature of tongue dorsum movement during [k] closures such as these is the frequently observed 'looping' trajectory, in which the tongue slides forward on the palate (Mooshammer *et al.*, 1995; Kuehn and Moll, 1976; Hardcastle *et al.*, 1996).

Details of articulatory kinematics such as those represented in this illustration are important features of speech production, and need to be incorporated into any comprehensive model of the process. The following sections will outline some of the features of articulatory kinematics, biomechanics and sensorimotor control in the speech production system. The focus will be supralaryngeal structures.

Articulatory kinematics

Articulatory organs interact with one another to create vocal tract shapes that result in the different acoustic events having linguistic significance in the communication process. It is important to consider the ways in which the different organs combine in the oral region to obtain a fully comprehensive view of the speech production process. Such an overview requires the recording of a number of different organs, or of different parts of the same organ simultaneously. Unfortunately, however, there are still considerable technical difficulties in tracking a number of different articulations simultaneously in the oral region (see later in this chapter for a review of different methodologies). Most published work on articulatory kinematics has focused on individual organs, and these have tended to be the more accessible ones such as the lips and mandible. However, other articulators such as the tongue, velum and pharynx have also been investigated, and some data are available.

Activities of the supraglottal articulations during speech have been described generally in terms of the distance they move (e.g. maximum amplitude of displacement), duration of the movement, location of the movement end-points within the vocal tract, and peak velocity and acceleration of the movement (Perkell, 1997). Weismer (1988) has a useful summary of the main published kinematic data for articulators, arranged under the main headings of displacement, duration, velocity and acceleration. The speech material used in the different studies is quite variable, as is the methodology, so it is not surprising that there are considerable differences in the values of the different measures. There is evidence that a variety of speech features influence the kinematic variables. These include:

prosodic features such as stress, rhythm etc. (Beckman and Edwards, 1994)
different syntactic structures
the speaking rate (Kuehn and Moll, 1976; Adams *et al.*, 1993; Shaiman *et al.*, 1997)
the particular vocal tract dimensions of a speaker – e.g. narrow or wide hard palate, etc. (Perkell, 1997)
the style of speech
the characteristics of different classes of consonants (Gracco, 1994)
different directions of movements (e.g. opening versus closing gestures of the mandible for bilabial sounds (Smith and Gartenberg, 1984) and
the phonetic context (Parush *et al.*, 1983).

Given the influence of these features on articulatory kinematics, it is not surprising to find in the table in Weismer (1988) considerable variability in, for example, the values of velocity for a given articulator. Some investigators have identified a unifying characteristic in the relationship between velocity and displacement (commonly referred to as articulator 'stiffness'), which appears to remain relatively stable across all the above-mentioned speech variables (Kent and Moll, 1972). In addition, a number of researchers have found this ratio varies in an inverse curvilinear way with movement duration (Ostry and Munhall, 1985; Gracco and Abbs, 1989; Vatikiotis-Bateson and Kelso, 1993). Similar relationships have been used to account for limb motor control (Freund and Büdingen, 1978, as quoted by Weismer, 1988).

The velocity/displacement relationship is central to the so-called action theory of speech production, where the relationship is said to remain invariant despite differences in rate and stress (see Kelso *et al.*, 1985). Ostry *et al.* (1983), however, observed systematic rate and stress effects on the peak velocity-to-displacement relationship.

Detailed observation of the velocity profiles of articulators during speech production has been the subject of a number of recent studies (e.g. Shaiman *et al.*, 1997), and such observations can throw valuable light on the type of motor control processes that may be involved in the process. Shaiman *et al.* (1997) examined velocity profiles of lip protrusion across different rates: slow, normal and fast, using a head-mounted strain gauge transduction system (see later in this chapter). The profiles for upper lip protrusion showed less symmetry at slow speaking rates, but greater symmetry at normal and fast rates (Figure 12.7). Such rate-dependent changes in velocity symmetry have also been noted in limb movements (e.g. Bullock and Grossberg, 1988; Ostry *et al.*, 1987; Nagasaki, 1989). Shaiman *et al.* (1997) suggest that such asymmetry is a learned strategy used for approaching a target as quickly as possible before making corrective movements closer to the target. As movement speed decreases, feedback mechanisms are increasingly incorporated into the movement (see below in discussion of sensorimotor control). Faster movements may have no time for on-line sensory feedback.

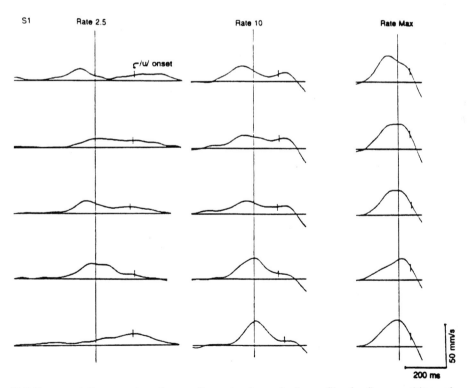

Figure 12.7 Representative samples of upper lip protrusion velocity profiles for five repetitions of one subject's production of part of the utterance 'I see two and I see tea again', spoken at increasing rates of speech. The vertical line indicates the /t/ release in 'two' and the mark, the acoustic onset of /u/. Other subjects showed similar trends (from Shaiman *et al.*, 1997)

Speech as goal-directed behaviour

As seen in the example shown in Table 12.1, different speech articulators are closely co-ordinated in time to produce meaningful speech utterances. One way of viewing speech utterances from the production point of view is to postulate that they consist of a string of speech segments, themselves consisting of ensembles for articulatory movements or gestures. There is evidence that gestures form synergies or ensembles that are closely co-ordinated with each other (Bernstein, 1967). These co-ordinated structures serve to simplify the high degrees of freedom problem mentioned above. Thus, the production of a bilabial stop such as [b] will involve a closing gesture, which is a co-ordinated activity involving the lips (mainly in fact the lower lip) and an accompanying jaw raising movement. It appears that there is a reciprocal relationship between the lower lip and the mandible in achieving a gesture such as the bilabial closure. Perturbation experiments have been carried out to explore the nature of this reciprocity further (Gracco and Abbs, 1985; Kelso *et al.*, 1984; Folkins and Abbs, 1975). In Kelso *et al.* (1984), a transient and unpredictable perturbation in the form of a downward drag is applied to the lower jaw while it is moving upward for the final [b] and [z] in words such as [bæb] and [bæz]. The perturbation is compensated for almost immediately (within 20–30 ms) in a task specific manner, for example by increasing upper lip activity, which would enable the lip closure to be completed. Similar examples of goal-directed behaviour have been explored using the so-called bite-block paradigm. In these experiments, customized bite-blocks of varying thicknesses are placed between the upper and lower molar teeth and subjects are able to compensate for the abnormal spatial relationships in the oral region almost immediately in achieving an accurate acoustic target for a vowel sound (Lindblom *et al.*, 1979).

These experiments show clearly that there are trading relationships between articulators, which ensure that the same goal is reached in more than one way and from more than one initial starting point. For example, a target alveolar stop (tip/blade of tongue contacting alveolar ridge) can be achieved in both the words 'eat' [i:t] and 'art' [a:t], although the initial starting points of the tongue for the two vowels are very different. In the first case, [i:], the tongue body is already raised forwards and upwards in the vocal tract, and in the [a:] vowel it lies flat and retracted towards the back wall of the pharynx. The goal itself may be articulatory in terms of spatial configurations of the speech structures, or acoustic in terms of an auditory target.

Biomechanical and sensorimotor properties

All speech movements are constrained by the inherent properties of the speech structures themselves, and any comprehensive model of speech production must take into account such constraints. Biomechanical properties of the speech motor system that need to be considered are discussed in detail by Abbs (1996). He groups the main biomechanical properties under three main categories;

1. Those pertaining to active muscle properties
2. Those related to variations in muscle force translation systems
3. Passive mechanical properties.

Most information on biomechanical constraints has come from EMG studies, using both hooked-wire and surface electrodes (Folkins and Kuehn, 1982). Almost all the speech muscles, including the intrinsic laryngeal muscles, have been investigated with EMG techniques and many of the current physiological models of speech production are based on these studies. One of the problems with EMG studies of the speech musculature is the interpretation of the details of motor neuron firing in terms of the actual force exerted by the muscle, and the eventual effect of such force in terms of movement of speech organs. Abbs (1996) points to the complexity of the relationship between innervation of the muscle and output force, and discusses intervening variables such as muscle length, rate of shortening/ lengthening, load against which the muscle is pulling (elastic, inertial or viscous), degree of fatigue and type of muscle fibre. Many of these biomechanical constraints operate in the limb musculature, but there are some interesting differences between the cranial nerve system that innervates the speech musculature and the spinal system responsible for limb musculature. For example many of the muscles in the oral region such as the intrinsic tongue muscles have very low innervation ratios (i.e. the number of muscle fibres innervated by a single motor unit), which enables greater neural control to be exerted over the structure as a whole.

Muscle elasticity appears to play an important role in speech motor control, and the relevance of this variable is exemplified by Abbs (1996) in a description of EMG activity in the orbicularis oris muscle during production of the bilabial stop [p]. The level of contraction in the lips (made up primarily of the orbicularis oris) increases during the closure of the stop, and one consequence of this is that the lips considerably stiffen. Abbs suggests this increase in stiffness is necessary for the lips to maintain an appropriate seal in the presence of the increase in intra-oral pressure during the stop closure. Just prior to release there is evidently a shutdown in EMG orbicularis oris activity, and the release of the stop appears to be implemented via control of inherent orbicularis oris elasticity rather than by a positive muscular force separating the lips.

Passive mechanical properties are also important to consider in models of speech motor control. A good example is the respiratory system, where passive elasticity stored in the thoracic structures (the ligaments and cartilages of the ribs) generate a decrease in volume and consequent outward flow of air as the basis for speech production. Full descriptions of how the speech production system utilizes these active and passive forces are currently lacking, but they are clearly important and of particular relevance given that speech organs such as the lips, tongue, vocal folds, velum, etc. consist largely of muscle and tissue.

Sensorimotor mechanisms

Perturbation experiments pioneered by Ewarts and colleagues (quoted by Abbs, 1996) raise the question of the role of sensorimotor mechanisms in the control of speech production. The speech production system is well-endowed with a wide variety of sensory receptor systems, which can potentially provide central neural regions with sensory information relating to mechanical pressure, timing and location of contact between articulators, etc. (Hardcastle, 1976; Smith, 1992). Three main sensory feedback channels have been identified as being potentially significant for speech motor control; a tactile feedback channel providing sensory information from mechanoreceptors situated in the superficial tissues of speech articulators, proprioceptive feedback from muscle spindle and tendon organs, and auditory feedback from the hair cells in the Organ of Corti in the inner ear. Table 12.2 summarizes some of the characteristics of these feedback channels. It

should be emphasized that the role of sensory receptors in speech motor control is at present highly speculative in the absence of solid experimental evidence (Smith, 1992).

Early work using sensory blocking techniques involving auditory masking noise and topical anaesthesia applied to the surface of organs such as the tongue or into the inferior alveolar nerve via a mandibular block (Scott and Ringel, 1971a, 1971b; Hardcastle, 1975) attempted to identify some of the functions of those sensory feedback channels. Despite methodological difficulties in interpreting the data, some robust quantifiable effects of the sensory blocking could be observed, including an increase of the area of tongue–palate contact for alveolar and post-alveolar fricative production following alteration to tactile feedback from the front two-thirds of the tongue (Hardcastle, 1975). These results were interpreted as evidence that some ongoing control of tongue contact precision may be exerted by tactile feedback from the tongue.

It seems reasonable to suggest that sensory receptors throughout the oral region may play some role in control of articulatory movements, either during the movement or after the movements have been executed. As articulators contact other moveable speech organs and fixed structures such as the hard palate and teeth, tissues are compressed and stretched, and such mechanical changes will be detected by the receptor organs situated in the ephithelial covering and in the lamina properia of tissues.

During the movement itself, ongoing sensory information will be available to the neural centres from muscle spindles and tendon organs distributed throughout the speech production apparatus. Muscle spindles respond to the change in length of a muscle and the rate of change in length, and have been located in all articulators except the lips (Abbs, 1996; Hardcastle, 1976). The response to rate of change in length means that predictive information would be available to the appropriate neural centres.

The precise role of the different sensory feedback channels during speech production is as yet unknown, but a number of possible functions of the channels have been suggested:

1. Prior to movement initiation, to determine state of motor system for programming the speech gesture (Gracco and Abbs, 1985)
2. Ongoing feedback monitoring during the course of a movement, and correction of any errors

Table 12.2 Main sensory feedback channels identified as being potentially significant for speech motor control

	Tactile	*Proprioceptive*	*Auditory*
Type of sensory receptors	(1) 'free' endings (2) 'complex' endings (e.g. Krause end-bulbs, Meissner corpuscles)	(1) muscle spindles (2) Golgi tendon organs (3) joint receptors	hair cells in Organ of Corti
Distribution of receptors	(1) superficial layers of oral mucosa (2) lamina propria, particularly deeper layers	(1) most speech muscles (2) tendons (3) capsules of joints	Organ of Corti in cochlea
Information sent to CNS	(1) and (2) { (a) localization of contact (b) pressure of contact (c) direction of movement (d) onset time of contact	(1) { (a) length of muscle fibre (b) velocity of stretch (c) direction of movement of muscle (2) { change of stretch on tendon by muscular contraction etc. (3) { (a) rate of joint movement (b) direction of joint movement (c) extent of joint movement	(a) intensity (b) frequency (c) direction of sounds (d) periodicity (e) duration
Main features of the feedback systems	(a) slower-acting than proprioceptive because (i) multisynaptic (ii) afferent fibres smaller (b) spatial projection of peripheral receptive surface preserved in sensory cortex and cerebellum (c) probably transmits information *after* the event (d) important for speech movements involving contact between articulators e.g. [t], [i] etc.	(a) fast-acting because (i) monosynaptic (ii) spindle afferent fibres largest in body (b) predictive information possible (c) provides information *during* the event (d) important for all articulations requiring precise positioning of articulatory structures	(a) slower-acting than tactile and proprioceptive because transmission of sound through air (for air conduction) (b) projection on auditory cortex preserves spatial characteristics of basilar membrane, also projections to other areas (c) supplies information *after* the event (d) important for open and back vowels (e.g. [a], [o]) (e) important for prosodic features such as pitch, duration, stress.

in the movement trajectory (particularly for slowed movements and newly learned movments)

3. Signalling to the central neural control system that a particular speech gesture has been completed and it is time to proceed to the next

4. Alerting the CNS that an error has been made (particularly auditory feedback channels), and confirming the correction.

Instrumental techniques for measuring orofacial functions

Most of our current knowledge of the functions of orofacial structures during speech production has come from investigations using a variety of specialized instrumental techniques. Some of these techniques have been designed specifically to record and analyse the movements of the lips, jaw, tongue and velum during speech. Other techniques for investigating aspects of laryngeal and respiratory function will not be covered here, but accounts can be found elsewhere (for example, Titze, 1994 for the larynx; Shadle, 1997 and Hixon *et al.*, 1987 for respiratory function; Baken, 1987 and Lass, 1996 for general surveys of instrumental techniques used in speech research).

Measurement of orofacial structures during speech can be quite problematic. Although some organs such as the lips and jaw are accessible to direct observation, many of the important speech organs such as the tongue, velum and pharynx are hidden from view. In the latter cases, previous investigation involved either potentially harmful X-ray techniques or inserting some type of probe or tracking device inside the mouth, with the accompanying possible interference with normal speech function. In general, measurement techniques must satisfy certain requirements if they are to be maximally useful for speech analysis:

1. They must be safe to use, and must not involve any potential hazard to the subject
2. They must be sensitive to articulatory motions – for example, measurements of the tongue should be able to detect movements as small as 1 mm – but not so sensitive that it is difficult to relate the measurement to the articulatory motion itself
3. The measurement technique should have an adequate frequency response. A response of 100–200 Hz seems appropriate for most purposes where direct tracking of articulatory organs is involved.

Table 12.3 summarizes the main instrumental techniques that have been developed for measuring articulatory activity during speech.

They may be divided into:

1. Techniques for acoustic analysis (providing indirect information on articulatory activity)
2. Techniques for articulatory movement analysis, including (a) imaging techniques, (b) movement transduction and point tracking, (c) techniques for measuring tongue–palate contacts and (d) aerodynamic transduction techniques (providing indirect indication of manner of articulation)
3. Techniques for neurophysiological analysis.

This list is not meant to be exhaustive, but is provided to illustrate the relatively wide range of instrumentation now available to the speech scientist. For the remainder of this chapter, the main techniques for measuring articulatory activity will

Table 12.3 Instrumental techniques for measuring articulatory activity during speech

1 Techniques for acoustic analysis (indirect)
- Spectrography: measures of formant frequencies, noise spectra, voicing, segment durations, rate and extent of formant transitions (indicating tongue position, velocity of movement, timing etc.)
- Wave-form analysis(from oscillograms): spirantization, periodicity, segment duration (indicating manner of articulation, voicing, articulatory timing, etc.)

2 Techniques for articulatory movement analysis
(a) Imaging techniques
- X-ray, including projection X-ray (video- and cinefluorography), xeroradiography, computerized tomography (CT scanning).
- Magnetic resonance imaging (MRI)
- Ultrasonics
(b) Movement transduction and point tracking
- Electromagnetic transduction techniques (e.g. EM(M)A 'electro-magnetic (mid-sagittal) articulometry)
- X-ray microbeam
- Opto-electronic systems (e.g. 'Selspot'; 'Optotrak')
- Strain-gauge transduction and mechanical systems
(c) Tongue–palate contacts
- Palatographic techniques (electropalatography (EPG); palatometry)
(d) Aerodynamic transduction techniques (indirect)
- Air pressure/air flow measurement (pneumotachograph, anemometer)

3 Neurophysiological analysis
- Electromyography (EMG)

be briefly described. (For a more detailed discussion see Lass, 1996; Hardcastle, 1996 and Ball and Code, 1997.) The discussion will focus on relatively direct measurement techniques, so will not include instruments that record acoustic and aerodynamic events.

Imaging techniques

X-ray

Up until relatively recently, by far the most common technique for imaging articulatory activity was X-ray (including cinefluorography, videofluorography, xeroradiography and computerized tomography (CT)).

The main advantage of X-ray techniques was that articulatory organs such as the tongue, lips, jaw and velum could be measured in relation to fixed structures such as the hard palate, teeth, back wall of the pharynx, etc. The most commonly used view was the sagittal section view (Figure 12.4), which remains the projection most favoured by phoneticians as the basis for their descriptions of place and manner of articulation associated with different speech sounds. Many of our current theories of speech sound production owe much to observation of X-ray images of speech (e.g. Moll, 1960).

However, the technique is severely limited by the potential danger of damage to soft tissues resulting from harmful radiation. This is indeed a serious limitation for speech analysis, which often requires the recording of relatively large amounts of data.

A specialized X-ray facility has been developed, the X-ray microbeam facility, which is now available at the University of Wisconsin (Nadler *et al.*, 1988; Kiritani *et al.*, 1975). By targeting small, well-defined areas of the vocal tract using computer controlled X-ray beams, it is possible to restrict radiation appreciably. However, the equipment required is complex and extremely expensive to run, and is so far available in only one centre.

For this reason, there has been a concentrated effort in recent times to develop a safe alternative to X-ray suitable for imaging articulatory structures. MRI (magnetic resonance imaging) is a very promising method involving the use of a body sectioning principle like the CT scan, but instead of X-rays it uses a magnetic field and radio waves to image the tissue (Stone, 1996; Baer *et al.*, 1991). Very clear images can be obtained with MRI, but at present its usefulness in speech research is rather limited because the sampling rate is too low, with a few seconds needed for each scan if the resolution is to remain high. However, new developments are taking place at present and it is hoped that, before long, real-time MRI scanning will be a possibility.

Ultrasound

Ultrasound is another technique which avoids the problems of X-rays, and it has the added advantage of offering a scanning rate (of 30–47 scans/s) that is suitable for analysing at least some aspects of speech dynamics (Stone, 1996).

One significant advantage of ultrasound is that it is possible to obtain coronal section views of organs, such as the tongue, which are very important for compiling three-dimensional representations. Figure 12.8 shows coronal section views of the tongue surface during two different articulations. There are, however, disadvantages in using ultrasound. When imaging the tongue, most of the ultrasound energy is reflected back to the probe at the air interface below the tongue tip (so no clear image of the surface of the tip is possible); also, outlines of other relevant hard structures within the oral region (such as the hard palate, jaw etc.) cannot easily be imaged. However, ultrasound technology is advancing rapidly, and the technique offers many obvious advantages for speech research.

Movement transduction and point tracking systems

The third main group of techniques comprises various movement transduction and point tracking systems. This group includes the most significant systems as far as investigating tongue, jaw and lip kinematics is concerned.

Most work has concentrated on the lips and jaw as the most accessible organs. The tongue and

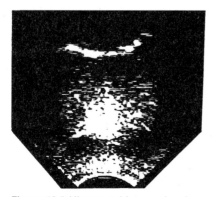 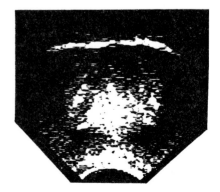

Figure 12.8 Ultrasound image showing coronal section views of the tongue dorsum, for two different articulations, /a/ (left) and /l/ (right). The outline of the tongue surface can clearly be seen as the white line at the top of each image (photographs courtesy of Maureen Stone)

velum, being relatively inaccessible, present special problems for movement transduction systems.

Systems utilizing electromagnetic transduction have been used for a variety of purposes, including measurement of the chest wall (Hixon *et al.*, 1976). For measuring articulatory organs in the orofacial region, the Articulograph AG100 (manufactured by Carstens) uses a specially-made helmet housing three electromagnets. Small coils attached to the midline of various articulatory structures such as the tongue, lips and mandible are tracked as they move through the electromagnetic fields. A crucial problem with many of these systems is possible artifacts caused by tilt of the coils, and measures to counteract these problems are now incorporated into the calibration systems and software (Hoole *et al.*, 1993; Perkell *et al.*, 1992 and Engelke *et al.*, 1989). After transferring the digitized data onto a PC, X, Y co-ordinates of the movements of the individual coils can be displayed in various different ways (see Figure 12.6 above for a sample EMA display). The system remains an extremely useful method of studying articulatory kinematics.

Other movement transduction systems used for studying speech kinematics include various opto-electronic and strain gauge systems. Optical systems are particularly suitable for tracking movements of the more accessible articulatory organs such as the lips and jaw. They usually involve attaching light sources or reflectors to various points on the articulatory structures, and tracking their trajectories with either television or optoelectronic detectors (Baken, 1987).

A commercially available Selsport system can be used to obtain a three-dimensional representation of lip and jaw movement (Lindholm, 1974). The technique uses active light emitting diodes as infrared light sources attached to various structures, and photodetectors are located in the focal plane of an optical lens. Signals from the photodetectors are processed by computer, and three-dimensional data can be produced in the form of tables or graphs. Another commercially available marker-tracking system is OPTOTRAK, which can be used to represent three-dimensional jaw motion. New developments using a special system for measuring side-to-side movements of the jaw as well as anteroposterior and supero-inferior movements are described by Vatikiotis-Bateson and Ostry (1992).

One articulator organ which is particularly difficult to track is the velum, and various opto-electronic systems have been developed to measure the area of opening of the velopharyngeal port (Ohala, 1971) or the movement of the velum from above. One technique for indirect indication of movement involves inserting a probe containing both light source and sensor element into the nasal cavity. Light from the source is reflected back from the moving velum, and the proximity detected by the sensor (Künzel, 1979). The latter system, called a velograph, has been used in therapy for speakers with velopharyngeal incompetence as a biofeedback device indicating movement of the velum (Künzel, 1982).

Another widely used technique is palatography, a traditional technique designed to record location of contact between the tongue and hard palate during speech (Abercrombie, 1957). This location of contact is important phonetically because many speech sounds are differentiated by such contact patterns (e.g. /t/ versus /k/, /s/ versus /ʃ/, etc.). Newer developments in palatography, called electropalatography, record the dynamic aspects of tongue contact – that is, the changing positions of contact on speaking (Hardcastle *et al.*, 1991a, 1991b; Hardcastle and Gibbon, 1997).

In electropalatography, the subject wears a thin artificial palate made of acrylic with a number of gold or silver electrodes (usually 60–90) embedded in the surface to detect lingual contact. A small sinusoidal signal passes through the subject's body and lingual–palatal contact is identified by the presence of this signal on a given palatal electrode. The output can be displayed on a computer screen, and printouts of sequences of palatal contacts can be obtained. Figure 12.9 shows a printout of a normal speaker's production of the word 'tactics'. The printout reveals many details of articulatory activity. Full contact with the palate is indicated for the /t/ (frames 43–60), with a horseshoe-shaped configuration (complete contact down the lateral margins of the palate and across the alveolar ridge). Velar closure involving the back part of the tongue begins at frame 82, and briefly overlaps with anterior contact for the second /t/ from frames 92–96. The timing of this alveolar–velar gesture overlap is quite precisely controlled, and the releases take place in the correct sequence (for example, the velar release at frame 97 occurs before the alveolar release of frame 109 and not vice versa). The contact for the second /k/ (132–144) is noticeably more extensive than for the first /k/, reflecting the influence of the preceding close vowel [i]. At the end of the word, the pattern for /s/ shows a grooved configuration in

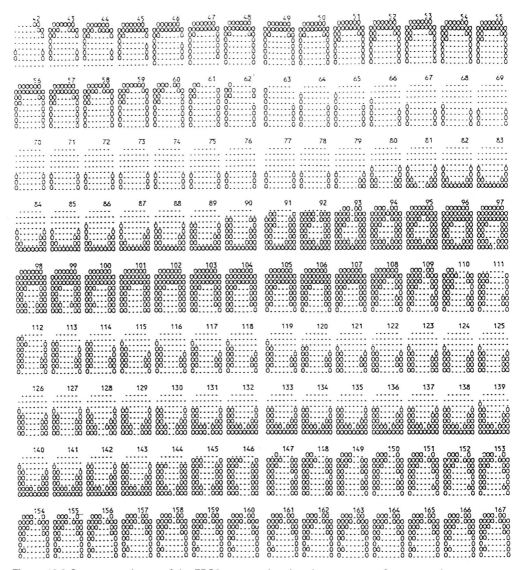

Figure 12.9 Computer printout of the EPG3 system showing the sequence of tongue-palate contact patterns for a speaker's production of the word 'tactics'. Each individual palate diagram shows the presence of contact as zero with the alveolar region at the top and the velar region at the bottom. Sampling interval is 10 ms

the anterior part of the tongue with a narrow channel down the midline.

The patterns of contact can be processed in various ways including a so-called 'totals' display, which sums the number of activated electrodes in a given area of the palate and expresses these as a function of time (see EPG display in Figure 12.6, which shows totals for the front half and rear half of the palate). Various methods of data reduction for EPG are discussed at length in Hardcastle *et al.* (1991a). The technique has been particularly useful

for studying lingual co-articulatory effects (Hardcastle, 1994) in identifying different patterns of contact for particular speech sounds depending on the phonetic environment in which they occur. There have also been applications in speech pathology, particularly in the assessment and treatment of disorders of articulation (Hardcastle *et al.* 1991b). The direct real-time display of contact patterns has been very useful in treatment, as subjects are able to monitor and change their abnormal articulatory patterns according to a prescribed normal pattern (see Hardcastle and Gibbon, 1997).

EPG records details of tongue contact only, so provides only indirect information on articulatory kinematics. There is no direct information on the proximity of the tongue to the palate; nor is there any way of directly measuring precisely which part of the tongue is making the contact. When used in conjunction with electromagnetic articulography, however (Figure 12.6), these drawbacks can largely be overcome. Increasingly, equipment for the analysis of speech production is adapting to a multisensor approach, in which a number of different organs or a number of different measurements of the same organ are acquired simultaneously.

The final technique to be discussed here is electromyography, which has a relatively long history in speech research (Basmajian and De Luca; 1985; Gentil and Moore, 1997; Baken, 1987; Stone, 1996). EMG techniques aim to detect electrical discharges associated with muscle activity, and have been applied to muscles in the respiratory, laryngeal and supralaryngeal systems. The technique is commonly used in physiology, particularly in the diagnosis of a wide range of pathological neuromuscular conditions. For speech purposes it has been used mainly to detect the onset and offset of electrical activity in a muscle, and the relative amplitude of the signal. For detailed investigation of speech dynamics, special types of micro-electrodes ('hooked-wire' electrodes) are commonly used. These are fine wires inserted into the target muscle by means of a hypodermic needle. Small hooks in the end of the wires retain the position in the body of the muscle, and they can be withdrawn by a gradual pull on the wire. Most of the speech muscles in the orofacial region have been investigated with hooked-wire electrodes, including the velopharyngeal muscles (Kuehn and Moon, 1994), the tongue muscles (Baer *et al.*, 1988) and the lips (Folkins *et al.*, 1988; Kennedy and Abbs, 1979; Blair and Muller, 1987). Surface electrodes are also used, particularly where the aim is to record responses from a relatively large number of motor units in a muscle or from muscles immediately below the electrodes. They have been particularly useful for investigating lip activity associated with speech (Wohlert and Goffman, 1994; Goffman and Smith, 1994).

EPG is an important technique in speech research because it remains the only way of directly monitoring activity in particular muscles. Much of our current knowledge of the speech musculature in fact comes from carefully controlled investigations using the technique. However, due to the complexity of the speech system, the interpretation of EMG signals in terms of actual patterns of movement of specific articulators remains problematic (Abbs, 1996). For this reason EMG is usually used in conjunction with other instrumental techniques such as the specialized movement transducers discussed above, which monitor relatively directly the movement of the particular organs.

We can anticipate that, in the future, multisensor systems will become more widely used in speech research in the quest for comprehensive models of the complex speech motor system, including a clearer understanding of orofacial kinematics.

References

Abbs, J. H. (1996). Mechanisms of speech motor execution and control. *In Principles of Experimental Phonetics* (N. J. Lass, ed.), pp. 93–111. Mosby.

Abercrombie, D. (1957). Direct palatography. *Z. Phonetik.*, **10**, 21–5.

Adams, S. G., Weismer, G. and Kent, R. D. (1993). Speaking rate and speech movement velocity profiles. *J. Speech Hearing Res.*, **36**, 41–54.

Baer, T., Alfonso, P. and Honda, K. (1988). Electromyography of the tongue muscles during vowels in /ə pVp/ environment. *Ann. Bull.* 22, pp. 7–20. Research Institute Logopedics and Phoniatrics, University of Tokyo.

Baer, T., Gore, J. C., Gracco, L. C. and Nye, P. W. (1991). Analysis of vocal tract shape and dimensions using magnetic resonance imaging. *J. Acoust. Soc. Am.*, **90**, 799–828.

Baken, R. J. (1987). *Clinical Measurement of Speech and Voice.* College Hill.

Ball, M. and Code, C. (eds.) (1997). *Instrumental Clinical Phonetics.* Whurr.

Basmajian, J. V. and De Luca, C. J. (1985). *Muscles Alive: Their Functions Revealed by Electromyography* (5th edn.). Williams & Wilkins.

Beckman, M. E. and Edwards, J. (1994). Articulatory evidence for differentiating stress categories. *Phonological Structure and Phonetic Form: Papers in Laboratory Phonology II* (P. A. Keating, ed.). Cambridge University Press.

Bernstein, N. (1967). *The Co-ordination and Regulation of Movements.* Pergamon.

Blair, C. and Muller, E. (1987). Functional identification of the perioral neuromuscular system: A signal flow diagram. *J. Speech Hearing Res.*, **30**, 60–70.

Bullock, D. and Grossberg, S. (1988). Neural dynamics of planned arm movements; emergent invariants and speech accuracy properties during trajectory formation. *Psychol. Rev.*, **95**, 49–90.

Crystal, D. (1997). *The Cambridge Encyclopedia of Language* (2nd edn.). Cambridge University Press.

Denes, P. B. and Pinson, E. M. (1993). *The Speech Chain: The Physics and Biology of Spoken Language*. Freeman.

Engelke, W., Schönle, P. W., Kring, R. A. and Richter, C. (1989). Zur Untersuchung orofazialer Bewegungsfunktionen mit der elektromagnetischen Articulographie. *Deutsche Zahnärzliche Zeitschrift*, **44**, 618–22.

Folkins, J. W., and Abbs, J. H. (1975). Lip and jaw motor control during speech; responses to resistive loading of the jaw. *J. Speech Hearing Res.*, **18**, 207–20.

Folkins, J. W. and Kuehn, D. P. (1982). Speech production. *In Speech, Language and Hearing, Volume 1 Normal Processes* (N. J. Lass, L. V. McReynolds, J. L. Northern and D. E. Yoder, eds.), p. 246. W.B. Saunders.

Folkins, J. W., Linville, R. N., Garrett, J. D. and Brown, C. K. (1988). Interactions in the labial musculature during speech. *J. Speech Hearing Res.*, **31**, 253–64.

Fowler, C. A. (1980). Co-articulation and theories of extrinsic timing. *J. Phonetics*, **8**, 113–33.

Freund, H. J. and Büdingen, H. J. (1978). The relationship between speed and amplitude of the fastest voluntary contractions of human arm muscles. *Exp. Brain Res.*, **31**, 1–12.

Gentil, M. and Moore, W. H. Jnr. (1997). Electropalatography. In *Instrumental Clinical Phonetics* (M. J. Ball and C. Code, eds.), pp. 87–118. Whurr.

Goffman, L. and Smith, A. (1994). Motor unit territories in the human perioral musculature. *J. Speech Hearing Res.*, **37**, 975–84.

Gracco, V. L. (1994). Some organizational characteristics of speech movement control. *J. Speech Hearing Res.*, **37**, 4–27.

Gracco, V. L. and Abbs, J. H. (1985). Dynamic control of the perioral system during speech: kinematic analyses of autogenic and nonautogenic sensorimotor processes. *J. Neurophysiol.*, **54**, 418–32.

Gracco, V. L. and Abbs, J. H. (1989). Sensorimotor characteristics of speech motor sequences. *Exp. Brain Res.*, **75**, 586–98.

Hardcastle, W. J. (1975). Some aspects of speech production under controlled conditions of oral anaesthesia and auditory masking. *J. Phonetics*, **3**, 197–214.

Hardcastle, W. J. (1976). *Physiology of Speech Production; An introduction for Speech Scientists*. Academic Press.

Hardcastle, W. J. (1994). Assimilations of alveolar stops and nasals in connected speech. In *Studies in General and English Phonetics* (in Honour of Professor J. D. O'Connor) (J. Windsor-Lewis, ed.), pp. 49–67. Routledge.

Hardcastle, W. J. (1996). Current developments in instrumentation for studying supraglottal structures. In *Advances in Clinical Phonetics* (M. J. Ball and M. Duckworth, eds.), pp. 27–50. John Benjamins.

Hardcastle, W. J. and Gibbon, F. E. (1997). Electropalatography and its clinical applications. In *Instrumental Clinical Phonetics* (M. Ball and C. Code, eds.), pp. 151–95. Whurr.

Hardcastle, W. J., Gibbon, F. E. and Nicolaidis, K. (1991a). EPG data reduction methods and their implications for studies of lingual coarticulation. *J. Phonetics*, **19**, 251–66.

Hardcastle, W. J., Gibbon, F. E. and Jones, W. (1991b). Visual display of tongue–palate contact: electropalatography in the assessment and remediation of speech disorders. *Br. J. Disorders Comm.*, **26**, 41–74.

Hardcastle, W. J., Vaxelaire, B., Gibbon, F. *et al.* (1996). EMA/EPG study of lingual coarticulation in /kl/ clusters. In *Proc. 4th Speech Production Seminar*, Autrans, France, pp. 35–56. ESCA, CNRS, ICP.

Hixon, T. J. *et al.* (1987). *Respiratory Function in Speech and Song*. College Hill Press.

Hixon, T. J., Mead, J. and Goldman, M. (1976). Dynamics of the chest wall during speech production: function of the thorax, rib cage, diaphragm and abdomen. *J. Speech Hearing Res.*, **19**, 297–356.

Hoole, P., Kühnert, B., Mooshammer, T. and Tillmann, H. G. (eds.) (1993). *Proceedings of the ACCOR Workshop on Electromagnetic Articulography in Phonetic Research*. Forschungsberichte des Instituts für Phonetik und sprachliche Kommunikation der Universität München (FIPKM) 31.

Kelso, J. A. S., Tuller, B., Vatikiotis-Bateson, E. and Fowler, C. A. (1984). Functionality-specific articulatory co-operation adaptation to jaw perturbations during speech. Evidence for co-ordinative structures. *J. Exp. Psychol. Hum. Percept. Perf.*, **10**, 812–32.

Kelso, J. A. S., Vatikiotis-Bateson, E., Saltzman E. L. and Kay, B. (1985). A qualitative dynamic analysis of reiterant speech production: phase portraits, kinematics and dynamic modeling. *J. Acoust. Soc. Am.*, **77**, 266–80.

Kennedy, J. G. III and Abbs, J. H. (1979). Anatomical studies of the perioral motor system. Foundations for studies of speech physiology. In *Speech and Language: Advances in Basic Research and Practice*, Vol. 1 (N. J. Lass, ed.). Academic Press, pp. 212–267.

Kent, R. D. and Moll, K. L. (1972). Cinefluorographic analysis of selected lingual consonants. *J. Speech Hearing Res.*, **15**, 453–73.

Kent, R. D. and Minifie, F. D. (1977). Co-articulation in speech production models. *J. Phonetics*, **5**, 115–33.

Kent, R. D., Adams, S. G. and Turner, G. S. (1996). Models of speech production. In *Principles of Experimental Phonetics* (N. J. Lass, ed.), pp. 3–45. Mosby.

Kier, W. M. and Smith, K. K. (1985). Tongues, tentacles and trunks: the biomechanics of movement in muscular hydrostats. *Zoolog. J. Linnean Soc.*, **83**, 307–24.

Kiritani, S., Itoh, K. and Fujimura, O. (1975). Tongue-pellet tracking by a computer controlled X-ray microbeam system. *J. Acoust. Soc. Am.*, **57**, 1516–20.

Kuehn, D. P. and Moll, K. L. (1976). A cineradiographic study of VC and CV articulatory velocities. *J. Phonetics*, **4**, 303–20.

Kuehn, D. P. and Moon, J. B. (1994). Levator veli palatini muscle activity in relation to intraoral air pressure variation. *J. Speech Hearing Res.*, **37**, 1260–70.

Künzel, H. J. (1979). Some observations on velar movement in plosives. *Phonetica*, **36**, 384–404.

Künzel, H. J. (1982). First applications of a biofeedback device for the therapy of velopharyngeal incompetence. *Folia Phoniatrica*, **34**, 92–100.

Lass, N. J. (ed.) (1996). *Principles of Experimental Phonetics*. Mosby.

Lindblom, B. E. F., Lubker, J. F. and Gay, T. (1979). Formant frequencies of some fixed-mandible vowels and a model of speech motor programming by predictive simulation. *J. Phonetics*, **7**, 147–61.

Lindholm, L. E. (1974). An optoelectronic instrument for remote on-line movement monitoring. In *Biomechanics IV* (R. C. Nelson and C. A. Moorehouse, eds.), pp. 510–12. University Park Press.

Moll, K. L. (1960) Cinefluorographic techniques in speech research. *J. Speech Hearing Res.*, **3**, 227–41.

Mooshammer, C., Hoole, P. and Kühnert, B. (1995). On loops. *J. Phonetics*, **23**, 3–21.

Nadler, R. D., Robl, E. P. , Wahl, D. J. *et al.* (1988). Wisconsin X-ray microbeam system: articulatory pellet tracking specifications. *J. Acoust. Soc. Am.*, **83**, 112.

Nagasaki, H. (1989). Asymmetric velocity and acceleration profiles of human arm movements. *Exp. Brain Res.*, **68**, 37–46.

Ohala, J. J. (1971). Monitoring soft palate movements in speech. *J. Acoust. Soc. Am.*, **50**, 140A.

Ohala, J. J. (1983). The origin of sound patterns in vocal tract constrains. *In The Production of Speech* (P. F. MacNeilage, ed.). Springer.

Ostry, D. J. and Munhall, K. G. (1985): Control of rate and duration of speech movements. *J. Acoust. Soc. Am.*, **77**, 640–48.

Ostry, D. J., Keller, E. and Parush, A. (1983). Similarities in the control of the speech articulators and the limbs: kinematics of tongue dorsum movements in speech. *J. Exp. Psychol: Hum. Percept. Perf.*, **9**, 622–36.

Ostry, D. J., Cooke, J. D. and Munhall, K. G. (1987). Velocity curves of human arm and speech movements. *Exp. Brain Res.*, **68**, 37–46.

Parush, A., Ostry, D. J. and Munhall, K. G. (1983). A kinematic study of lingual co-articulation in VCV sequences. *J. Acoust. Soc. Am.*, **74**, 1115–25.

Perkell, J. S. (1997): Articulatory processes. In *Handbook of Phonetic Sciences* (W. J. Hardcastle and J. Laver, eds.), pp. 333–70. Blackwells.

Perkell, J. S., Cohen, M. H., Svirsky, M. *et al.* (1992). Electromagnetic midsagittal articulometric (EMMA) systems for transducing speech articulatory movements. *J. Acoust. Soc. Am.*, **92**, 3078–96.

Scott, C. M. and Ringel, R. L. (1971a). Articulation without oral sensory control. *J. Speech Hearing Res.*, **14**, 804–18.

Scott, C. M. and Ringel, R. L. (1971b). The effect of motor and sensory disruptions on speech; a description of articulation. *J. Speech Hearing Res.*, **14**, 819–28.

Seikel, J. A., King, D. W. and Drumwright, D. G. (1997). *Anatomy and Physiology for Speech and Language*. Singular.

Shadle, C. H. (1997). The aerodynamics of speech. In *The Handbook of Phonetic Sciences* (W. J. Hardcastle and J. Laver, eds.), pp. 33–64. Blackwells.

Shaiman, S., Adams, S. G. and Kimelman, M. D. Z. (1997). Velocity profiles of lip protrusion across changes in speaking rate. *J. Speech Lang. Hear. Res.*, **40**, 144–58.

Shattuck-Hufnagel, S. (1987). The role of word-onset consonants in speech production planning: new evidence from speech error patterns. In *Motor and Sensory Processes of Language* (E. Keller and M. Gopnik, eds.), pp. 17–51. Erlbaum.

Smith, A. (1992). The control of orofacial movements in speech. *Crit. Rev. Oral Biol. Med.*, **3**, 233–67.

Smith, B. L. and Gartenberg, T. E. (1984). Initial observations concerning developmental characteristics of labiomandibular kinematics. *J. Acoust. Soc. Am.*, **75**, 1599–1605.

Stevens, K. N. (1997). Articulatory–acoustic–auditory relationships. In *Handbook of Phonetic Sciences* (W. J. Hardcastle and J. Laver, eds.), pp. 462–506. Blackwells.

Stevens, K. N. (1989). On the quantal nature of speech. *J. Phonetics*, **17**, 3–46.

Stone, M. (1996). Investigation for the study of speech physiology. In *Principles of Experimental Phonetics* (N. J. Lass, ed.), pp. 495–524. Mosby.

Stone, M. and Lundberg, A. (1996). Three-dimensional tongue surface shapes of English consonants. *J. Acoust. Soc. Am.*, **99**, 3728–37.

Titze, I. (1994). *Principles of Voice Production*. Prentice-Hall.

Vatikiotis-Bateson, E. and Ostry, D. J. (1992). Rigid body reconstruction of jaw motion in speech. *J. Acoust. Soc. Jpn.*, **4(10)**, 281–83.

Vatikiotis-Bateson, E. and Kelso, J. A. S. (1993). Rhythm type and articulatory dynamics in English, French and Japanese. *J. Phon.*, **21**, 231–65.

Weismer, G. (1988). Speech production. In *Handbook of Speech – Language Pathology and Audiology* (N. J. Lass, L. V. McReynolds, J. L. Northern and D. E. Yoder, eds.). Mosby.

Wohlert, A. B. and Goffman, L. (1994). Human perioral muscle activation patterns. *J. Speech Hearing Res.*, **37**, 1032–40.

13 Balance

W. De Weerdt and A. Spaepen

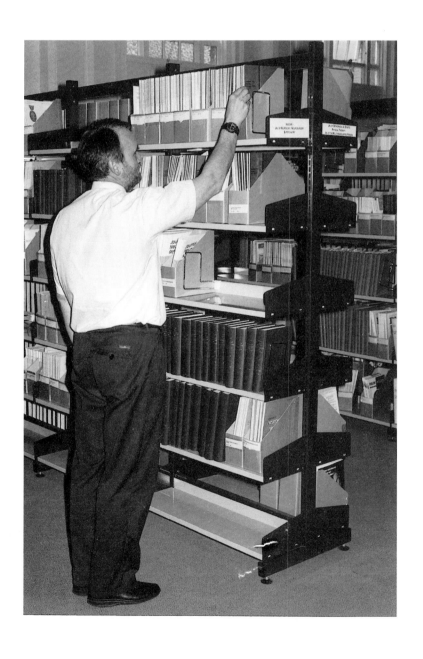

Introduction

The sense of balance is not prominent in our consciousness, but we can perceive a loss of balance or dizziness when we are spun around. Evidence exists that supports the contention that the vestibular system has some sensation of its own: this is in the form of recordings of cortical-evoked potentials, sensation reports induced by stimulation of cortical areas and dysfunction produced by cortical lesions (Guedry, 1974). The sense of balance is essential for the co-ordination of motor responses, eye movements and postural adjustments. Disruption of the sense of balance leads to vertigo, nausea, disorganized balance reactions and autonomic signs such as pallor, sweating, vomiting and hypotension, and we soon become conscious of these feelings.

The mechanism of balance is based on an intrinsic co-operation between the vestibular system, proprioceptive and tactile information, and vision. Balance not only depends on the integrity of these systems, but also on the sensory integration within the central nervous system, visual and spatial perception, effective muscle tone which adapts rapidly to change, muscle strength and joint flexibility (Andrews, 1987).

External causes of falls and cardiovascular disorders associated with balance problems will not be discussed in this chapter.

The maintenance of balance

Role of the vestibular system

The vestibular system refers to the vestibule of the inner ear, which mainly contains the peripheral organs. Within this cavity is the membranous labyrinth, which consists of three directionally-sensitive and more or less mutually perpendicular semicircular ducts and a pair of swellings called the utricle and saccule.

When the head is rotated, the force exerted by the inertia of the fluid in the semicircular ducts acts against the cupula. This action produces a displacement of the sensory hairs on the receptor cells, and alters the level of activity in the nerve fibres innervating them. The receptor system of the vestibular apparatus is so sensitive, it can respond to angular accelerations or decelerations as small as $0.1° \, s^{-2}$. The dynamic function, mediated principally by the semicircular ducts, enables us to track the rotation of the head in space and is important for the reflex control of eye movements (Kelly, 1991).

A portion of the floor of the utricle is also thickened and contains hair cells. The macula of the utricle lies roughly in the horizontal plane when the head is held erect, so that the otoliths rest directly upon it. If the head is tilted or undergoes linear acceleration, the otoliths deform the gelatinous mass, which in turn bends the hairs of the receptor cells.

The saccule also has a macula. This is oriented vertically when the head is in a normal position. It also detects the position of the head in space, and responds selectively to vertically-directed linear force. The static function, mediated principally by the utricle and saccule, enables us to monitor the absolute position of the head in space, and this plays a pivotal role in the control of posture. The utricle and saccule also detect linear accelerations; therefore they have both a static and dynamic function.

The information from the peripheral end organs is relayed by the vestibular portion of the eighth nerve to the vestibular nuclei in the brain stem and the flocculo-nodular lobe, the vestibular portion of the cerebellum. The vestibular hair cell may either depolarize or hyperpolarize, depending upon the direction of the head movement or tilt. The bidirectional nature of the hair cell response, along with the co-ordination of inputs from the bilateral labyrinths, provides the central nervous system with multiple indications of head movement and position.

The whole system functions to keep the body balanced, to co-ordinate head and body movements and, most remarkably, to keep the eyes fixed on a point in space even when the head is moving (Kelly, 1991).

The postural disturbance of someone with acute vestibular failure demonstrates the potential importance of vestibular function in the maintenance of balance. The vestibular influence is exerted via various channels.

Vestibulospinal reflex

From the lateral vestibular nucleus (Deiters' nucleus), secondary neurons descend in the ipsilateral ventral white column and end by synapsing onto lower motor neurons. The lateral vestibulospinal tract has a pronounced facilitatory effect on both alpha and gamma motor neurons, which innervate muscles in the limbs. This tonic excitation of the extensors of the leg and the flexors of the arm enables us to maintain an upright body posture (Liebman and Tadmor, 1991). The vestibulospinal reflex contracts the limb muscles for landing during falls.

Vestibular and neck reflex

Vestibular reflexes are evoked by changes in the position of the head. Neck reflexes are triggered by tilting, bending or turning the neck. Both reflexes produce co-ordinated effects on muscles of the arms, legs and neck.

The medial, superior and inferior vestibular nuclei give rise to the medial vestibulospinal tract, which terminates bilaterally in the cervical region of the cord. The axons in this tract make monosynaptic connections with motor neurons innervating the neck muscles. This tract participates in the reflex control of neck movements so that the position of the head can be maintained accurately and is correlated with eye movements. Vestibular reflexes acting on the neck (vestibulocollic reflexes) and vestibulospinal reflexes are primarily static (Ghez, 1991a; Kelly, 1991; Liebman and Tadmor, 1991).

Vestibulo-oculomotor reflex

From the medial, superior and inferior nuclei, crossed and uncrossed neurons descend via the medial vestibulospinal tract. Just before descending, these neurons branch and give off axons which ascend to the pons and midbrain, where they synapse with the sixth (abducens), fourth (trochlear) and third (oculomotor) nuclei, which are all concerned with eyeball muscle movement. In order to make sure that the object of visual fixation is seen by the area of the retina with maximal resolution and best colour perception (the macula), the position of the eyes must be maintained despite movement of the head. If the head is tilted to one side, the eyes rotate in the opposite direction. The vestibulo-ocular reflex circuit changes the head velocity signal into an eye velocity signal, which helps to maintain the visual field in the horizontal plane. Adjustment of the gain of the vestibulo-ocular reflex involves the cerebellar flocculus (Downton, 1992; Goldberg *et al.*, 1991; Kelly, 1991).

Role of the pontine and medullary reticular formation

The reticular formation is a central core of diffusely organized nuclei. Two groups of these nuclei, in the pons and the medulla, are involved in the control of posture. These nuclei project through the medial and lateral reticulospinal tract at all levels of the spinal cord.

The aforementioned connections from the reticular formation enable the co-ordination of posture and movement by integrating vestibular and other sensory inputs with commands from the cerebral cortex (Ghez, 1991a).

Role of the cerebellum

Lesions of the cerebellum disrupt co-ordination of limb and eye movements, impair balance and decrease muscle tone. The cerebellum is organized into three functional regions: the vestibulocerebellum, the spinocerebellum and the cerebrocerebellum.

The vestibulocerebellum

The vestibulocerebellum corresponds to the flocculonodular lobe. This region receives its input from the vestibular nuclei in the medulla, and projects directly back to them.

The vestibulocerebellum governs the axial and proximal limb muscles, which are used to maintain balance during stance and gait. It also controls eye movements, and co-ordinates movements of the head and eyes.

A lesion of the flocculonodular lobe causes disturbance of equilibrium, including ataxic gait, a compensatory wide-base standing position and nystagmus. When the patient moves while lying down, no deficits are seen.

The spinocerebellum

The spinocerebellum is so named because a major source of its input arises in the spinal cord. The spinocerebellum controls the medial and lateral components of the descending motor systems, and thus plays a major role in controlling the ongoing execution of limb movement. It also regulates muscle tone (Ghez, 1991b).

The cerebrocerebellum

The input of the cerebrocerebellum comes exclusively from the pontine nuclei, which relay information from the cerebral cortex. Its output is conveyed by the dentate nucleus to the thalamus, and from there to the motor and premotor cortices. The cerebrocerebellum is thought to play a special role in the planning and initiation of movement. It is particularly important in multi-joint movements and fractionated digit movements, and hence these movements are most impaired following lesions of the dentate nucleus (Ghez, 1991b).

Role of vision

The universal finding that sway is greater with eyes closed than with eyes open demonstrates the importance of vision in the maintenance of balance. Numerous people experience the hallucination of movement that may occur when sitting in a stationary train watching the moving train on the next platform. Experiments using a 'hanging room', in which visual information is misleading, have shown that such conditions induce loss of balance. Vision seems to be particularly important when other sensory input is reduced or impaired (Dornan *et al*., 1978; Lee and Lishman, 1975). Elderly fallers have been shown to have more errors in visual perception of verticality and horizontality than non-fallers (Tobis, 1981).

Role of proprioception

Proprioception is the sense that enables one to know exactly and at all times where the parts of the body are in space and in relation to one another. Somatosensory input is often underestimated as an element of normal and defective postural control. Vital information about the position of the body in space and the relative position of various body parts is constantly being transmitted by muscle and joint proprioceptors, especially those in the lower limbs and the neck. Proprioceptors in the cervical spine are particularly important but information from the postural muscles also contributes, as does information from skin receptors (Downton, 1992; Liebman and Tadmore, 1991).

Postural adjustment

Posture represents the overall position of the body and limbs relative to one another, and their orientation in space. Postural adjustments are necessary for all motor tasks and need to be integrated within voluntary movements. They support the head and body against gravity and other external forces, and maintain the centre of body mass aligned and balanced over the base of support. They stabilize supporting parts of the body during movements. Postural adjustments are achieved by means of anticipatory and feedback mechanisms.

Anticipatory mechanism

The anticipatory, or feed forward, mechanisms predict disturbances and produce pre-programmed responses that maintain stability. The key role of anticipatory responses is to generate postural adjustments before voluntary movements occur. The trigger for the anticipatory pre-emptive action is the recognition of a developing trend in the

afferent input. In this way the destabilizing effect of the movement is anticipated, and, as a result, the conditions never develop to the point at which an adequate stimulus becomes detectable, and the related reflex response is consequently not elicited. An individual's postural response to perturbing stimuli is shaped and modified by experience. Its effectiveness improves with practice, and depends on the context. The result is great improvement in the smoothness of the stabilizing effect of motor activity. The feed forward control makes it necessary to include assessment of postural responses preceding voluntary limb movements when measuring postural movement strategies (Ghez, 1991a; Ragnarsdóttir, 1996; Roberts, 1995).

Feedback mechanism

Compensatory or feedback responses are evoked by sensory events following a change of the centre of gravity. These automatic postural adjustments, typically produced by body sway, are extremely rapid. Like reflexes, they have a relatively stereotyped spatiotemporal organization. Unlike reflexes, postural adjustments are refined continuously by practice and learned much like skilled voluntary movements (Ghez, 1991a). Nashner (1976) found that swaying movements induced by moving a platform on which a patient was standing elicited rapid and highly stereotyped postural responses in a characteristic distal-to-proximal sequence. Responses based on muscle stretch have latencies that are half as slow as responses based exclusively on either vestibular or visual inputs.

The motor learning process

The cerebellum compares the intended movement (internal feedback) with the actual movement (external feedback). Several lines of evidence now support the idea that cerebellar circuits are modified by experience, and these changes are important for motor learning. To generate corrective signals, the cerebellum computes errors. The corrective adjustments take the form of feedback and feed forward controls, which operate on the descending motor system of the brain stem and cortex. Lesions of the cerebellum produce error in the planning and execution of movements.

Interaction between proprioception and cerebellum

The normal functions of the cerebellum are critically dependent upon its afferent input, particularly the proprioceptive part. Titubations that occur following lesions of the cerebellum are due to a failure to correct movement or to a defective use of sensory inputs in feedback correction. Damage to sensory fibres, for example in a demyelinating neuropathy or to the dorsal column of the spinal cord, can result in sensory ataxia (Hardie, 1993). Ataxia is a crude term, and comprises a variety of abnormalities of movement such as dysmetria, dyssynergia, dysdiadochokinesia and decomposition of movement.

Changes in postural control with age

Age changes in the above-mentioned integrative mechanisms have been demonstrated. Cutaneous sensation and proprioception show increased thresholds for excitability with age. There is a reduction of sensation, especially to spatial stimuli and slow moving targets. In addition, vestibular function declines and spinal stretch reflexes deteriorate mildly, leading to a minor prolongation of latency (Downton, 1992). The elderly (and children) sway more on average when standing still than young and middle-aged adults. However the individual variability is high and there is overlap between the normal ranges for younger adults and the elderly.

Postural control as measured by sway is impaired in various pathological conditions of vision, hearing, vestibular function and muscle and joint proprioception (de Jong *et al.*, 1977; Eklund and Lofstedt, 1970; Juntunen *et al.*, 1987; Norré and Forrez, 1986; Stevens and Tomlinson, 1971). The increased average sway in the elderly may therefore be related to an accumulation of pathology.

Balance disturbances, especially when associated with falling, are some of the commonest causes of (re)admission to hospital. The prevalence of falls increases markedly with advancing age. For some reason the prevalence of falls is higher in women, the female-male ratio being 2:1. This difference narrows in very advanced age (Andrews, 1986; Andrews, 1987; Prudham and Evans, 1981). Age and sex-related normative data are therefore essential for postural sway (Ragnarsdóttir, 1996).

Summary

Input from the vestibular labyrinth upholds the head in a vertical position. Neck reflexes maintain the head aligned with the body. Vestibular and neck reflexes also act on limb muscles to cushion falls and stabilize the body in relation to the support face. The vestibulo-oculomotor reflex helps to sustain the visual field in the horizontal plane. Much of the neural circuitry which integrates posture, feedback control, feed forward control, motor programme control and voluntary movement is located in the brain stem, spinal cord and cerebellum. Vision and proprioception play a pivotal role in the maintenance of balance.

The measurement of human balance

Static equilibrium of the human body standing upright in fact does not exist. At any moment in time, small movements of the body can be detected. The main reason for these movements is twofold. On the one hand, because of the upright position of the non-rigid body, a continuous postural control of a number of more or less vertically aligned body segments above the support base is required. On the other hand, this control is executed by the central and peripheral nervous system, regulating the intensity of the activity of muscles involved in keeping the body segments aligned. Since even so-called 'static' force production, however, is a dynamic process of triggering activity in a continuously changing set of motor units, one can easily understand that maintaining equilibrium in an upright position is a dynamic process.

In balance control, two main different groups of parameters can be distinguished:

1. First, several techniques exist to measure kinematic quantities of body segments, mainly displacement, velocity or acceleration. Further, mostly automated processing of the measurements is needed to derive quantitative parameters describing the quality of different aspects of postural control at different levels (hip, trunk, head). In some cases, attempts are made to compute displacements or accelerations of the body centre of gravity (CG), since this point is of crucial importance in the mechanics of postural stability.
2. Secondly, the origin or cause of the small body movements is also observed by means of the measurement of forces acting on the body, mainly the feet, or by registration of the activity of muscles (EMG) directly involved in postural control. Further data processing normally includes the calculation of the centre of pressure (CP), which is the point of application of

the forces on the feet, and of the synchronization pattern between muscle activity (e.g. gastrocnemius and tibialis anterior) and displacements of the centre of pressure, e.g. in the sagittal direction.

Measurement techniques

Experimental or clinical test arrangements often include tasks where it becomes increasing difficult for the test subjects to maintain the upright position or stability. For example, the support of one foot is raised or lowered at different speeds (Willems and Vranken, 1964), and lateral movements of the body and of the CP are registered. Alternatively, the support base for both feet can be tilted laterally or in the fore–aft direction and the subject asked to keep the platform, as far as possible, in a horizontal position (Begbie, 1966). Angular deviations are measured in time, from which specific parameters (such as maximum deviation, mean value and standard deviation, number of zero crossings, etc.) are calculated. These tests will not be discussed further because they vary greatly in test set-up and protocol, leading to results that cannot be comparable. Further discussion is limited to test situations with a fixed support base.

Measurement of body movements is most often based on automated data-acquisition from video frames. To this end, reflective markers are fixed on body joints, and on-line digitization of the co-ordinates of those markers then leads to a two- or three-dimensional description of the motion. Further calculations allow determination of the segmental and body centres of gravity. Measurements are typically at a rate of 50 frames per second. Since this number exceeds the frequencies in movement patterns (up to 10 Hz) by a factor of greater than two, this measurement rate is quite sufficient. Specific care has to be taken to exploit the resolution of video-measurement systems as far as possible. Since the amplitude of body movements of upper segments (arms, head) is in the order of a few centimetres and markers are at a distance of up to 2 m from each other (from the top of the head to feet), movements are indicated on only a small percentage of the total screen. A camera system with a vertical resolution of 600 pixels per line will show amplitudes of movement in the order of 15 pixels only, and for this reason it is often preferred to focus on movements of just part of the body.

The velocity and acceleration of selected points on the body can be measured by means of ultrasonic transducers or piezo- or silicon-based accelerometers respectively. These measuring devices deliver analogue output signals, which then can be registered digitally by means of classic analogue to digital converters. Since the frequency content of the signals is higher than in measurements of displacements, a higher sampling rate (e.g. 100 Hz) is recommended. The physical connection of a set of electrical wires between the transducers on the subject and the data-acquisition system makes the use of these devices more cumbersome than a wireless measurement of the movements.

Data-acquisition of EMG signals imposes even higher requirements on the sampling frequency of the signal. Even when surface electrodes are applied, frequencies can easily mount up to 300 Hz. Depending on the filters applied in the amplifier and pre-amplifier of the EMG signal, a sampling rate of at least 500 Hz (and preferably 2 kHz) should be applied.

Finally, forces applied by the support base onto the feet can also be measured. To this end, force plates are used. These measuring devices (approximately 50×50 cm – 60×100 cm) are mounted into the floor, and enable the measurement of the three spatial components of the force applied to the plate, the point of application of the force (CP), and the torsion exerted simultaneously with the force. In the measurement of postural control, both this CP and the horizontal forces in the fore and aft and lateral directions are of great importance, since they explain the cause of the movements of the body.

The measurement transducers in force plates utilize electrical strain gauges or piezo crystals. The former allow for measurements over longer time periods (up to several hours), whereas the latter limits measurements to a few minutes, after which drift at the output of the charge amplifier becomes significant. On the other hand, piezo crystal-based plates have a higher rigidity and, correspondingly, a higher frequency response to force-changes, typically two to four times higher than strain gauge-based platforms. Progress in the mechanical design of commercially available plates and in the connecting electronic circuitry, however, allows measurement of forces up to several hundred hertz, which is certainly sufficient for applications in posturography. Although strain gauge platforms are often less sensitive than piezo ones, they have the advantage of allowing measurements over a greater period of time without noticeable drift.

Mechanical principles of postural control

The relationship between the two sets of measurements mentioned above will briefly be described here: on the one hand the movements of the body, and on the other, the forces on the feet. Although postural control is a complex issue of both sagittal and lateral displacements of the body at different segmental levels, the mechanics can be explained for a sagittal plane, assuming a rigid body rotating around the ankles (Figure 13.1). From this simplified example, the reader can further extend into more complex movements of a similar nature at different levels.

Free body diagrams for the feet and the rest of the body are drawn in Figures 13.2 and 13.3 respectively.

Since the feet are continuously in the same position, equations for static equilibrium are applicable:

$$-S_h + R_h = 0$$
$$-S_v + R_v = 0$$
$$-M_{res} + R_v.xp + R_h.xd = 0$$

In this case, the relatively small weight of the feet is neglected relative to the other large forces, almost equal to body weight. It can be demonstrated that the moments produced by R_h are at least ten times smaller than those generated by R_v.

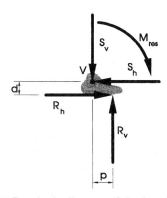

Figure 13.1 Postural control in the sagittal plane: basic oscillations of the body around the ankles

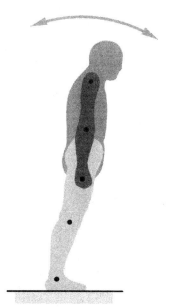

Figure 13.2 Free body diagram of the feet. M_{res} is the resultant moment of forces around the ankle joint. S_v and S_h are the vertical and horizontal components respectively of resultant force at the ankle. R_v and R_h are the vertical and horizontal components respectively of the contact force between the feet and floor. The weight of the feet is small in comparison with the other forces, and has been neglected

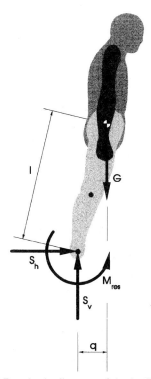

Figure 13.3 Free body diagram of the body (without feet) rotating around the ankles. G is equal to the weight of the body without the feet

The sum of moments can therefore be simplified as follows:

$$M_{res} = R_v xp$$

Equations of motion are used to express the relationship between forces, moments and movements of the body CG:

$$S_h = mx\,a_h$$

$$S_v - G = mx\,a_v$$

$$-Gxq + M_{res} = I_{ankle}\,x\alpha$$

where *m* is the mass of the body without feet and I_{ankle} is the moment of inertia of the body around the ankle.

Finally, since the horizontal acceleration of the CG (ah) is almost equal to the tangential component of the acceleration of a segment rotation around a fixed axis (the ankle), the following equation holds:

$$ah = -\alpha xl$$

From these equations, the following expression for the angular acceleration can be found:

$$\alpha = \frac{G(p - q)}{I_{ankle}}$$

This equation indicates that the angular acceleration (and thus also the acceleration of the CG) may be positive or negative, depending on the difference between p and q. As is explained in Figures 13.2 and 13.3, q indicates the horizontal distance between the ankle and the CG, whereas p is the distance between the same joint and the CP. Hence, if p−q is positive, the CP is in front of the CG and will generate a backward acceleration of the CG. If p−q is negative, the opposite direction of acceleration is generated and hence, if maintained for some time by proper action of plantar flexors or extensors, will produce forward velocity and, eventually, forward movement. In this way, the CP will always anticipate movements of the CG in stance. Furthermore, sways of the CP will

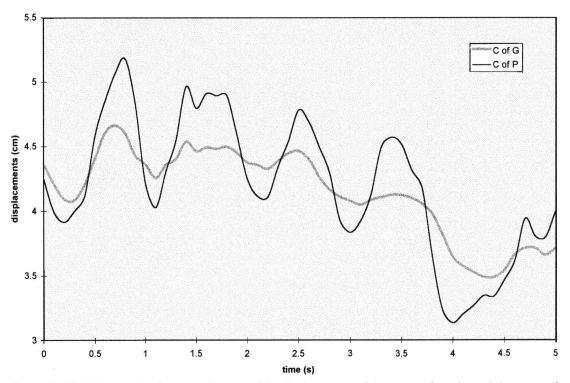

Figure 13.4 Typical example of measured curves of the displacements of the centre of gravity and the centre of pressure

always have larger amplitudes than those of the CG, since corrective movements are only possible on condition that the CP is in front of (for backward acceleration) or behind (for forward acceleration) the CG. This can clearly be seen in simultaneous measurements of sagittal displacements of both quantities, as illustrated in Figure 13.4 (Spaepen *et al.*, 1979).

Clinical evaluation theorem

A complicated neuromuscular system is in place to maintain the basically unstable upright position. For falls to occur during any activity at any age, postural control must be impaired relative to the amount by which it is stressed. Falls occurring during normal activities suggest a greater impairment of postural control (Downton, 1992).

Static and dynamic balance reactions

Static balance can be measured by the Romberg, sharpened Romberg, one-legged stance and sensory organization tests (quiet standing on a firm support during various visual conditions).

An ataxia meter produces a numerical or diagrammatic representation of sway in one or more directions (usually two directions at right angles). The body, however, does not move rigidly, and different body segments move in diverse ways and at various rates.

Fine control of posture is immensely complex. Maintaining static posture involves elaborate neuromuscular interaction, but its study has largely been conducted via measurement of postural sway during quiet standing (Figure 13.5). This may not

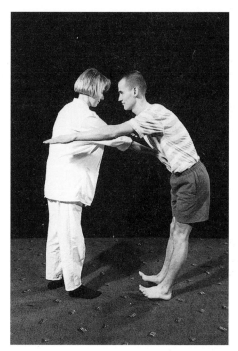

Figure 13.6 Use of a test that stresses static balance

be a particularly useful parameter to measure, and is perhaps analogous to the study of respiratory function by measuring vital capacity alone. If used, it might be better to resort to tests that stress static balance (Figures 13.6 and 13.7).

Effort might better be spent on the study of *dynamic balance*, either in the study of gait, walking along a beam or around a figure of eight, or in simple mobility assessments such as the 'get up and go' test (Mathias *et al.*, 1986) and the functional reach test (Duncan *et al.*, 1990). The latter assesses the subject's ability to reach forward with the arms at 90° of shoulder flexion. The distance of forward movement without losing balance is measured.

When balance is disturbed, various rescue mechanisms come into play to try to avoid loss of balance (Figure 13.8). Attempts are made by swaying to try to correct the initial derangement; staggering and sweeping movements may occur, and fall breaking reactions are invoked (Figures 13.6 and 13.8).

Although posturography has added very little to our understanding of the organization of posture and balance, in clinical practice simple assessments of posture can provide useful information about functional balance. The observation of

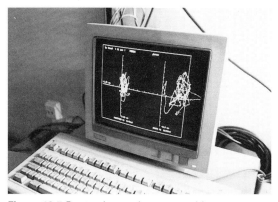

Figure 13.5 Postural sway is measured in two different ways: via the force platform (left on the screen) and via the displacement of a light placed on the shoulder of the patient (right on the screen). See also Figures 13.8 and 13.9

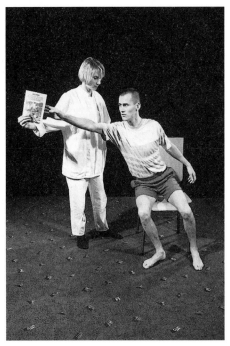

Figure 13.7 Balance reactions during reaching out

balance during quiet standing, a Romberg test and a sensitized Romberg test (Figure 13.9), the response to a minor balance stress, highlight areas of impairment.

Balance needs to be assessed in various postures and during movement from one posture to another (Figures 13.10 and 13.11). Having selected an assessment position suitable for each subject, adopt the following procedure:

Assess the amount of help subjects need to maintain the position

Apply pressure to the trunk in various directions, encouraging subjects to hold the position (or say 'don't let me move you')

Try the same approach when the subjects' eyes are closed.

Test the subjects' automatic reactions to balance disturbance by moving them; tilt them backwards, forwards and sideways and rotate them. Notice whether they move their head, trunk, upper limbs or lower limbs or all of them to maintain their equilibrium. Test their reactions when carrying out movements of a specific part of the body.

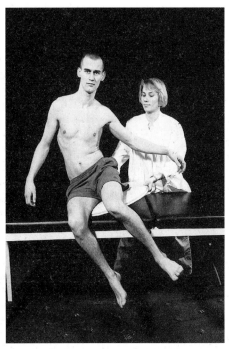

Figure 13.8 If balance is disturbed, various rescue mechanisms come into play to try to avoid loss of balance

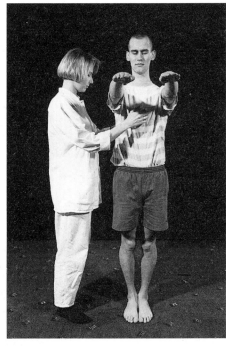

Figure 13.9 Assessment of static balance with the sensitized Romberg

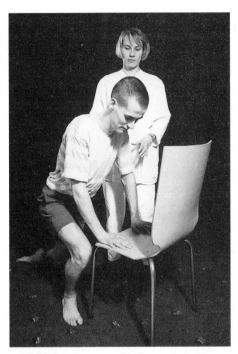

Figure 13.10 Assessment of balance during movement from one posture to another

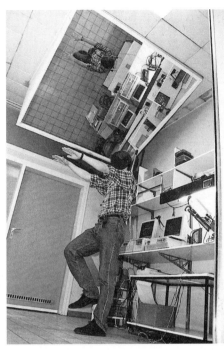

Figure 13.12 Dynamic balance assessment. Walk on the spot

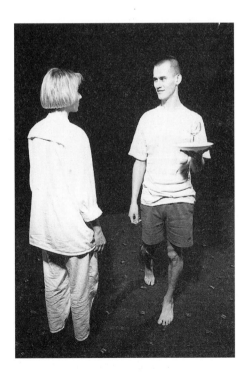

Figure 13.11 Maintenance of balance during dual tasking

To examine lateropulsion, specific tests can be performed – for example, a sensitized Romberg test (Figure 13.9), walking on the spot with the arms outstretched (Figures 13.12 and 13.13), or walking along a line (Figure 13.14). Patients with a unilateral functional loss of the vestibular system will deviate towards the side of the dysfunction (Figure 13.13).

Equilibrium reactions ensure proper body posture when a change occurs in the supporting surface. These reactions are essentially compensatory movements that render equilibrium possible. They have two components; first, an ability to bring the extremities into a proper position for equilibrium, and second, a sufficient supporting tonus.

The measurement technique is as follows. Place the subject supine, or sitting or standing on a tilting table. In supine, the initial observation is a stretching out of the extremities to the side to which the tipping is occurring, accompanied by a slight abduction. Gradually, compensatory abduction of the leg and arm to the opposite side takes place. Trunk and head turn to the direction of the tilt (Figure 13.15). In the sitting position, the same reactions occur. When standing, the trunk is shifted in the direction opposite to that of the tilt, the upper

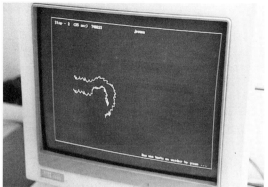

Figure 13.13 Registration of the displacement of a light fixed on the shoulder during walking on the spot

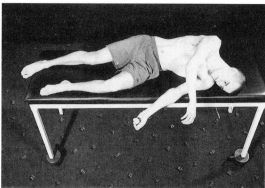

Figure 13.15 Equilibrium reactions occurring with a change in the supporting surface

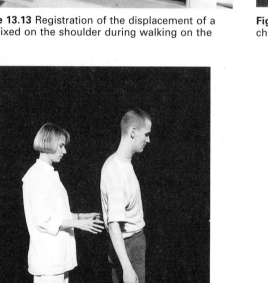

Figure 13.14 Assessment of walking along a line

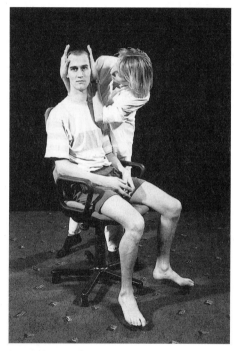

Figure 13.16 Assessment of cervicogenic vertigo and nystagmus

leg is bent at the knee and the other one extended (Atkinson, 1974; Downton, 1992).

Cervicogenic vertigo
Neck movements should be tested to see if they precipitate symptoms. One test is specifically designed to separate vestibular disease from cervicogenic vertigo (Figure 13.16). The patient is seated in a swivel chair, and the head immobilized with both hands. The chair is swivelled back and forth, and reproduction of the patient's symptoms, sometimes with nystagmus, is suggestive of cervical proprioceptive disease. Manual cervical manipulation may be indicated (Ferezy, 1992).

Dizziness, giddiness, vertigo
History-taking is a very important step. It is crucial to try to understand which type of sensation is described. Is it a sensation of rotation (self or environment), a feeling of being pushed to one

side, dysequilibrium, unsteadiness with or without falling, light-headedness, fainting, anxiety?

The duration of individual attacks is particularly useful if vertigo has occurred. Benign paroxysmal positional vertigo lasts for a few seconds to minutes. Ménière's disease causes episodes of vertigo lasting for a few hours. An attack lasting for days to weeks suggests vestibular neuronitis.

The effect on the symptoms of lying or sitting in specific positions should be examined. The assessment of the dizzy patient also includes a neurological examination, looking especially for evidence of brain-stem dysfunction, cerebellar problems, evidence of peripheral neuropathy or loss of proprioception (Figures 13.17–13.20).

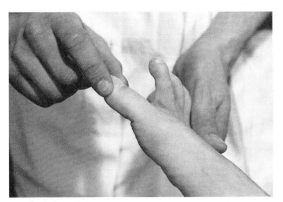

Figure 13.17 Balance reactions depend on intact proprioceptive sensation. Assessment of joint position sense

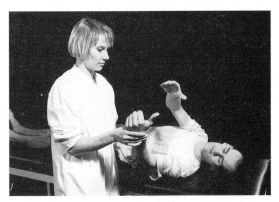

Figure 13.19 Thumb finding test

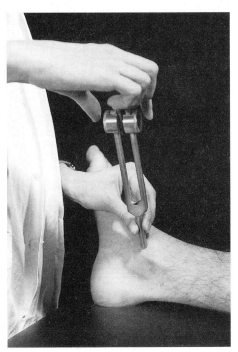

Figure 13.18 Assessment of vibration sense using a 128 Hz tuning fork

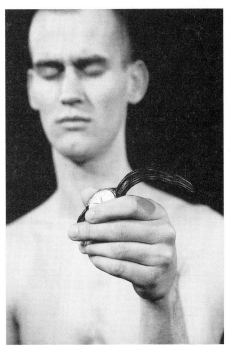

Figure 13.20 Stereognosis is impaired if touch and position senses are defective

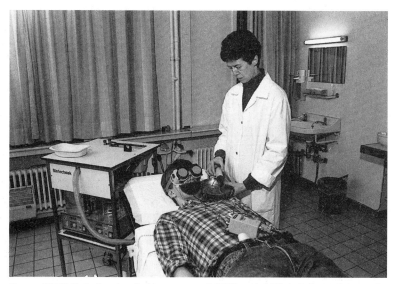

Figure 13.21 Caloric stimulation: water of 30°C and 44°C is irrigated through the external auditory meatus. This test stimulates one labyrinth at a time

Vegetative symptoms

Apart from the sensation of vertigo, patients may experience vegetative symptoms such as nausea, pallor, sweating, vomiting, hypotension and prostration. These symptoms are, as a rule, more marked in peripheral than in central vestibular lesions.

Vestibular examination

Tests currently available for evaluating vestibular function are the caloric stimulation and rotating tests (Figures 13.21 and 13.22). They stimulate the horizontal semicircular canals, leaving the two other canals and otolith organs untested.

Nystagmus

Observation of nystagmus is of paramount importance in detecting vestibular diseases (Figures 13.23, 13.24). Nystagmus is labelled in descriptive terms such as horizontal, rotatory, vertical, fast, long-lasting.

Physiotherapists should specifically be alert for positional nystagmus. Patients should be moved around in various positions, and movements in the sagittal plane are particularly important. The Hallpike manoeuvres are part of the standard examination (Figure 13.25). The patient sits on the examining table with the head turned to one side, and is tipped back abruptly to lie with the head

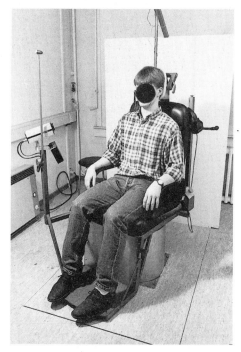

Figure 13.22 The rotational test: the chair is rotated at various speeds. When rotation to one side has stopped, the endolymph continues to flow in that direction. The result is a nystagmus in the opposite direction. This test stimulates the labyrinths on both sides

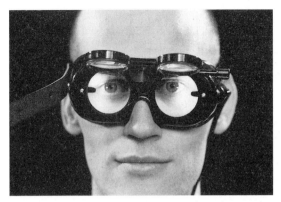

Figure 13.23 Observation of positional nystagmus with visual fixation

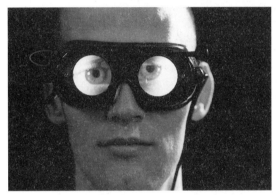

Figure 13.24 Observation of positional nystagmus without visual fixation with the use of Frenzel glasses (glasses with +20 dioptre biconvex lenses enclosed with a source of illumination so as to abolish optic fixation and facilitate observation of the subject's eyes)

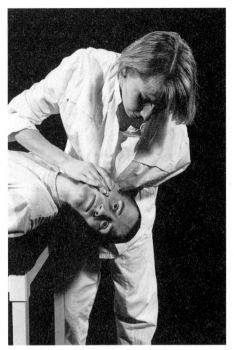

Figure 13.25 The Hallpike manoeuvres are part of the standard examination

extended over the end of the table. Observe the nystagmus as well as reproduced symptoms such as vertigo and neurovegetative reactions (Ferezy, 1992).

Oscillopsia

Disturbance of the vestibular pathways can give rise to oscillopsia, which is a visual perception of rapid to-and-fro movement of the outside world due to excessive slip of images of stationary objects upon the retina. Mechanisms to deal with increased retinal slip due to reduced vestibulo-ocular reflexes include potentializing of the cervico-ocular reflex, perceptual adaptation, and pre-programming of compensatory slow eye movements in anticipation of head movements.

Vision

All too often a patient's visual complaints are dismissed because Snellen acuity (or the tumbling E test) is normal and the visual fields to confrontation are full. Poor progress can result from an undetected visual disturbance. Further tests to be considered are the contrast sensitivity test, colour vision, computerized perimetry and, in some cases, visual-evoked potentials.

Hyperventilation

It is good practice to have the patient hyperventilate for a period, as many patients confuse hyperventilation with vertigo. If hyperventilation reproduces the patient's symptoms, vestibular disease is much less likely (Ferezy, 1992).

Postural hypotension

Blood pressure should be measured in the lying, sitting and standing positions. Hypotension can be an associated autonomic sign of vestibular dysfunction; however, it can also be the basis of aspecific symptoms. Postural hypotension is traditionally defined as a drop in systemic systolic blood pressure of 20 mmHg from that measured when lying after standing for two minutes. The problem with this definition is that patients who have symptomatic postural hypotension cannot stand for two minutes; they fall, owing to decreased cerebral blood flow. Symptoms are probably related to the ability of the cerebral circulation to respond to the changes in systemic blood pressure – some patients with just a slight drop in systemic blood pressure feel dizzy or light-headed, whilst for others the cerebral blood circulation responds quickly to a marked drop in systemic blood pressure and symptoms are not produced (Andrews, 1987).

Conclusion

Postural adjustments occur as a result of both sensory feedback and feed forward in anticipation or preparation. There is no unambiguous appraisal of the contribution of the diverse sensory and motor factors in the maintenance of posture and balance. Because of the ability of the central nervous system to adapt for the loss of function, a given pathology may not be apparent until the patient is temporarily deprived of the compensating system (Winter, 1995). This means that interpreting problems with postural stability or anticipating difficulties caused by sensory or motor damage is difficult. For posture, gait and functional activities, the measurable difference from normal is the effect of what remains after the system has compensated for the inadequacy, and is not a measure of the defect itself.

References

Andrews, K. (1986). The relevance of readmission to hospital. *J. Am. Geriatr. Soc.*, **34**, 5–11.

Andrews, K. (1987). *Rehabilitation of the Older Adult*. Edward Arnold.

Atkinson, H. W. (1974). Developmental background to physiotherapy. In *Neurology for Physiotherapists*. (J. Cash, ed.), pp. 38–53. Faber and Faber.

Begbie, G. H. (1966). Effects of alcohol and varying amount of visual information on balancing tests. *Ergonomics*, **9**, 325–33.

de Jong, P. T., de Jong, J. M., Cohen, B. and Jongkees, L. B. (1977). Ataxia and nystagmus induced by injection of local anaesthetics in the neck. *Ann. Neurol.*, **1**, 240–46.

Dornan, J., Fernie, G. R. and Holliday, P. J. (1978). Visual input: its importance in the control of postural sway. *Arch. Phys. Med. Rehabil.*, **59**, 586–91.

Downton, J. H. (1992). *Falls in the Elderly*. Edward Arnold.

Duncan, P. W., Weiner, D. K., Chandler, J. and Studenski, S. (1990). Functional reach: a new clinical measure of balance. *J. Geront.*, **45**, 192–7.

Eklund, G. and Lofstedt, L. (1970). Biomechanical analysis of balance. *Biomed. Eng.*, **5**, 333–7.

Ferezy, J. S. (1992). *The Chiropractic Neurological Examination*. Aspen Publishers.

Ghez, C. (1991a). Posture. In *Principles of Neural Science*, 3rd edn. (E. R. Kandal, J. H. Schwartz and T. M. Jessell, eds.), pp. 596–607. Prentice Hall International.

Ghez, C. (1991b). The cerebellum. In *Principles of Neural Science*, 3rd edn. (E. R. Kandal, J. H. Schwartz and T. M. Jessell, eds.), pp. 626–46. Prentice Hall International.

Goldberg, M. E., Egger, H. M. and Gouras, P. (1991). The ocular motor control. In *Principles of Neural Science*, 3rd edn. (E. R. Kandal, J. H. Schwartz and T. M. Jessell, eds.), pp. 626–46. Prentice Hall International.

Guedry, F. E. (1974). Psychophysics of vestibular sensation. In *Handbook of Sensory Physiology – Vestibular System* (H. H. Kornhuber, ed.), pp. 3–154. Springer Verlag.

Hardie, R. J. (1993). Tremor and ataxia. In *Neurological Rehabilitation* (R. Greenwood, M. P. Barnes, T. M. McMillan and D. C. Ward, eds.), pp. 173–8. Churchill Livingstone.

Juntunen, J., Matikainen, E., Ylikoski, J. *et al.* (1987). Postural body sway and exposure to high-energy impulse noise. *Lancet*, **2**, 261–4.

Kelly, J. P. (1991). The sense of balance. In *Principles of Neural Science*, 3rd edn. (E. R. Kandal, J. H. Schwartz and T. M. Jessell, eds.), pp. 500–511. Prentice Hall International.

Lee, D. N. and Lishman, J. R. (1975). Visual proprioceptive control of stance. *J. Hum. Move. Stud.*, **1**, 87–95.

Liebman, M. and Tadmor, R. (1991). *Neuroanatomy made Easy and Understandable*. Aspen Publishers.

Mathias, S., Nayak, U. S. and Isaacs, M. D. (1986). Balance in elderly patients: the 'get-up-and-go' test. *Arch. Phys. Med. Rehabil.*, **67**, 387–9.

Nashner, L. M. (1976). Adapting reflexes controlling the human posture. *Exp. Brain Res.*, **26**, 59–72.

Norré, M. E. and Forrez, G. (1986). Posture testing (posturography) in the diagnosis of peripheral vestibular pathology. *Arch. Otorhinolaryngol.*, **243**, 186–9.

Prudham, D. and Evans, J. G. (1981). Factors associated with falls in the elderly: a community study. *Age and ageing*, **10**, 141–6.

Ragnarsdóttir, M. (1996). The concept of balance. *Physiotherapy*, **82**, 368–75.

Roberts, T. (1995). *Understanding Balance. The Mechanics of Posture and Locomotion*. Chapman and Hall.

Spaepen, A. J., Peeraer, L. and Willems, E. J. (1979). Centre of gravity and centre of pressure in stabilometric studies. A comparison with film analysis. *Agressologie*, **20B**, 117–18.

Stevens, D. L. and Tomlinson, G. E. (1971). Measurement of human postural sway. *Proc. R. Soc. Med.*, **64**, 653–5.

Tobis, J. S., Nayak, U. S. L. and Hoehler, F. (1981). Visual perception of verticality and horizontality amongst elderly fallers. *Arch. Phys. Med. Rehabil.*, **62**, 619–22.

Willems, E. J. and Vranken, M. S. (1964). Postural reaction of man on a slowly moving base. In *Biomechanics IV* (R. C. Nelson and C. A. Morehouse, eds.), pp. 60–72. University Park Press.

Winter, D. A. (1995). Human balance and posture control during standing and walking. *Gait and Posture*, **3**, 193–214.

14 Measurement and analysis of functional human movement – the state of the art

B. R. Durward, P. J. Rowe and G. D. Baer

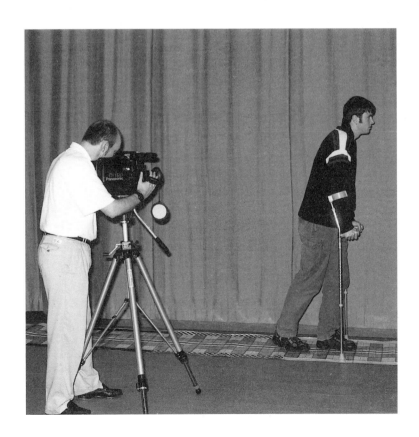

Introduction

In designing this book it was intended to draw together, in one volume, the many and diverse measurement methods available to record functional human movement and to compile a series of reviews which indicate the current state of knowledge related to common human activities. The chapters in this book reveal the measurement 'tool kit' available to those wishing to investigate functional human movement and provide an introduction to the current understanding and knowledge related to specific tasks. This process has enabled reflection on the field as a whole, and a consideration of the many issues that have been raised. In this way, an opinion has been formed of the current 'state of the art' in measuring functional human movement. This chapter contains an analysis of the current state of development and outlines future avenues for exploration.

The most fundamental question to be asked is, why measure functional human movement?

Why do healthcare professionals need to measure human movement?

The professional perspective

The therapy literature abounds with statements that indicate the need for measurement by health professionals. Currier (1990) states that 'A profession is an occupation whose members must possess a body of knowledge that is both identifiable and different from that of others, and the members must assume responsibility for adding to that body of knowledge'. Likewise, Rothstein (1985) argues that 'Without a scientific basis for the assessment (and measurement) process, we face the future as independent practitioners unable to communicate with one another, unable to document efficacy and unable to claim scientific credibility for our profession'.

There is much to recommend the sentiments outlined in these quotations. Implicit within these statements is the premise that a professional is someone who accepts the obligation and responsibility to measure the outcome and effectiveness of intervention. Traditionally, professional respectability has been based upon clinical skills and techniques. While it is recognized that without these abilities health care professionals could not deliver therapy, it has not been widely accepted that measurement skills and techniques are equally important in delivering therapy and therefore in defining a health care profession. Professionals should advocate that the value placed on measurement skills is equal to that placed on therapeutic skills.

If it is accepted that health care incorporates a scientific process, then it becomes inevitable that measurement becomes an essential component of patient care. An examination of therapy reveals many instances where measurement is a key feature. For example, the therapist–patient interaction requires the identification of problems, diagnosis, treatment planning, progress monitoring and treatment modification. In each case, to reach a decision, the therapist must collect and assimilate data that informs the management of the patient. Similarly, measurement data are required in order to communicate with patients, carers and other health care professionals. Finally, measurement data can be used to compare individuals within a group, patients with healthy normal subjects, different types of patient groups and different treatment options. In all these ways the measurement process and the data it provides facilitate clinical decision-making. Without this process, clinical decisions will continue to be based on belief rather than knowledge.

It has been argued that a profession will only survive if it accepts the obligation to base judgements on knowledge. Taking a more positive perspective, a profession is a body of people who take responsibility for the integrity of knowledge in their field and who are active in developing and expanding this knowledge base. On an individual level, a professional in health care is one who not only values the quality of the treatment delivered, but also the quality of the outcome measures that can demonstrate effectiveness. At present, the consideration given to intervention and evaluation is unequal. To redress this imbalance, health care professionals need to invest in an exploration of appropriate measurement techniques to produce suitable measures.

The political perspective

Ultimately, whether health care professions are proactive in this process or not, society will increasingly insist on the presentation of evidence in support of therapeutic intervention. Over recent years, the public has become more aware of the deficiencies and inadequacies of the scientific basis for many health care interventions. This awareness has occurred at the same time as concerns have developed over financial constraints on health care budgets. Inevitably, therefore, the cost and effectiveness of health care have been questioned. The desire for value for money has expressed itself in recent years with the emergence of concepts such as 'evidence-based medicine' and 'clinical effectiveness'. These external factors, while changing in name and form, are unlikely to disappear, and it therefore seems inevitable that the professions will need to respond to these demands.

The educational perspective

The measurement process has inherent benefits of its own, regardless of the data it provides. In order to plan a study, it is necessary to articulate a question or hypothesis that is relevant and relates to an area of uncertainty. In order to achieve this it is necessary to develop an understanding of the current knowledge base, the underlying assumptions and theories related to treatments, and the conventions prevalent within practice. The process of forming this understanding, based on an open and unbiased enquiry into the literature, allows the identification of fundamental principles or foundations of practice, areas of consensus and disagreement, conflicts in theory and the recognition that practice, in some instances, is based on belief rather than knowledge. This systematic enquiry combined with the adoption of a sceptical approach to the literature will ensure that appropriate research questions are developed and that clinicians base clinical decisions on the best available knowledge.

A fundamental product of the process of measurement is the acceptance of the unknown. Once it is accepted that there are areas of uncertainty in practice, the professional is able to engage in more open-minded and critical consideration of the issues. In this sense, the professional is freed from the restraints of accumulated prejudice and is able to form judgements on scientific evidence alone.

The ethical perspective

Typically, ethical considerations are considered of prime importance when planning and carrying out research in the clinical setting. This need for ethical consideration in research is not disputed. However, it is appropriate to ask whether it is ethical to apply treatment without evidence of effectiveness. If it is impossible to provide the recipients of a treatment with evidence that they will benefit from it, should they be expected to agree to it?

The clinical perspective

Issues related to the restoration of movement are central to many of the physical interventions carried out by health care professionals in the course of their work. The ability to measure movement is therefore crucial in establishing the clinical effectiveness of these professions.

An examination of current assessment and measurement methods used in clinical practice reveals a dependence on a wide range of clinical rating scales and simple timed functional tests. While of interest, these tools have many limitations when used to measure movement. They are inherently subjective in nature and therefore depend upon the judgement and experience of the rater, leaving them open to bias and prejudice. In addition, they have often been developed with reference to a particular treatment approach and are therefore contaminated; they seek what they expect to find and ignore that which they do not perceive as relevant.

Subjective rating scales often rely on classification of the subjects ability to perform a task using labels (e.g. 'able', 'unable', 'able with minimal assistance', or 'walks 3 m alone', 'walks 5 m with no aid in 15 s'). These scores serve to provide an overview of functional ability, but cannot be said to measure the performance of movement. They do not include information as to the quality, range, pattern or timing of movement. A major characteristic of these rating tools is a dependency on crude intervals that attempt to differentiate levels of ability. In this context these scales are a compromise in that they limit the number of levels to ensure reasonable reliability. This limitation often leads to 'floor' and 'ceiling' effects, and an inability to differentiate levels of performance. While many of these scales have been tested to establish levels of reliability, the establishment of validity is often problematic. The behaviour rated by these scales is often undefined, which leads to difficulties in establishing concurrent validity with data from another validated tool.

Many of the methods and tools described in this book have much to offer physical therapists in establishing the effectiveness of their treatment. The adoption of some of these techniques would provide the clinician with a range of benefits. The objective nature of these measurement techniques means that the data are less likely to be affected by recorder bias, and they provide a level of description substantially better than subjective rating scales or techniques dependent upon visual observation. This objective description of movement frequently contradicts the expectations and perceptions of the clinician. In revealing contradictions, these descriptions help the clinician to re-evaluate practice and outcome, and hence form a new understanding of patient problems. This scientific evaluation of movement provides an analytical insight that facilitates the development of practice.

In order for the evaluation of practice to progress from a dependency on subjective and insensitive measures to more accurate and revealing objective measurement systems, a period of development is required. The acceptance by professionals that this transition is required and desirable is the first step, but this should then be followed by investment in education, training and resources. Clinicians will need to understand the range of techniques available, their strengths, weaknesses and limitations, and issues related to implementation such as data reduction and analysis. Clinicians will need to be trained to operate these systems and understand the difficulties associated with their use in the clinical environment. Finally, resources, in terms of time and money, will be required to purchase and use these measurement systems routinely in clinical practice.

If a high value is placed on the development and implementation of effective therapeutic techniques, then it follows that a high value should also be placed on the measures available to demonstrate effectiveness. It is precisely because clinicians value clinical skills and their potential to aid and improve the quality of life in the population that they should be committed to the continued development of quality measurements of human functional performance.

The movement measurement systems – are they fit for purpose?
The nature of the systems

This book illustrates the diversity of measurement systems currently available. While they offer considerable potential to improve clinical measurement, they currently possess a number of limitations. Many of the systems are controlled and operated using a computer, and for some individuals this feature creates fear and apprehension, which is exacerbated by software that is difficult to use and often restrictive in its ability to provide meaningful clinical data. The instructions for use, provided by the manufacturer, are often unclear, and are peppered throughout with technical jargon. When problems occur, the user often fails to obtain suitable assistance from the manufacturers.

Modern measurement systems are impressive in that they are constructed to appear sophisticated and technologically advanced. Unfortunately, this can lead to a false sense of security regarding the validity of the data produced and an inability to comprehend the methods by which these data are acquired. As a result, many of these systems are poorly validated by investigators other than the designers or manufacturers. This problem exists despite the relative ease with which the issues of validity could be addressed.

Many of these systems have been developed in parallel with other technological advances. Currently, movement science remains a relatively small and under-utilized field and, consequently, movement measurement systems tend to be expensive and under developed. The widespread adoption of these new movement measurement techniques by the clinical community will lead to the possibility of mass production. As with the car, high-volume production will inevitably lead to reductions in cost, increased user-friendliness and the requirement for manufacturers to consider the needs of the purchaser. We can expect many of the current shortcomings with existing systems to reduce in the foreseeable future.

Use of the systems

On face value, modern movement measurement systems often appear to be simple to use. However, when used with a human subject, difficulties in application can arise.

For example, a stopwatch appears a simple and easy to use tool; however, on attempting to measure the time taken by a stroke patient to rise to stand, difficulties are encountered immediately. The human recorder needs to decide when movement begins and ends by visual observation in order to start and stop the stopwatch. Likewise, the time recorded will exclude the initial reaction time when starting the watch, and include the terminal reaction time at the end of the movement. A true recording of the time taken to stand is only obtained if these two reaction times are equal.

Attempts to automate the initiation and termination of data collection by means of switches or other kinds of event marker can also be problematic. They can be triggered by movement artifacts, such as preparatory body adjustments prior to the initiation of the movement, and can fail to be triggered at the end of the task due to the stabilizing movements that occur. The definition of the start and end of a functional movement requires careful consideration before a valid measure of performance can be made. In some circumstances suitable events can be defined, thus allowing this process to be automated.

The measurement of functional human movement may require the attachment of measuring transducers or body markers directly to the body surface, giving rise to further complications. These systems often behave in a predictable and testable manner when bench-tested using a calibration rig; however, when these systems are attached to the body, care must be taken to ensure that the output remains valid.

An initial consideration is the definition of suitable anatomical planes and axes of movement that reflect the complex three-dimensional movements exhibited by joints and body segments. Current clinical definitions of joint motion lack clarity and scientific rigour, which makes it difficult to develop an appropriate protocol for the attachment of measuring devices such that they record faithfully the motion being investigated. The techniques adopted to attach measurement systems directly to the body should also be selected with care. This is important to ensure that the measuring device remains correctly aligned throughout the potential range of movement, and that the device itself remains in a correct configuration at each point of the measurement range. For example, knee joint angle can be measured with a television system using three markers attached to the greater trochanter, the lateral aspect of the knee joint and the lateral malleolus. However, this protocol will fail if skin movement occurs to the extent that the markers move in relation to the initial anatomical landmarks. Likewise, bulging of the soft tissues around the knee may cause the knee marker to become displaced or detached. Careful bench-testing of the device can reveal appropriate and inappropriate modes of operation. When devising an attachment system, care must be taken to ensure that only appropriate modes of operation occur during the performance of the functional movement. Finally, it can be difficult to demonstrate on the human subject (unlike a bench test) that the data recorded (the dependent variable) are correct. This is mainly due to the inability to prescribe predictable movements (the independent variable) or to measure the movement with reference to a suitable gold standard.

Some movements may not be amenable to measurement, and this may be due to the nature of the task, the design of the equipment or the environment in which the task would normally be performed. For example, it is difficult to see how rolling could be measured with equipment attached to the body surface. In this example, the equipment could either be damaged or interfere with the motion. If skin markers and cameras were used to record the rolling motion they would be obscured for substantial parts of the movement, and the analysis would fail. Other examples of problems include trailing cables, surface wires, arm-swing obscuring body motion, and the inability to transport equipment to various settings such as the outdoors, home or school.

Attempts to standardize human movement have led to the development of test protocols that require the performance of movements in such a way that they are constrained and may be abnormal. This standardization is done in an attempt to reduce the influence of potential confounding variables, and to aid data processing and analysis. Examples during rising to stand include carrying out the movement with the arms folded across the chest, positioning the feet prior to motion and completing the task while looking at a target in a standardized position. When considering standardization, there is a balance to be struck between preserving the essence of the task while limiting the confounding variables and facilitating analysis.

The communication and interpretation of results is often made difficult due to uncertainty surrounding important definitions and testing protocols. For example, what is balance? Measures of balance include:

1. Variables related to the centre of pressure – mean position over 10 s, the limits of stability and postural sway
2. Body posture – angle of upper body and variation in angle of the upper body
3. Symmetry of weight distribution – percentage of weight borne on one leg, symmetry indices and variation in the symmetry index. (Durward and Rowe, 1991).

An example of uncertainty in the protocols used for testing is illustrated by the 10 m walking test.

While many authors now advocate this simple test of walking ability, the literature offers little guidance as to the protocol by which to measure a subject. What determines the start and end of motion? Should the subject 'warm-up', walk barefoot, in shoes or slippers? Should the data be normalized with reference to height or leg length?

A number of practical restraints can arise when using measurement systems. Some systems reported in the literature are not commercially available, and require considerable technical knowledge in order to recreate them. The use of many measurement tools can be limited by cost, access to a suitable testing space, the need for technical support and the design limitations inherent within much of the software required to operate these systems. Additional constraints include the need to gain ethical approval before testing in order to ensure that subjects are protected in terms of privacy, discomfort, use of time, and safety. Inevitably testing subjects (particularly those who are vulnerable or in pain) has a cost to the individual, and steps must be taken to ensure that the data obtained have value in that they add to existing knowledge.

In an ideal world, the design of measurement studies should be guided by the research question. In forming the question, the researcher should identify appropriate dependent variables or outcome measures that can be used to provide an answer to the question posed. In reality, it is often the case that the researcher intending to investigate movement has a limited knowledge of the potential measurement tools, restricted access to these tools, and little financial support with which to purchase them. As a consequence, knowledge of and access to measurement systems tends to dominate the planning process. This leads to research that is driven more by the available measurement systems than by the desire to produce outcome measures of clinical relevance.

Data from the systems

A further complication with the use of measurement systems is the lack of a comprehensive normal database in the literature. This means that, for most studies of subjects with a certain pathology, comparative normal data are unavailable and hence must be recorded by the investigator. The normal database currently available in the literature has a number of limitations. The normal subjects recruited are primarily young, fit and active males; typically students associated with physical education, sports science or physical therapy, members of the armed forces, astronauts or convicts. It would appear that these groups are readily available to the researcher and are prepared to give informed consent.

Females, the middle-aged and the elderly and those with impairments or disabilities do not feature prominently in the groups of normal subjects reported in the literature. Therefore, current normal databases cannot be considered to represent typical populations because the inclusion of the physically fit and the exclusion of the unfit leads to the formation of normal values that have an inherent bias. This is well illustrated by a consideration of the elderly, in which group it would be unusual to find subjects without physical limitations. If inclusion criteria for studies are prohibitive they can lead to the situation where only the super-fit elderly subject, without any physical limitation, is selected. This gives rise to the formation of a super-normal group, and data which give a false representation of normal performance in the elderly.

Conversely, exclusion criteria that are too lenient may lead to the recruitment of a group of subjects with considerable medical problems that again cannot be considered as representative of the population. In studies of normal functional human movement, where the sample size is limited, care should be given to the selection of appropriate inclusion and exclusion criteria. There is also a need to establish a comprehensive and well-defined database of agreed normal population values (parameters) for a range of functional human activities. The design of this normal database should include population values for males and females over a range of ages, heights and weights.

To ensure that this database is of general use, the movement science community must establish suitable protocols for the collection, processing, analysis and presentation of the data. Once these protocols have been agreed, it will be possible to share data and communicate effectively within the discipline.

Where to now?

The chapters in this text present a review of the 'toolkit' currently available for the measurement of functional human movement. Collectively, they demonstrate the range and scope of evaluative methods that can be used to analyse important human functional tasks. This 'toolkit' has the potential to address many of the difficult functional measurement issues observed in clinical practice. The measurement techniques illustrated in this book have much to offer both the patient and the health care professional in that they provide the possibility of basing decision-making on scientific principles.

Further development of the 'toolkit' is required. In this chapter an attempt has been made to discuss the key development issues from both clinical and measurement perspectives. A consideration of both sets of issues reveals that continued development cannot be within the province of a single profession. For example, if responsibility for development of these systems rests solely with engineers and manufacturers, then it is likely that the tools will fail to meet the needs of clinicians. Conversely, most health care professionals do not have sufficient technical ability to design and commission appropriate tools for the objective measurement of human functional ability.

There is also a need to develop and incorporate suitable methods of data recording, processing and analysis. Inevitably these tasks would involve the skills of software engineering, information science and statistics. For these reasons, development must involve a multidisciplinary team with contributions from patients, clinicians, engineers, manufacturers, statisticians, software specialists and information scientists. For all of these disciplines there is a need for strategic professional development and the opportunity to gain an understanding of the skills and requirements of others in the team.

There is a danger that the technology illustrated in this book might drive both our scientific enquiry and the development of measurement techniques for recording functional human movement. A clear articulation of the research question and the potential for benefit to health care provision should be the starting point for study design, and must precede the selection of appropriate measurement techniques. Only in this way is it possible to gather data that will address clinical issues in an appropriate manner.

Once the clinical question has been articulated with clarity, it is possible to consider which tools from the diversity of measures available would be appropriate to shed light on this question. At this point a choice of measures is often available. The investigator may select a simple, quick, 'low-tech' tool or a complex, analytical, 'hi-tech' tool, depending on the nature of the study. Both tools may be appropriate, but if the simple tool provides data of sufficient quality to address the question then it should be given preference. In the situation where complex and analytical evaluations are required to address the question, it may be necessary to utilize the more complex tools. These 'hi-tech' systems can also be particularly useful in validating the simple, 'low-tech' measures.

Inevitably, many of these measurement methods will be developed as part of the research process. However, it would be inappropriate to view them as relevant only to the researcher. Many measurement techniques used routinely in other fields of clinical practice were developed as part of research, and a similar trend in the measurement of functional human movement should be expected. It is therefore artificial to categorize measurement methods as either 'clinical' or 'research'. Good measurement methods, developed in the course of research, should be adopted as part of clinical practice. The process of measurement should have scientific integrity and relevance, irrespective of the context in which it is carried out. Measurement should ultimately be classified as either scientific or unscientific, and not as clinical or research.

The way forward, then, involves a concerted team approach to explore and enhance our understanding of functional human movement. There is a need to improve our knowledge of functional tasks, to develop suitable methods for measuring these tasks and to produce theories that attempt to explain the effects of therapeutic intervention on the restoration of function. The achievement of these objectives will enable the testing, modification and extension of theory, and hence allow the development of practice that is based on scientific evidence.

References

Currier, D. P. (1990). *Elements of Research in Physical Therapy* (3rd edn.). Williams & Wilkins.

Durward, B. R. and Rowe, P. J. (1991). Symmetry not so simple. *Proc. 11th Int. Cong. World Confed. Phys. Ther.*, *London*, 447–449.

Rothstein, J. M. (1985). *Measurement in Physical Therapy*. Churchill Livingstone.

Index